2017 Classic Shirt-Pocket Edition

LARGE PRINT EDITION

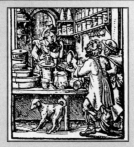

31ST EDITION

"Desire to take medicines ... distinguishes man from animals."
— Sir William Osler

Editor-in-Chief
Richard J. Hamilton, MD, FAAEM, FACMT, FACEP
Professor and Chair, Department of Emergency Medicine
Drexel University College of Medicine
Philadelphia, PA

JONES & BARTLETT
L E A R N I N G

World Headquarters
Jones & Bartlett Learning
5 Wall Street
Burlington, MA 01803
978-443-5000
info@jblearning.com
www.jblearning.com

Jones & Bartlett Learning books and products are available through most bookstores and online booksellers. To contact Jones & Bartlett Learning directly, call 800-832-0034, fax 978-443-8000, or visit our website www.jblearning.com.

The information in the *Pocket Pharmacopoeia* is compiled from sources believed to be reliable, and exhaustive efforts have been put forth to make the book as accurate as possible. The *Pocket Pharmacopoeia* is edited by a panel of drug information experts with extensive peer review and input from more than 50 practicing clinicians of multiple specialties. Our goal is to provide health professionals focused, core-prescribing information in a convenient, organized, and concise fashion. We include FDA-approved dosing indications and those off-label uses that have a reasonable basis to support their use. *However, the accuracy and completeness of this work cannot be guaranteed.* Despite our best efforts, this book may contain typographical errors and omissions. The *Pocket Pharmacopoeia* is intended as a quick and convenient reminder of information you have already learned elsewhere. The contents are to be used as a guide only, and healthcare professionals should use sound clinical judgment and individualize therapy to each specific patient care situation. This book is not meant to be a replacement for training, experience, continuing medical education, or studying the latest drug prescribing literature. This book is sold without warranties of any kind, expressed or implied, and the publisher and editors disclaim any liability, loss, or damage caused by the contents. Although drug companies purchase and distribute our books as promotional items, the Tarascon editorial staff alone determines all book content.

ISSN: 1945-9076
ISBN: 978-1-284-11893-3
6048
Printed in the United States of America
20 19 18 17 16   10 9 8 7 6 5 4 3 2 1

Production Credits

VP of Content Architecture and Production:
Paul Belfanti

V.P., Manufacturing and Inventory Control:
Therese Connell

Manufacturing and Inventory Control Supervisor:
Amy Bacus

Executive Editor:
Nancy Anastasi Duffy

Production Manager:
Daniel Stone

Rights and Media Specialist:
Wes DeShano

Marketing Manager:
Lindsay White

Composition: Cenveo

Text and Cover Design:
Kristin E. Parker

Printing and Binding:
Cenveo

Cover Printing: Cenveo

If you obtained your *Pocket Pharmacopoeia* from a bookstore, please send your address to info@tarascon.com. This allows you to be the first to hear of updates! (We don't sell or distribute our mailing lists, by the way.)

The cover woodcut is *The Apothecary* by Jost Amman, Frankfurt, 1574.

Remember from last year that we puzzled over a patient on an experimental regimen that requires two very expensive medications – pill X and pill Y. Every day at the same time, the patient must take one X and one Y pill. One morning, while putting his medication into a pill cup, the patient accidentally puts in one X and two Y pills. Unfortunately, X and Y are both the same exact size and weight and are white, scored, uncoated tablets with no markings and they are indistinguishable from each other. The pills are expensive so he cannot just throw them out and start over and they MUST be taken together at the exact dose. What can the patient do to make sure that he only takes one X and one Y pill from these three pills? The answer was to is to add a second X pill to the cup – then you would have two X and two Y pills. Next, cut each pill in half and take one half, leaving the other half in the cup. No matter what order you take them in, you will end up taking two ½ tabs of X and Y each and leave the same for tomorrow's dose!

This year's puzzler is about a weird soda machine in the hospital basement. It is labeled as selling only cans of cola, diet cola, or random (sometimes gives cola, sometimes diet). A soda costs $1. You are about to put your money in and get a cola when the security guard walks by and says, "Don't do it Doc, every label on that machine is wrong!" How much money do you have to spend and how many buttons do you press to figure out which button really gets you which soda?

CONTENTS

PAGE INDEX FOR TABLES

TARASCON POCKET PHARMACOPOEIA EDITORIAL STAFF*

EDITOR-IN-CHIEF

Richard J. Hamilton, MD, FAAEM, FACMT, FACEP, Professor and Chair, Department of Emergency Medicine, Drexel University College of Medicine, Philadelphia, PA

ASSOCIATE EDITORS

Jill E. Allen, PharmD, BCPS, Drug Information Consultant, Pin Oak Associates, Salt Lake City, UT

Kim K. Birtcher, MS, PharmD, BCPS, Clinical Professor, University of Houston College of Pharmacy, Houston, TX

Jill S. Borchert, PharmD, BCACP, BCPS, FCCP, Professor and Vice Chair, Pharmacy Practice, Director, PGY2 Ambulatory Care Residency Program, Midwestern University Chicago College of Pharmacy, Downers Grove, IL

Marie Cottman, PharmD, Owner, Pacific Compounding Pharmacy and Consultations, Inc., Lecturer, Department of Pharmaceutics and Medicinal Chemistry, Thomas J. Long School of Pharmacy and Health Sciences, University of the Pacific, Stockton, CA

Deborah A. Hass, PharmD, BCOP, BCPS, Oncology Pharmacist, Mt. Auburn Hospital, Cambridge, MA

William A. Kehoe, Pharm.D., MA, FCCP, BCPS, Professor of Pharmacy Practice and Psychology, Chairman, Department of Pharmacy Practice, University of the Pacific, Stockton, CA

Neeta Bahal O'Mara, PharmD, BCPS, Coldstream Consulting LLC, Skillman, NJ

Jeffrey T. Sherer, MPH, PharmD, BCPS, Clinical Associate Professor, University of Houston College of Pharmacy, Houston, TX

William Terneus Jr., Pharm.D, BCPS Martin Health System-Tradition Medical Center, Port St. Lucie, FL

*Affiliations are given for information purposes only, and no affiliation sponsorship is claimed.

PREFACE TO THE TARASCON POCKET PHARMACOPOEIA®

The *Tarascon Pocket Pharmacopoeia®* arranges drugs by clinical class with a comprehensive index in the back. Trade names are italicized and capitalized. Drug doses shown in mg/kg are generally intended for children, while fixed doses represent typical adult recommendations. Brackets indicate currently available formulations, although not all pharmacies stock all formulations. The availability of generic, over-the-counter, and scored formulations is mentioned. We have set the disease or indication in red for the pharmaceutical agent. It is meant to function as an aid to find information quickly. Codes are as follows:

▶ **METABOLISM & EXCRETION: L** = primarily liver, **K** = primarily kidney, **LK** = both, but liver > kidney, **KL** = both, but kidney > liver.

♀ **SAFETY IN PREGNANCY:** Prior FDA system **A** = Safety established using human studies, **B** = Presumed safe based on animal studies, **C** = Uncertain safety; no human studies and animal studies show an adverse effect, **D** = Unsafe - evidence of risk that may in certain clinical circumstances be justifiable, **X** = Highly unsafe - risk of use outweighs any possible benefit. As of June 2015, the FDA no longer uses letter categories to describe pregnancy risk. New drugs do not have a letter category, and letter categories will be gradually removed from product labeling for older drugs. We have developed the Tarascon Safety in Pregnancy Classification System to describe the safety of drugs in pregnancy. We apply this rating system to new drugs and to older drugs when the prior FDA letter is removed from the product label. Our system assigns the following risk category to each trimester of pregnancy (1st/2nd/3rd):

 X: Risk outweighs benefit or contraindicated

 O: Benefit outweighs risk; use in pregnancy as indicated.

 ?: Risk vs. benefit is unclear; consider alternatives.

For example, the Tarascon pregnancy classification of X/X/X for isotretinoin indicates that use is unsafe in all trimesters of pregnancy. The classification of O/O/X for naproxen indicates that use in the third trimester of pregnancy is unsafe. The trimester risk categories may also be followed by a comment. For example, the pregnancy category for asenapine is: ?/?/?R withdrawal and EPS in neonates exposed in 3rd trimester.

"R" denotes that the drug has a pregnancy exposure registry. Prescribers are encouraged to enroll patients in pregnancy exposure registries; contact information is available in product labeling.

▶ **SAFETY IN LACTATION:** + Generally accepted as safe, ? Safety unknown or controversial, − Generally regarded as unsafe. Many of our "+" listings are from the AAP policy "The Transfer of Drugs and Other Chemicals Into Human Milk" (see www.aap.org) and may differ from those recommended by the manufacturer.

© **DEA CONTROLLED SUBSTANCES: I** = High abuse potential, no accepted use (e.g., heroin, marijuana), **II** = High abuse potential and severe dependence liability (e.g., morphine, codeine, hydromorphone, cocaine, amphetamines, methylphenidate, secobarbital). Some states require triplicates. **III** = Moderate dependence liability (e.g., *Tylenol #3, Vicodin*), **IV** = Limited dependence liability (benzodiazepines, propoxyphene, phentermine), **V** = Limited abuse potential (e.g., *Lomotil*).

§ **RELATIVE COST:** Cost codes used are "per month" of maintenance therapy (e.g., antihypertensives) or "per course" of short-term therapy (e.g., antibiotics). Codes are calculated using average wholesale prices (at press time in US dollars) for the most common indication and route of each drug at a typical adult dosage. For maintenance therapy, costs are calculated based upon a 30-day supply or the quantity that

Code	Cost
$	< $25
$$	$25 to $49
$$$	$50 to $99
$$$$	$100 to $199
$$$$$	≥ $200

might typically be used in a given month. For short-term therapy (i.e., 10 days or less), costs are calculated on a single treatment course. When multiple forms are available (e.g., generics), these codes reflect the least expensive generally available product. When drugs don't neatly fit into the classification scheme above, we have assigned codes based upon the relative cost of other similar drugs. *These codes should be used as a rough guide only*, as (1) they reflect cost, not charges, (2) pricing often varies substantially from location to location and time to time, and (3) HMOs, Medicaid, and buying groups often negotiate quite different pricing. Check with your local pharmacy if you have any questions.

✦ **CANADIAN TRADE NAMES:** Unique common Canadian trade names not used in the US are listed after a maple leaf symbol. Trade names used in both nations or only in the US are displayed without such notation.

■ **BLACK BOX WARNINGS:** This icon indicates that there is a black box warning associated with this drug. Note that the warning itself is not listed.

ABBREVIATIONS IN TEXT

AAP	American Academy of Pediatrics	**cap**	capsule
ACCP	American College of Chest Physicians	**cm**	centimeter
ACR	American College of Rheumatology	**CMV**	cytomegalovirus
ACT	activated clotting time	**CNS**	central nervous system
ADHD	attention deficit hyperactivity disorder	**COPD**	chronic obstructive pulmonary disease
AHA	American Heart Association	**CrCl**	creatinine clearance
Al	aluminum	**CV**	Cardiovascular
ANC	absolute neutrophil count	**CVA**	stroke
ASA	aspirin	**CYP**	cytochrome P450
BMI	body mass index	**D5W**	5% dextrose
BP	blood pressure	**dL**	deciliter
BPH	benign prostatic hyperplasia	**DM**	diabetes mellitus
BUN	blood urea nitrogen	**DMARD**	disease-modifying drug
Ca	calcium	**DPI**	dry powder inhaler
CAD	coronary artery disease	**DRESS**	drug rash eosinophilia and systemic symptoms

(cont.)

ABBREVIATIONS IN TEXT (*continued*)

ECG	electrocardiogram	**INR**	international normalized ratio
EPS	extrapyramidal symptoms	**IU**	international units
ET	endotracheal	**IV**	intravenous
g	gram	**JIA**	juvenile idiopathic arthritis
GERD	gastroesophageal reflux disease	**kg**	kilogram
gtts	drops	**lb**	pound
GU	genitourinary	**LFT**	liver function test
h	hour	**LV**	left ventricular
HAART	highly active antiretroviral therapy	**LVEF**	left ventricular ejection fraction
Hb	hemoglobin	**m^2**	square meters
HBV	hepatitis B virus	**MAOI**	monoamine oxidase inhibitor
HCTZ	hydrochlorothiazide	**mcg**	microgram
HCV	hepatitis C virus	**MDI**	metered dose inhaler
HIT	heparin-induced thrombocytopenia	**mEq**	milliequivalent
HPV	human papillomavirus	**mg**	milligram
HSV	herpes simplex virus	**Mg**	magnesium
HTN	hypertension	**MI**	myocardial infarction
IM	intramuscular	**min**	minute

(cont.)

ABBREVIATIONS IN TEXT (*continued*)

mL	milliliter	RA	rheumatoid arthritis
mo	months old	RSV	respiratory syncytial virus
MRSA	methicillin-resistant *Staphylococcus aureus*	SC	subcutaneous
ng	nanogram	sec	second
NHLBI	National Heart, Lung, and Blood Institute	soln	solution
NPH	neutral protamine hagedorn	supp	suppository
NS	normal saline	susp	suspension
N/V	nausea/vomiting	tab	tablet
NYHA	New York Heart Association	TB	tuberculosis
OA	osteoarthritis	TCA	tricyclic antidepressant
oz	ounce	TNF	tumor necrosis factor
pc	after meals	TPN	total parenteral nutrition
PO	by mouth	UTI	urinary tract infection
PR	by rectum	wt	weight
prn	as needed	y	year
PTT	partial thromboplastin time	yo	years old
q	every		

THERAPEUTIC DRUG LEVELS

Drug	Level	Optimal Timing
carbamazepine trough	4–12 mcg/mL	Just prior to next dose
cyclosporine trough	50–300 ng/mL	Just prior to next dose
digoxin	0.8–2.0 ng/mL	Just prior to next dose
ethosuximide trough	40–100 mcg/mL	Just prior to next dose
lidocaine	1.5–5 mcg/mL	12–24 hours after start of infusion
lithium trough	0.6–1.2 meq/l	Just prior to first morning dose
NAPA	10–30 mcg/mL	Just prior to next procainamide dose
phenobarbital trough	15–40 mcg/mL	Just prior to next dose

(cont.)

(cont.)

phenytoin trough	10–20 mcg/mL	Just prior to next dose
primidone trough	5–12 mcg/mL	Just prior to next dose
procainamide	4–10 mcg/mL	Just prior to next dose
quinidine	2–5 mcg/mL	Just prior to next dose
theophylline	5–15 mcg/m	8–12 hours after once daily dose
valproate trough (epilepsy)	50–100 mcg/mL	Just prior to next dose
valproate trough (mania)	45–125 mcg/mL	Just prior to next dose
vancomycin trough[1]	10–20 mg/L	Just prior to next dose
zonisamide[2]	10–40 mcg/mL	Just prior to dose

THERAPEUTIC DRUG LEVELS *(continued)*

Drug	Level	Optimal Timing
Aminoglycoside Conventional Dosing		
amikacin peak	20–35 mcg/mL	30 minutes after infusion
amikacin trough	<5 mcg/mL	Just prior to next dose
gentamicin peak	5–10 mcg/mL	30 minutes after infusion
gentamicin trough	<2 mcg/mL	Just prior to next dose
tobramycin peak	5–10 mcg/mL	30 minutes after infusion
tobramycin trough	<2 mcg/mL	Just prior to next dose

(cont.)

Aminoglycoside Once Daily Dosing[3]		
amikacin peak	35–60 mcg/mL	30 minutes after infusion
amikacin trough	<4 mcg/mL	Just prior to next dose
gentamicin peak	15–20 mcg/mL	30 minutes after infusion
gentamicin trough	<1 mcg/mL	Just prior to next dose
tobramycin peak	15–20 mcg/mL	30 minutes after infusion
tobramycin trough	<1 mcg/mL	Just prior to next dose

[1]Maintain vancomycin trough >10 mg/L to avoid resistance; optimal trough for complicated infections is 15–20 mg/L
[2]Ranges not firmly established but supported by clinical trial results
[3]Peak or trough levels may not be routinely monitored.

OUTPATIENT PEDIATRIC DRUGS

med	strength	*Age*	*2mo*	*4mo*	*6mo*	*9mo*	*12mo*	*15mo*	*2yo*	*3yo*	*5yo*
		Kg	5	6½	8	9	10	11	13	15	19
		lbs	11	15	17	20	22	24	28	33	42
		freq	**teaspoons of liquid per dose** *(1 tsp = 5 mL)*								
Tylenol (mg)		q4h	80	80	120	120	160	160	200	240	280
Tylenol (tsp)	160/t	q4h	½	½	¾	¾	1	1	1¼	1½	1¾
ibuprofen (mg)		q6h	--	--	75†	75†	100	100	125	150	175
ibuprofen (tsp)	100/t	q6h	--	--	¾t	¾t	1	1	1¼	1½	1¾
amoxicillin or	125/t	bid	1	1¼	1½	1¾	1¾	2	2¼	2¾	3½
Augmentin	200/t	bid	½	¾	1	1	1¼	1¼	1½	1¾	2¼
(not otitis media)	250/t	bid	½	½	¾	¾	1	1	1¼	1¼	1¾
	400/t	bid	¼	½	½	½	¾	¾	¾	1	1
amoxicillin,	200/t	bid	1	1¼	1¾	2	2	2¼	2¾	3	4
(otitis media)‡	250/t	bid	¾	1¼	1½	1½	1¾	1¾	2¼	2½	3¼
	400/t	bid	½	¾	¾	1	1	1¼	1½	1½	2

(cont.)

Auamentin ES‡	600/t	bid	?	½	½	¾	¾	¾	1	1¼	1½
azithromycin*§	100/t	qd	¼†	½†	½	½	½	½	¾	¾	1
(5-day Rx)	200/t	qd	--	¼†	¼	¼	¼	¼	½	½	½
Bactrim/Septra	---	bid	½	¾	1	1	1	1¼	1½	1½	2
cefaclor*	125/t	bid	1	1	1¼	1½	1½	1¾	2	2½	3
"	250/t	bid	½	½	¾	¾	¾	1	1	1¼	1½
cefadroxil	125/t	bid	½	¾	1	1	1¼	1¼	1½	1¾	2¼
"	250/t	bid	¼	½	½	½	¾	¾	¾	1	1
cefdinir	125/t	qd	--	¾†	1	1	1	1¼	1½	1¾	2
cefixime	100/t	qd	½	½	¾	¾	¾	1	1	1¼	1½
cefprozil*	125/t	bid	--	¾†	1	1	1¼	1½	1½	2	2¼
"	250/t	bid	--	½†	½	½	¾	¾	¾	1	1¼
cefuroxime	125/t	bid	--	¾	¾	1	1	1	1½	1¾	2¼
cephalexin	125/t	qid	--	½	¾	¾	1	1	1¼	1½	1¾
"	250/t	aid	--	¼	¼	½	½	½	¾	¾	1

(cont.)

clarithromycin	125/t	bid	½[†]	½	½	½	¾	¾	¾	1	1¼
"	250/t	bid	--	--	--	¼	½	½	½	½	¾
dicloxacillin	62½/t	qid	½	¾	1	1	1¼	1¼	1½	1¾	2
nitrofurantoin	25/t	qid	¼	½	½	½	½	¾	¾	¾	1
penicillin V**	250/t	bid-tid	--	1	1	1	1	1	1	1	1
cetirizine	5/t	qd	--	--	½	½	½	½	½	½	½
Benadryl	12.5/t	q6h	½	½	¾	¾	1	1	1¼	1½	2
prednisolone	15/t	qd	¼	½	½	¾	¾	¾	1	1	1¼
prednisone	5/t	qd	1	1¼	1½	1¾	2	2¼	2½	3	3¾
Robitussin	---	q4h	--	--	¼[†]	¼[†]	½	½	¾	¾	1
Tylenol w/ codeine[¶]		q4h	--	--	--	--	--	--	--	1	1

(cont.)

*Dose shown is for otitis media only; see dosing in text for alternative indications.

†Dosing at this age/weight not recommended by manufacturer.

‡AAP now recommends high dose (80–90 mg/kg/d) for all otitis media in children; with Augmentin used as ES only.

§Give a double dose of azithromycin the first day.

**AHA dosing for streptococcal pharyngitis. Treat for 10 days.

¶AAP recommends against the use of codeine in children; FDA is considering the issue.

tsp/t = teaspoon; q = every; h = hour; kg = kilogram; Lbs = pounds; ml = mililiter;
bid = two times per day; qd = every day; qid = four times per day; tid = three times per day

PEDIATRIC VITAL SIGNS AND INTRAVENOUS DRUGS

Age		Pre-matr	New-born	2m	4m	6m	9m	12m	15m	2y	3y	5y
Weight	(kg)	2	3½	5	6½	8	9	10	11	13	15	19
	(lbs)	4¼	7½	11	15	17	20	22	24	28	33	42
Maint fluids	(mL/h)	8	14	20	26	32	36	40	42	46	50	58
ET tube	(mm)	2½	3/3½	3½	3½	3½	4	4	4½	4½	4½	5
Defib	(Joules)	4	7	10	13	16	18	20	22	26	30	38
Systolic BP	(high)	70	80	85	90	95	100	103	104	106	109	114
	(low)	40	60	70	70	70	70	70	70	75	75	80
Pulse rate	(high)	145	145	180	180	180	160	160	160	150	150	135
	(low)	100	100	110	110	110	100	100	100	90	90	65
Resp rate	(high)	60	60	50	50	50	46	46	30	30	25	25
	(low)	35	30	30	30	24	24	20	20	20	20	20
adenosine	(mg)	0.2	0.3	0.5	0.6	0.8	0.9	1	1.1	1.3	1.5	1.9
atropine	(mg)	0.1	0.1	0.1	0.13	0.16	0.18	0.2	0.22	0.26	0.30	0.38
Benadryl	(mg)	-	-	5	6½	8	9	10	11	13	15	19
bicarbonate	(meq)	2	3½	5	6½	8	9	10	11	13	15	19

(cont.)

dextrose	(g)	1	2	5	6½	8	9	10	11	13	15	19
epinephrine	(mg)	.02	.04	.05	.07	.08	.09	.1	.11	.13	.15	.19
lidocaine	(mg)	2	3/2	5	6½	8	9	10	11	13	15	19
morphine	(mg)	0.2	0.3	0.5	0.6	0.8	0.9	1	1.1	1.3	1.5	1.9
mannitol	(g)	2	3½	5	6½	8	9	10	11	13	15	19
naloxone	(mg)	.02	.04	.05	.07	.08	.09	.1	.11	.13	.15	.19
diazepam	(mg)	0.6	1	1.5	2	2.5	2.7	3	3.3	3.9	4.5	5
fosphenytoin*	(PE)	40	70	100	130	160	180	200	220	260	300	380
lorazepam	(mg)	0.1	0.2	0.3	0.35	0.4	0.5	0.5	0.6	0.7	0.8	1.0
phenobarb	(mg)	30	60	75	100	125	125	150	175	200	225	275
phenytoin*	(mg)	40	70	100	130	160	180	200	220	260	300	380
ampicillin	(mg)	100	175	250	325	400	450	500	550	650	750	1000
ceftriaxone	(mg)	-	-	250	325	400	450	500	550	650	750	1000
cefotaxime	(mg)	100	175	250	325	400	450	500	550	650	750	1000
gentamicin	(mg)	5	8	12	16	20	22	25	27	32	37	47

*Loading doses; fosphenytoin dosed in "phenytoin equivalents."

CONVERSIONS

Temperature:
F = (1.8) C + 32
C = (F − 32)/1.8

Liquid:
1 fluid ounce = 30 mL
1 teaspoon = 5 mL
1 tablespoon = 15 mL

Weight:
1 kilogram = 2.2 lbs
1 ounce = 30 g
1 grain = 65 mg

INHIBITORS, INDUCERS, AND SUBSTRATES OF CYTOCHROME P450 ISOZYMES

The cytochrome P450 (CYP) inhibitors and inducers below do not necessarily cause clinically important interactions with substrates listed. We exclude in vitro data which can be inaccurate. Refer to other resources for more information if an interaction is suspected based on this chart. A drug that inhibits CYP subfamily activity can block the metabolism of substrates by that enzyme, which can lead to substrate accumulation and toxicity. CYP inhibitors are classified by how much they increase the area-under-the-curve (AUC) of a substrate: weak (1.25- to 2-fold), moderate (2- to 5-fold), or strong (≥5 fold). A drug that induces CYP subfamily activity increases substrate metabolism, which can lead to reduced substrate efficacy. CYP inducers are classified by how much they decrease the AUC of a substrate: weak (20 to 50%), moderate (50 to 80%) and strong (>80%). A drug is considered a sensitive substrate if a CYP inhibitor increases the AUC of that drug by ≥ 5-fold. While AUC increases of >50% often do not affect patient response, smaller increases can be important if the drug has a narrow therapeutic range (eg, theophylline, warfarin, cyclosporine). This table may be incomplete since new evidence about drug metabolism is continually being identified.

INHIBITORS, INDUCERS, AND SUBSTRATES OF CYTOCHROME P450 ISOZYMES (*continued*)

CYP1A2

Inhibitors. *Strong:* ciprofloxacin, fluvoxamine. ***Moderate:*** methoxalan, mexiletine, oral contraceptives, vemurafenib, zileuton. ***Weak:*** acyclovir, allopurinol, caffeine, cimetidine, deferasirox, disulfiram, echinacea, famotidine, propafenone, propranolol, simeprevir, terbinafine, ticlopidine, verapamil. ***Unclassified:*** amiodarone, atazanavir, citalopram, clarithromycin, estradiol, isoniazid, peginterferon alfa-2a and 2b.

Inducers. *Moderate:* montelukast, phenytoin, smoking. ***Weak:*** omeprazole, phenobarbital. ***Unclassified:*** carbamazepine, charcoal-broiled foods, rifampin, ritonavir, tipranavir-ritonavir.

Substrates. *Sensitive:* caffeine, duloxetine, melatonin, ramelteon, tizanidine. ***Unclassified:*** acetaminophen, amitriptyline, asenapine, bendamustine, cinacalcet, clomipramine, clozapine, cyclobenzaprine, erlotinib, estradiol, fluvoxamine, haloperidol, imipramine, loxapine, mexiletine, mirtazapine, naproxen, olanzapine, ondansetron, pomalidomide, propranolol, rasagiline, riluzole, roflumilast, ropinirole, ropivacaine, R-warfarin, tasimelteon, theophylline, zileuton, zolmitriptan.

(cont.)

CYP2B6

Inhibitors. *Weak:* clopidogrel, prasugrel. *Unclassified:* voriconazole.

Inducers. *Moderate:* efavirenz, rifampin. *Weak:* isavuconazole, nevirapine, artemether (in *Coartem*). *Unclassified:* baicalin (in *Limbrel*), ritonavir.

Substrates. *Sensitive:* bupropion, efavirenz. *Unclassified:* cyclophosphamide, ketamine, meperidine, methadone, nevirapine, prasugrel, propofol.

CYP2C8

Inhibitors. *Strong:* clopidogrel, gemfibrozil. *Moderate:* deferasirox. *Weak:* atazanavir, fluvoxamine, ketoconazole, pazopanib, trimethoprim.

Inducers. *Moderate:* rifampin. *Unclassified:* barbiturates, carbamazepine, rifabutin, ritonavir.

Substrates. *Sensitive:* repaglinide. *Unclassified:* amiodarone, carbamazepine, dabrafenib, dasabuvir (in *Viekira Pak, Viekira XR*), enzalutamide, ibuprofen, imatinib, isotretinoin, loperamide, montelukast, paclitaxel, pioglitazone, rosiglitazone, selexipag, treprostanil.

(cont.)

INHIBITORS, INDUCERS, AND SUBSTRATES OF CYTOCHROME P450 ISOZYMES (*continued*)

CYP2C9

Inhibitors. *Moderate:* amiodarone, fluconazole, miconazole, oxandrolone. *Weak:* capecitabine, cotrimoxazole, etravirine, fluvastatin, fluvoxamine, metronidazole, oritavancin, tigecycline, voriconazole, zafirlukast. *Unclassified:* cimetidine, fenofibrate, fenofibric acid, fluorouracil, imatinib, isoniazid, leflunomide, ritonavir.

Inducers. *Moderate:* carbamazepine, enzalutamide, rifampin. *Weak:* aprepitant, bosentan, elvitegravir, phenobarbital, St John's wort. *Unclassified:* dabrafenib, rifapentine, ritonavir.

Substrates. *Sensitive:* celecoxib. *Unclassified:* azilsartan, bosentan, chlorpropamide, diclofenac, etravirine, fluoxetine, flurbiprofen, fluvastatin, formoterol, glimepiride, glipizide, glyburide, ibuprofen, irbesartan, lesinurad, losartan, mefenamic acid, meloxicam, montelukast, naproxen, nateglinide, ospemifene, phenytoin, piroxicam, ramelteon, ruxolitinib, sildenafil, tolbutamide, torsemide, vardenafil, voriconazole, S-warfarin, zafirlukast, zileuton.

(cont.)

(cont.)

CYP2C19

Inhibitors. *Strong*: fluconazole, fluvoxamine. ***Moderate*:** esomeprazole, fluoxetine, moclobemide, omeprazole, voriconazole. ***Weak*:** armodafinil, carbamazepine, cimetidine, etravirine, felbamate, human growth hormone, ketoconazole, oral contraceptives, oritavancin. ***Unclassified*** : chloramphenicol, eslicarbazepine, isoniazid, modafinil, oxcarbazepine.

Inducers. *Moderate*: enzalutamide, rifampin. ***Unclassified*:** efavirenz, ritonavir, St John's wort, tipranavir.

Substrates. *Sensitive*: lansoprazole, omeprazole. ***Unclassified*:** amitriptyline, bortezomib, brivaracetam, carisoprodol, cilostazol, citalopram, clobazam, clomipramine, clopidogrel, clozapine, cyclophosphamide, desipramine, dexlansoprazole, diazepam, escitalopram, esomeprazole, etravirine, flibanserin, formoterol, imipramine, lacosamide, methadone, moclobamide, nelfinavir, pantoprazole, phenytoin, progesterone, proguanil, propranolol, rabeprazole, sertraline, tofacitinib, voriconazole, R-warfarin.

INHIBITORS, INDUCERS, AND SUBSTRATES OF CYTOCHROME P450 ISOZYMES (*continued*)

CYP2D6

Inhibitors. *Strong:* bupropion, fluoxetine, paroxetine, quinidine. ***Moderate:*** cinacalcet, dronedarone, duloxetine, mirabegron, rolapitant, terbinafine. ***Weak:*** amiodarone, asenapine, celecoxib, cimetidine, desvenlafaxine, diltiazem, diphenhydramine, echinacea, escitalopram, febuxostat, gefitinib, hydralazine, hydroxychloroquine, imitinib, methadone, oral contraceptives, pazopanib, propafenone, ranitidine, ritonavir, sertraline, telithromycin, venlafaxine, vemurafenib, verapamil. ***Unclassified:*** abiraterone, chloroquine, clobazam, clomipramine, cobicistat, darunavir-ritonavir, fluphenazine, haloperidol, lorcaserin, lumefantrine (in *Coartem*), metoclopramide, moclobamide, panobinostat, peginterferon alfa-2b, perphenazine, quinine, ranolazine, thioridazine, tipranavir-ritonavir.

Inducers. None known.

Substrates. *Sensitive:* atomoxetine, desipramine, dextromethorphan, metoprolol, nebivolol, perphenazine, tolterodine, venlafaxine. ***Unclassified:*** amitriptyline, aripiprazole, brexpiprazole, carvedilol, cevimeline, chlorpheniramine, chlorpromazine, clozapine, cinacalcet, clomipramine, codeine*, darifenacin, dihydrocodeine, dolasetron, donepezil, doxepin, duloxetine, fesoterodine,

(cont.)

flecainide, fluoxetine, formoterol, galantamine, haloperidol, hydrocodone, iloperidone, imipramine, loratadine, loxapine, maprotiline, methadone, methamphetamine, metoclopramide, meclizine, mexiletine, mirtazapine, morphine, nortriptyline, ondansetron, paroxetine, pimozide, primaquine, promethazine, propafenone, propranolol, quetiapine, risperidone, ritonavir, tamoxifen, tamsulosin, tetrabenazine, thioridazine, timolol, tramadol*, trazodone, trimipramine, vortioxetine.

* Metabolism by CYP2D6 required to convert to active analgesic metabolite; analgesia may be impaired by CYP2D6 inhibitors.

CYP3A4

Inhibitors. *Strong*: clarithromycin, cobicistat, conivaptan, indinavir, itraconazole, ketoconazole, lopinavir-ritonavir, nefazodone, nelfinavir, posaconazole, ritonavir, saquinavir, telithromycin, voriconazole. ***Moderate:*** aprepitant, atazanavir, ciprofloxacin, crizotinib, darunavir-ritonavir, diltiazem, dronedarone, erythromycin, fluconazole, fosamprenavir, grapefruit juice (variable), imatinib, isavuconazole, netupitant (in *Akynzeo*), verapamil. ***Weak:*** alprazolam, amiodarone, amlodipine, atorvastatin, bicalutamide, cilostazol, cimetidine, cyclosporine, everolimus, fluoxetine, fluvoxamine, ginko, goldenseal, isoniazid, ivacaftor, lapatinib, lomitapide,

(cont.)

INHIBITORS, INDUCERS, AND SUBSTRATES OF CYTOCHROME P450 ISOZYMES (*continued*)

nilotinib, oral contraceptives, pazopanib, ranitidine, ranolazine, simeprevir, ticagrelor, tipranavir–ritonavir zileuton. *Unclassified:* danazol, miconazole, palbociclib, quinine, quinupristin–dalfopristin, sertraline.

Inducers. *Strong:* carbamazepine, enzalutamide, lumacaftor (in *Orkambi*),mitotane, phenytoin, rifampin, rifapentine, St Johns wort. ***Moderate:*** bosentan, efavirenz, etravirine, modafinil, nafcillin. ***Weak:*** aprepitant, armodafinil, clobazam, echinacea, fosamprenavir, lesinurad, oritavancin, pioglitazone, rufinamide. ***Unclassified:*** artemether (in *Coartem*), barbiturates, bexarotene, dabrafenib, dexamethasone, eslicarbazepine, ethosuximide, griseovulvin, nevirapine, oxcarbazepine, primidone, rifabutin, ritonavir, tocilizumab, vemurafenib.

Substrates. Sensitive: alfentanil, aprepitant, budesonide, buspirone, conivaptan, darifenacin, darunavir, dasatinib, dronedarone, eletriptan, eplerenone, everolimus, felodipine, fluticasone, ibrutinib, indinavir, isavuconazole, ivacaftor, lomitapide, lopinavir (in *Kaletra*), lovastatin, lurasidone, maraviroc, midazolam, nisoldipine, quetiapine, saquinavir, sildenafil, simvastatin, sirolimus, tipranavir, tolvaptan, triazolam, vardenafil. *Unclassified:* alfuzosin, aliskiren,

(cont.)

almotriptan, alprazolam, amiodarone, amlodipine, apixaban, apremilast, aripiprazole, armodafinil, artemether (in *Coartem*), atazanavir, atorvastatin, avanafil, axitinib, bedaquiline, bortezomib, bosentan, bosutinib, brentuximab, brexpiprazole, bromocriptine, buprenorphine, cabazitaxel, cabozantinib, carbamazepine, cariprazine, carbamazepine, ceritinib, cevimeline, cilostazol, cinacalcet, cisapride, citalopram, clarithromycin, clobazam, clomipramine, clonazepam, lopidogrel, clozapine, cobicistat, colchicine, corticosteroids, crizotinib, cyclophosphamide, cyclosporine, dabrafenib, daclatasvir, dapsone, desogestrel, desvenlafaxine, dexamethasone, dexlansoprazole, diazepam, dihydroergotamine, diltiazem, disopyramide, docetaxel, dofetilide, dolasetron, domperidone, donepezil, doxorubicin, dutasteride, efavirenz, elbasvir (in *Zepatier*), elvitegravir, enzalutamide, ergotamine, erlotinib, erythromycin, escitalopram, esomeprazole, eszopiclone, ethinyl estradiol, ethosuximide, etoposide, etravirine, exemestane, fentanyl, fesoterodine, finasteride, flibanserin, fosamprenavir, fosaprepitant, galantamine, gefitinib, grazoprevir (in *Zepatier*) guanfacine, haloperidol, hydrocodone, hydroxychloroquine, imatinib, imipramine, irinotecan, isradipine, itraconazole, ivacaftor, ivadrabine, ixabepilone, ketamine, ketoconazole, lansoprazole, lapatinib, letrozole, levonorgestrel, lidocaine, loratadine, loxapine, lumefantrine (in *Coartem*), macitentan, methylergonovine, mifepristone, mirtazapine,

INHIBITORS, INDUCERS, AND SUBSTRATES OF CYTOCHROME P450 ISOZYMES (*continued*)

modafinil, mometasone, naloxegol, nateglinide, nefazodone, nelfinavir, netupitant (in *Akynzeo*), nevirapine, nicardipine, nifedipine, nilotinib, nimodipine, nintedanib (minor), olaparib, ondansetron, ospemifene, oxybutynin, oxycodone, paclitaxel, panobinostat, pantoprazole, paritaprevir (in *Viekira Pak*, *Viekira XR*), palbociclib, paricalcitol, pazopanib, pimozide, pioglitazone, pomalidomide, ponatinib, prasugrel, praziquantel quinidine, quinine, rabeprazole, ramelteon, ranolazine, regorafenib, repaglinide, rifabutin, rifampin, riociguat, ritonavir, rivaroxaban, roflumilast, romidepsin, ruxolitinib, saxagliptin, sertraline, silodosin, solifenacin, sonidegib, sufentanil, sunitinib, tacrolimus, tadalafil, tamoxifen, tamsulosin, tasimelteon, telithromycin, temsirolimus, testosterone, tiagabine, ticagrelor, tinidazole, tofacitinib, tolterodine, tramadol, trazodone, venetoclax, verapamil, vilazodone, vinblastine, vincristine, vinorelbine, vorapaxar, voriconazole, R-warfarin, zaleplon, ziprasidone, zolpidem, zonisamide.

INHIBITORS, INDUCERS, AND SUBSTRATES OF P-GLYCOPROTEIN

The p-glycoprotein (P-gp) inhibitors and inducers listed below do not necessarily cause clinically important interactions with P-gp substrates. We exclude in vitro data which can be inaccurate. Refer to other resources for more information if an interaction is suspected based on this chart. P-gp is an efflux transporter that pumps drugs out of cells. In the gut, P-gp reduces drug absorption by pumping drugs into the gut lumen. In the kidney, it increases drug excretion by pumping drugs into urine. P-gp inhibitors can increase exposure to P-gp substrates, potentially increasing their risk of toxicity. P-gp inducers can reduce exposure to P-gp substrates, potentially increasing the risk of treatment failure. Some drugs are dual inhibitors of P-gp and CYP3A4 (e.g., clarithromycin, dronedarone, erythromycin, itraconazole, ketoconazole, verapamil), while others are dual inducers of P-gp and CYP3A4 (e.g., carbamazepine, phenytoin, rifampin, St John's wort). Potent P-gp inhibitors are defined here as drugs that increase the area-under-the-curve (AUC) of a P-gp substrate (digoxin or fexofenadine) by ≥1.5-fold. This table may be incomplete since new evidence about drug interactions is continually being identified.

INHIBITORS, INDUCERS, AND SUBSTRATES OF P-GLYCOPROTEIN (continued)

Inhibitors. *Potent:* amiodarone, clarithromycin, cyclosporine, dronedarone, flibanserin, itraconazole, lapatinib, lopinavir-ritonavir, ranolazine, ritonavir, verapamil. ***Unclassified:*** atorvastatin, azithromycin, captopril, carvedilol, cobicistat, conivaptan, daclatasvir, darunavir-ritonavir, diltiazem, dipyridamole, erythromycin, etravirine, everolimus, felodipine, indinavir, isavuconazole, isradipine, ivacaftor, ketoconazole, ledipasvir, lomitapide, naproxen, nifedipine, nilotinib, posaconazole, quinidine, rolapitant, saquinavir-ritonavir, simeprevir, telmisartan, ticagrelor, velpatasvir (in *Epclusa*).

Inducers: carbamazepine, fosamprenavir, phenytoin, rifampin, St John's wort, tipranavir-ritonavir*. *Tipranavir induces CYP3A4 and P-gp, while ritonavir inhibits both pathways. This makes it difficult to predict the effect of ritonavir-boosted tipranavir on substrates of P-gp.

(cont.)

Substrates: afatinib, aliskiren, ambrisentan, apixaban, boceprevir, ceritinib, clobazam, clopidogrel, colchicine, cyclosporine, dabigatran, dasabuvir (in Viekira Pak, Viekira XR), digoxin, diltiazem, docetaxel, dolutegravir, edoxaban, etoposide, everolimus, fexofenadine, fosamprenavir, imatinib, indinavir, lapatinib, ledipasvir (in Harvoni), linagliptin, loperamide, lovastatin, maraviroc, morphine, nadolol, naloxegol, nilotinib, nintedanib, ombitasvir (in Viekira Pak, Viekira XR), paclitaxel, paliperidone, paritaprevir (in Viekira Pak, Viekira XR), pomalidomide, posaconazole, pravastatin, propranolol, quinidine, ranolazine, rifaximin, ritonavir, rivaroxaban, romidepsin, saquinavir, saxagliptin, silodosin, simeprevir, sirolimus, sitagliptin, sofosbuvir, tacrolimus, tenofovir, ticagrelor, tolvaptan, topotecan, velpatasvir (in *Epclusa*) vinblastine, vincristine.

DRUG THERAPY REFERENCE WEBSITES (selected)

Professional societies or governmental agencies with drug therapy guidelines

AAP	American Academy of Pediatrics	www.aap.org
ACC	American College of Cardiology	www.acc.org
ACCP	American College of Chest Physicians	www.chestnet.org
ACCP	American College of Clinical Pharmacy	www.accp.com
ACR	American College of Rheumatology	www.rheumatology.org
ADA	American Diabetes Association	www.diabetes.org
AHA	American Heart Association	www.heart.org
AHRQ	Agency for Healthcare Research and Quality	www.ahcpr.gov
AIDSinfo	HIV Treatment, Prevention, and Research	www.aidsinfo.nih.gov
AMA	American Medical Association	www.ama-assn.org
APA	American Psychiatric Association	www.psych.org
APA	American Psychological Association	www.apa.org
ASHP	Amer. Society Health-Systems Pharmacists	www.ashp.org/shortages
	Drug Shortages Resource Center	
ATS	American Thoracic Society	www.thoracic.org
CDC	Centers for Disease Control and Prevention	www.cdc.gov
CDC	CDC bioterrorism and radiation exposures	www.bt.cdc.gov
IDSA	Infectious Diseases Society of America	www.idsociety.org
MHA	Malignant Hyperthermia Association	www.mhaus.org

(cont.)

Other therapy reference sites

Cochrane library	www.cochrane.org
Emergency Contraception Website	www.not-2-late.com
Immunization Action Coalition	www.immunize.org
QTDrug lists	www.crediblemeds.org
Managing Contraception	www.managingcontraception.com

ANALGESICS

OPIOID EQUIVALENCY*

Opioid	PO	IV/SC/IM
buprenorphine	n/a	0.3–0.4 mg
butorphanol	n/a	2 mg
codeine	130 mg	75 mg
fentanyl	?	0.1 mg
hydrocodone	20 mg	n/a
hydromorphone	7.5 mg	1.5 mg
levorphanol	4 mg	2 mg

Opioid	PO	IV/SC/IM
meperidine	300 mg	75 mg
methadone	5–15 mg	2.5–10 mg
morphine	30 mg	10 mg
nalbuphine	n/a	10 mg
oxycodone	20 mg	n/a
oxymorphone	10 mg	1 mg
pentazocine	50 mg	30 mg

*Approximate equianalgesic doses as adapted from the 2003 American Pain Society (www.ampainsoc.org) guidelines and the 1992 AHCPR guidelines. n/a = Not available. See drug entries themselves for starting doses. Many recommend initially using lower than equivalent doses when switching between different opioids. IV doses should be titrated slowly with appropriate monitoring. All PO dosing is with immediate-release preparations. Individualize all dosing, especially in the elderly, children, and in those with chronic pain, opioid naïve, or hepatic/renal insufficiency.

ANALGESICS—NSAIDs

Salicylic acid derivatives	ASA, diflunisal, salsalate, Trilisate
Propionic acids	flurbiprofen, ibuprofen, ketoprofen, naproxen, oxaprozin
Acetic acids	diclofenac, etodolac, indomethacin, ketorolac, nabumetone, sulindac, tolmetin
Fenamates	meclofenamate
Oxicams	meloxicam, piroxicam
COX-2 inhibitors	celecoxib

Note: If one class fails, consider another.

Muscle Relaxants

BACLOFEN (✱*Lioresal, Lioresal D.S.*) Spasticity related to MS or spinal cord disease/injury: Start 5 mg PO three times per day, then increase by 5 mg/dose q 3 days until 20 mg PO three times per day. Max dose 20 mg four times per day. [Generic only: Tabs 10, 20 mg.] ▶K ♀C ▶+ $

CARISOPRODOL (*Soma*) Acute musculoskeletal pain: 350 mg PO three to four times per day. Abuse potential. [Generic/Trade: Tabs 250, 350 mg.] ▶LK ♀? ▶− ⊚IV $

CHLORZOXAZONE (*Parafon Forte DSC, Lorzone, Remular-S*) Musculoskeletal pain: 500 to 750 mg PO three to four times per day to start. Decrease to 250 mg three to four times per day. [Generic/Trade: Tabs 500 mg (Parafon Forte DSC 500 mg tabs, scored). Trade only: Tabs 250 mg (Remular-S), 375, 750 mg (Lorzone).] ▶LK ♀C ▶? $

CYCLOBENZAPRINE (*Amrix, Flexeril, Fexmid*) Musculoskeletal pain: Start 5 to 10 mg PO three times per day, max 30 mg/day or 15 to 30 mg (extended-release) PO daily. Not recommended in elderly. [Generic/Trade: Tabs 5, 7.5, 10 mg. Extended-release caps 15, 30 mg ($$$$$).] ▶LK ♀B ▷? $

DANTROLENE (*Dantrium, Revonto, Ryanodex*) Chronic spasticity related to spinal cord injury, CVA, cerebral palsy, MS: 25 mg PO daily to start, up to max of 100 mg two to four times per day if necessary. Malignant hyperthermia: 2.5 mg/kg rapid IV push q 5 to 10 min continuing until symptoms subside or to a max total dose of 10 mg/kg (Dantrium, Revonto). Minimum of 1 mg/kg IV push with additional doses administered if necessary up to a total max dose of 10 mg/kg (Ryanodex). Prevention of malignant hyperthermia in patients at high risk: 2.5 mg/kg over a period of at least 1 min approximately 75 min before surgery (Ryanodex). Additional doses may be given if surgery is prolonged. [Generic/Trade: Caps 25, 50, 100 mg. Trade only: Vials 20 mg (Dantrium, Revonto), 250 mg (Ryanodex).] ▶LK ♀C ▷— $$$$ ■

METAXALONE (*Skelaxin*) Musculoskeletal pain: 800 mg PO three to four times per day. [Generic/Trade: Tabs 800 mg, scored. Generic only: Tabs 400 mg.] ▶LK ♀? ▷? $$$$

METHOCARBAMOL (*Robaxin, Robaxin-750*) Acute musculoskeletal pain: 1500 mg PO four times per day or 1000 mg IM/IV three times per day for 48 to 72 h. Maintenance: 1000 mg PO four times per day, 750 mg PO q 4 h, or 1500 mg PO three times per day. Tetanus: Specialized dosing. [Generic/Trade: Tabs 500, 750 mg. OTC in Canada.] ▶LK ♀C ▷? $

ORPHENADRINE (*Norflex*) Musculoskeletal pain: 100 mg PO two times per day. 60 mg IV/IM two times per day. [Generic only: 100 mg extended-release. OTC in Canada.] ▶LK ♀C ▷? $$

TIZANIDINE (*Zanaflex*) Muscle spasticity due to MS or spinal cord injury: 4 to 8 mg PO q 6 to 8 h prn, max 36 mg/day. [Generic/Trade: Tabs 4 mg, scored. Caps 2, 4, 6 mg. Generic only: Tabs 2 mg.] ▶LK ♀C ▷? $$$$

Non-Opioid Analgesic Combinations

ASCRIPTIN (acetylsalicylic acid + aluminum hydroxide + magnesium hydroxide + calcium carbonate)   Multiple strengths. 1 to 2 tabs PO q 4 h. [OTC Trade only: Tabs 325 mg aspirin/50 mg magnesium hydroxide/50 mg Al hydroxide/50 mg Ca carbonate (Ascriptin and Aspir-Mox). 500 mg aspirin/33 mg magnesium hydroxide/33 mg Al hydroxide/237 mg Ca carbonate (Ascriptin Maximum Strength).] ▶♀D ▶? $

BUFFERIN (acetylsalicylic acid + calcium carbonate + magnesium oxide + magnesium carbonate) 1 to 2 tabs/caps PO q 4 h. Max 12 tabs/caps/caps in 24 h. [OTC Trade only: Tabs/caps 325 mg aspirin/158 mg Ca carbonate/63 mg of magnesium oxide/34 mg of magnesium carbonate. Bufferin ES: 500 mg aspirin/222.3 mg Ca carbonate/88.9 mg of magnesium oxide/55.6 mg of magnesium carbonate.] ▶K ♀D ▶? $

ESGIC (acetaminophen + butalbital + caffeine) 1 to 2 tabs or caps PO q 4 h. Max 6 in 24 h. [Generic only: Tabs/caps, 325 mg acetaminophen/50 mg butalbital/40 mg caffeine. Oral soln 325/50/40 mg per 15 mL. Generic/Trade: Tabs (Esgic Plus) 500/50/40 mg.] ▶LK ♀C ▶? $

EXCEDRIN MIGRAINE (acetaminophen + acetylsalicylic acid + caffeine) 2 tabs/caps/geltabs PO q 6 h while symptoms persist. Max 8 tabs/caps/geltabs in 24 h. [OTC Generic/Trade: Tabs/caps/geltabs 250 mg acetaminophen/250 mg aspirin/65 mg caffeine.] ▶LK ♀D ▶? $

FIORICET (acetaminophen + butalbital + caffeine) 1 to 2 caps PO q 4 h. Max 6 caps in 24 h. [Generic/Trade: Tabs 325 mg acetaminophen/50 mg butalbital/40 mg caffeine.] ▶LK ♀C ▶? $

GOODY'S EXTRA STRENGTH HEADACHE POWDER (acetaminophen + acetylsalicylic acid + caffeine) 1 powder PO followed with liquid, or stir powder into a glass of water or other liquid. Repeat in 4 to 6 h prn. Max 4 powders in 24 h. [OTC trade only: 260 mg acetaminophen/520 mg aspirin/32.5 mg caffeine per powder paper.] ▶LK ♀D ▶? $

NORGESIC (orphenadrine + acetylsalicylic acid + caffeine) Multiple strengths; write specific product on Rx. Norgesic: 1 to 2 tabs PO three to four times per day. Norgesic Forte: 1 tab PO three to four times per day. [Generic only: Tabs 25 mg orphenadrine/385 mg aspirin/30 mg caffeine (Norgesic). Tabs 50/770/60 mg (Norgesic Forte).] ▶KL ♀D ▶? $$$

PHRENILIN (acetaminophen + butalbital) Tension or muscle contraction headache: 1 to 2 tabs PO q 4 h. Max 6 in 24 h. [Generic/Trade: Tabs 325 mg acetaminophen/50 mg butalbital (Phrenilin). Caps, 650/50 mg (Phrenilin Forte).] ▶LK ♀C ▶? $

SEDAPAP (acetaminophen + butalbital) 1 to 2 tabs PO q 4 h. Max 6 tabs in 24 h. [Generic only: Tabs 650 mg acetaminophen/50 mg butalbital.] ▶LK ♀C ▶? $

SOMA COMPOUND (carisoprodol + acetylsalicylic acid) 1 to 2 tabs PO four times per day. Abuse potential. [Generic only: Tabs 200 mg carisoprodol/325 mg aspirin.] ▶LK ♀D ▶– ©IV $$$

FIORINAL (acetylsalicylic acid + butalbital + caffeine, ✦Tecnal, Trianal) 1 to 2 tabs PO q 4 h. Max 6 tabs in 24 h. [Generic/Trade: Caps 325 mg aspirin/ 50 mg butalbital/40 mg caffeine.] ▶KL ♀D ▶– ©III $$

ULTRACET (tramadol + acetaminophen, ✦Tramacet) Acute pain: 2 tabs PO q 4 to 6 h prn (up to 8 tabs/day for no more than 5 days). Adjust dose in elderly and renal dysfunction. Avoid in opioid-dependent patients. Seizures may occur if concurrent antidepressants or seizure disorder. [Generic/Trade: Tabs 37.5 mg tramadol/325 mg acetaminophen.] ▶KL ♀C ▶– ©IV $$

Non-Steroidal Anti-Inflammatories—COX-2 Inhibitors

CELECOXIB (*Celebrex*) OA, ankylosing spondylitis: 200 mg PO daily or 100 mg PO two times per day. RA: 100 to 200 mg PO two times per day. Familial adenomatous polyposis: 400 mg PO two times per day with food. Acute pain, dysmenorrhea: 400 mg single dose, then 200 mg two times per day prn. An additional 200 mg dose may be given on day 1 if needed. JRA: Give 50 mg PO two times per day for age 2 to 17 yo and wt 10 to 25 kg,

(cont.)

give 100 mg PO two times per day for wt greater than 25 kg. Contraindicated in sulfonamide allergy. [Generic/Trade: Caps 50, 100, 200, 400 mg.] ▶L ♀C (D in 3rd trimester) ▶? $$$$$ ■

Non-Steroidal Anti-Inflammatories—Salicylic Acid Derivatives

ACETYLSALICYLIC ACID (*Ecotrin, Empirin, Halfprin, Bayer, Anacin, ZORprin, aspirin, ✦Asaphen, Entrophen, Novasen*) Analgesia: 325 to 650 mg PO/PR q 4 to 6 h. Platelet aggregation inhibition: 81 to 325 mg PO daily. [Generic/Trade (OTC): Tabs 325, 500 mg; chewable 81 mg; enteric-coated 81, 162 mg (Halfprin), 81, 325, 500 mg (Ecotrin), 650, 975 mg. Trade only: Tabs, controlled-release 650, 800 mg (ZORprin, Rx). Generic only (OTC): Supps 60, 120, 200, 300, 600 mg.] ▶K ♀D ▶? $

CHOLINE MAGNESIUM TRISALICYLATE (*Trilisate*) RA/OA: 1500 mg PO two times per day. [Generic only: Tabs 500, 750, 1000 mg. Soln 500 mg/5 mL.] ▶K ♀C (D in 3rd trimester) ▶? $$

DIFLUNISAL (*Dolobid*) Pain: 500 to 1000 mg initially, then 250 to 500 mg PO q 8 to 12 h. RA/OA: 500 mg to 1 g PO divided two times per day. [Generic only: Tabs 500 mg.] ▶K ♀C (D in 3rd trimester) ▶– $$$ ■

SALSALATE (*Salflex, Disalcid, Amigesic*) RA/OA: 3000 mg/day PO divided q 8 to 12 h. [Generic only: Tabs 500, 750 mg, scored.] ▶K ♀C (D in 3rd trimester) ▶? $$ ■

Non-Steroidal Anti-Inflammatories—Other

ARTHROTEC (diclofenac + misoprostol) OA: One 50/200 tab PO three times per day. RA: One 50/200 tab PO three to four times per day. If intolerant, may use 50/200 or 75/200 PO two times per day. Misoprostol is an abortifacient. [Generic/Trade: Tabs 50 mg/200 mcg, 75 mg/200 mcg, diclofenac/misoprostol.] ▶LK ♀ X ▶– $$$$$ ■

DICLOFENAC (*Voltaren, Voltaren XR, Flector, Zipsor, Cambia, Zorvolex, ✦Voltaren Rapide*) Multiple strengths; write **(cont.)**

specific product on Rx. Immediate- or delayed-release: 50 mg PO two to three times per day or 75 mg PO two times per day. Extended-release (Voltaren XR): 100 to 200 mg PO daily. Patch (Flector): Apply 1 patch to painful area two times per day. Gel: 2 to 4 g to affected area four times per day. Acute migraine with or without aura: 50 mg single dose (Cambia). [Generic/Trade: Tabs, extended-release (Voltaren XR) 100 mg. Topical gel (Voltaren) 1% 100 g tube. Generic only: Tabs, immediate-release: 25, 50 mg. Generic only: Tabs, delayed-release: 25, 50, 75 mg. Trade only: Patch (Flector) 1.3% diclofenac epolamine. Trade only: Caps, liquid-filled (Zipsor) 25 mg. Caps (Zorvolex) 18, 35 mg. Trade only: Powder for oral soln (Cambia) 50 mg.] ▶L ♀B (D in 3rd trimester) ▶– $$$ ■

DUEXIS (ibuprofen + famotidine) OA, RA: One 800/26.6 mg ibuprofen/famotidine tablet PO three times per day. [Trade only: tabs: 800/26.6 mg ibuprofen/famotidine.] ▶LK ♀– Avoid NSAID use after 30 weeks gestation. ▶ Ibuprofen and famotidine are present in breast milk in small amounts. Effects on milk production or infant are unknown. ■

ETODOLAC Multiple strengths; write specific product on Rx. Immediate-release: 200 to 400 mg PO two to three times per day. Extended-release: 400 to 1200 mg PO daily. [Generic only: Caps, immediate-release: 200, 300 mg. Tabs, immediate-release: 400, 500 mg. Tabs, extended-release: 400, 500, 600 mg.] ▶L ♀C (D in 3rd trimester) ▶– $ ■

FLURBIPROFEN (Ansaid) 200 to 300 mg/day PO divided two to four times per day. [Generic/Trade: Tabs, immediate-release 50, 100 mg.] ▶L ♀B (D in 3rd trimester) ▶+ $$$ ■

IBUPROFEN (Motrin, Advil, Nuprin, Rufen, NeoProfen, Caldolor) 200 to 800 mg PO three to four times per day. Peds older than 6 mo: 5 to 10 mg/kg PO q 6 to 8 h. GI perforation and necrotizing enterocolitis has been reported with NeoProfen. [OTC: Caps/Liqui-Gel caps 200 mg. Tabs 100, 200 mg. Chewable tabs 100 mg. Susp (infant gtts) 50 mg/1.25 mL (with calibrated dropper), 100 mg/5 mL. Rx Generic/Trade: Tabs 400, 600, 800 mg.] ▶L ♀B (D in 3rd trimester) ▶+ ■

INDOMETHACIN (*Indocin, Indocin SR, Indocin IV*) Multiple strengths; write specific product on Rx. Immediate-release preparations: 25 to 50 mg cap PO three times per day. Sustained-release: 75 mg cap PO one to two times per day. [Generic only: Caps, immediate-release 25, 50 mg. Caps, sustained-release 75 mg. Trade only: Supp 50 mg. Oral susp 25 mg/5 mL (237 mL)] ▶L ♀B (D in 3rd trimester) ▶+ $ ■

KETOPROFEN (*Orudis, Orudis KT, Actron, Oruvail*) Immediate-release: 25 to 75 mg PO three to four times per day. Extended-release: 100 to 200 mg cap PO daily. [Rx Generic only: Caps, extended-release 200 mg. Caps, immediate-release 50, 75 mg.] ▶L ♀B (D in 3rd trimester) ▶– $$$ ■

KETOROLAC (*Toradol*) Moderately severe acute pain: 15 to 30 mg IV/IM q 6 h or 10 mg PO q 4 to 6 h prn. Combined duration IV/IM and PO is not to exceed 5 days. Moderately severe, acute pain, single-dose treatment: 60 mg IM or 30 mg IV if patient younger than 65 yo, 30 mg IM or 15 mg IV if patient 65 yo or older, has renal impairment, or wt < 50 kg. [Generic only: Tabs 10 mg.] ▶L ♀C (D in 3rd trimester) ▶+ $ ■

MECLOFENAMATE Mild to moderate pain: 50 mg PO q 4 to 6 h prn. Max dose 400 mg/day. Menorrhagia and primary dysmenorrhea: 100 mg PO three times per day for up to 6 days. RA/OA: 200 to 400 mg/day PO divided three to four times per day. [Generic only: Caps 50, 100 mg.] ▶L ♀B (D in 3rd trimester) ▶– $$$ ■

MEFENAMIC ACID (*Ponstel, ✱Ponstan*) Mild to moderate pain, primary dysmenorrhea: 500 mg PO initially, then 250 mg PO q 6 h prn for no more than 1 week. [Generic/Trade: Caps 250 mg.] ▶L ♀D ▶– $$$$$ ■

MELOXICAM (*Mobic, ✱Mobicox*) RA/OA: 7.5 mg PO daily. JRA, age 2 yo or older: 0.125 mg/kg PO daily. [Generic/Trade: Tabs 7.5, 15 mg. Generic only: Susp 7.5 mg/5 mL (1.5 mg/mL).] ▶L ♀C (D in 3rd trimester) ▶? $ ■

NABUMETONE (*Relafen*) RA/OA: Initial: Two 500 mg tabs (1000 mg) PO daily. May increase to 1500 to 2000 mg PO daily or divided two times per day. [Generic only: Tabs 500, 750 mg.] ▶L ♀C (D in 3rd trimester) ▶– $$ ■

NAPROXEN (*Naprosyn, Aleve, Anaprox, EC-Naprosyn, Naprelan, Prevacid NapraPAC*) Immediate-release: 250 to 500 mg PO two times per day. Delayed-release: 375 to 500 mg PO two times per day (do not crush or chew). Controlled-release: 750 to 1000 mg PO daily. JRA: Give 2.5 mL PO two times per day for wt 13 kg or less, give 5 mL PO two times per day for 14 to 25 kg, give 7.5 mL PO two times per day for 26 to 38 kg. 500 mg naproxen equivalent to 550 mg naproxen sodium. [OTC Generic/Trade (Aleve): Tabs, immediate-release 200 mg. OTC Trade only (Aleve): Caps, Gelcaps, immediate-release 200 mg. Rx Generic/Trade: Tabs, immediate-release (Naprosyn) 250, 375, 500 mg. (Anaprox) 275, 550 mg. Tabs, delayed-release enteric-coated (EC-Naprosyn) 375, 500 mg. Tabs, controlled-release (Naprelan) 375, 500, 750 mg. Susp (Naprosyn) 125 mg/5 mL. Prevacid NapraPAC: 7 lansoprazole 15 mg caps packaged with 14 naproxen tabs 375 mg or 500 mg.] ▶L ♀B (D in 3rd trimester) ▶+ $$$ ■

OXAPROZIN (*Daypro*) 1200 mg PO daily. [Generic/Trade: Tabs 600 mg, trade scored.] ▶L ♀C (D in 3rd trimester) ▶– $$$ ■

PIROXICAM (*Feldene, Fexicam*) 20 mg PO daily. [Generic/Trade: Caps 10, 20 mg.] ▶L ♀B (D in 3rd trimester) ▶+ $$$

SULINDAC (*Clinoril*) 150 to 200 mg PO two times per day. [Generic/Trade: Tabs 200 mg. Generic only: Tabs 150 mg.] ▶L ♀B (D in 3rd trimester) ▶– $ ■

TOLMETIN (*Tolectin*) 200 to 600 mg PO three times per day. [Generic only: Tabs 200 (scored), 600 mg. Caps 400 mg.] ▶L ♀C (D in 3rd trimester) ▶+ $$$ ■

VIMOVO (naproxen + esomeprazole) OA, RA, ankylosing spondylitis: One 375/20 or 500/20 tab two times per day at least 30 minutes before meals. [Trade only: Delayed release tabs 375/20 and 500/20 mg naproxen/esomeprazole.] ▶L ♀ Avoid NSAID use after 30 weeks gestation. ▶ Naproxen present in breast milk at 1% of serum concentration. Esomeprazole is present in breast milk. Effects on milk production or infant are unknown. ■

Opioid Agonist-Antagonists

BUPRENORPHINE (*Probuphine, Buprenex, Butrans, Subutex*)
Analgesia: 0.3 to 0.6 mg IV/IM q 6 h prn. Treatment of opioid dependence (must undergo special training and be registered to prescribe for this indication): Induction 8 mg SL on day 1, 16 mg SL on day 2. Maintenance: 16 mg SL daily. Can individualize to range of 4 to 24 mg SL daily. Opioid dependence—Probuphine maintenance (if stable on 8 mg/day or less of transmucosal form): four implants in the inner aspect of one arm and left in place for 6 months and then removed. May repeat at 6 months in other arm one time only. Moderate to severe chronic pain: 5 to 20 mcg/h patch changed q 7 days. [Generic only: SL Tabs 2, 8 mg. Trade only (Butrans): Transdermal patches 5, 10, 20 mcg/h.] ▶L ♀C ▶– ⊚lll $ IV, $$$$$ SL ■

BUTORPHANOL (*Stadol, Stadol NS*) 0.5 to 2 mg IV or 1 to 4 mg IM q 3 to 4 h prn. Nasal spray (Stadol NS): 1 spray (1 mg) in 1 nostril q 3 to 4 h. Abuse potential. [Generic only: Nasal spray 1 mg/spray, 2.5 mL bottle (14 to 15 doses/bottle).] ▶LK ♀C ▶+ ⊚IV $$$ ■

NALBUPHINE (*Nubain*) 10 to 20 mg IV/IM/SC q 3 to 6 h prn. ▶LK ♀? ▶? $

PENTAZOCINE (*Talwin NX*) 30 mg IV/IM q 3 to 4 h prn (Talwin). 1 tab PO q 3 to 4 h. (Talwin NX = 50 mg pentazocine/0.5 mg naloxone). [Generic/Trade: Tabs 50 mg with 0.5 mg naloxone, trade scored.] ▶LK ♀C ▶? ⊚IV $$$ ■

Opioid Agonists

CODEINE 0.5 to 1 mg/kg up to 15 to 60 mg PO/IM/IV/SC q 4 to 6 h. Do not use IV in children. [Generic only: Tabs 15, 30, 60 mg. Oral soln: 30 mg/5 mL.] ▶LK ♀C ▶– ⊚lI $ ■

FENTANYL (*Ionsys, Duragesic, Actiq, Fentora, Sublimaze, Abstral, Subsys, Lazanda, Onsolis*) Transdermal (Duragesic): 1 patch q 72 h (some with chronic pain may require q 48 h dosing). May wear more than 1 patch to achieve the

(cont.)

FENTANYL TRANSDERMAL DOSE
(Dosing based on ongoing morphine requirement.)

Morphine* (IV/IM)	Morphine* (PO)	Transdermal fentanyl*
10–22 mg/d	60–134 mg/d	25 mcg/h
23–37 mg/d	135–224 mg/d	50 mcg/h
38–52 mg/d	225–314 mg/d	75 mcg/h
53–67 mg/d	315–404 mg/d	100 mcg/h

*For higher morphine doses, see product insert for transdermal fentanyl equivalencies.

correct analgesic effect. Transmucosal lozenge (Actiq) for breakthrough cancer pain: 200 to 1600 mcg, goal is 4 lozenges on a stick per day in conjunction with long-acting opioid. Buccal tab (Fentora) for breakthrough cancer pain: 100 to 800 mcg, titrated to pain relief. Buccal soluble film (Onsolis) for breakthrough cancer pain: 200 to 1200 mcg, titrated to pain relief. Sublingual tab (Abstral) for breakthrough cancer pain: 100 mcg, may repeat once after 30 minutes. Sublingual spray (Subsys) for breakthrough cancer pain: 100 mcg, may repeat once after 30 minutes. Nasal spray (Lazanda) for breakthrough cancer pain: 100 mcg. Adult analgesia/procedural sedation: 50 to 100 mcg slow IV over 1 to 2 min; carefully titrate to effect. Analgesia: 50 to 100 mcg IM q 1 to 2 h prn. [Generic/Trade: Transdermal patches 12, 25, 50, 75, 100 mcg/h. Actiq lozenges on a stick, berry-flavored 200, 400, 600, 800, 1200, 1600 mcg. Trade only: (Fentora) buccal tab 100, 200, 400, 600, 800 mcg, packs of 4 or 28 tabs. Trade only: (Onsolis) buccal soluble film 200, 400, 600, 800, 1200 mcg in child-resistant, protective foil, packs of 30 films. Trade only: (Abstral) SL tabs 100, 200, 300, 400, 600, 800 mcg, packs of 4 or 32 tabs. Trade only: (Subsys) SL spray 100,

(cont.)

200, 400, 600, 800, 1200, 1600 mcg blister packs in cartons of 10 and 30 (30 only for 1200 and 1600 mcg). Trade only: (Lazanda) nasal spray 100, 400 mcg/spray, 8 sprays/bottle.] ▶L ♀C ▶+ ⊚ll $ – varies by therapy ■

HYDROMORPHONE (*Dilaudid, Exalgo, ✦Hydromorph Contin*) Adults: 2 to 4 mg PO q 4 to 6 h. 0.5 to 2 mg IM/SC or slow IV q 4 to 6 h. 3 mg PR q 6 to 8 h. Titrate dose as high as necessary to relieve cancer or nonmalignant pain where chronic opioids are necessary. Peds age 12 yo or younger: 0.03 to 0.08 mg/kg PO q 4 to 6 h prn or give 0.015 mg/kg/dose IV q 4 to 6 h prn. Controlled-release tabs: 8 to 64 mg daily. [Generic/Trade: Tabs 2, 4, 8 mg (8 mg trade scored). Oral soln 5 mg/5 mL. Controlled-release tabs (Exalgo): 8, 12, 16, 32 mg.] ▶L ♀C ▶? ⊚ll $$ ■

LEVORPHANOL (*Levo-Dromoran*) 2 mg PO q 6 to 8 h prn. [Generic only: Tabs 2 mg, scored.] ▶L ♀C ▶? ⊚ll $$$$

MEPERIDINE (*Demerol, pethidine*) 1 to 1.8 mg/kg up to 150 mg IM/SC/PO or slow IV q 3 to 4 h. 75 mg meperidine IV/IM/SC is equivalent to 300 mg meperidine PO. [Generic/Trade: Tabs 50 (trade scored), 100 mg. Generic only: Syrup 50 mg/5 mL.] ▶LK ♀C but + ▶+ ⊚ll $$

METHADONE (*Diskets, Dolophine, Methadose, ✦Metadol*) Severe pain in opioid-tolerant patients: Initial dose is 2.5 mg IM/SC/PO q 8 to 12 h prn. Titrate up by 2.5 mg per dose q 5 to 7 days as necessary to relieve cancer or nonmalignant pain where chronic opioids are necessary. May start as high as 10 mg per dose if opioid-dependent patient and dosing is managed by experienced practitioner using an opioid conversion formula. Opioid dependence: Typical dose to prevent withdrawal is 20 mg PO daily but must be managed by an experienced practitioner. Treatment longer than 3 weeks is maintenance and only permitted in approved treatment programs. Opioid-naive patients: Not recommended in opioid-naive patients as 1st-line treatment of acute pain, mild chronic pain, postoperative pain, or as a prn medication. [Generic/Trade:

(cont.)

Tabs 5, 10 mg. Dispersible tabs 40 mg (for opioid dependence only). Oral concentrate (Intensol): 10 mg/mL. Generic only: Oral soln 5, 10 mg/5 mL.] ▶L ♀C ▶? ⊚ll $ ■

MORPHINE (*MS Contin, Kadian, Avinza, Roxanol, Oramorph SR, MSIR, DepoDur, ✦Statex, M.O.S., Doloral, M-Eslon*) Controlled-release tabs (MS Contin, Oramorph SR): Start at 30 mg PO q 8 to 12 h. Controlled-release caps (Kadian): 20 mg PO q 12 to 24 h. Extended-release caps (Avinza): Start at 30 mg PO daily. Do not break, chew, or crush MS Contin or Oramorph SR. Kadian and Avinza caps may be opened and sprinkled in applesauce for easier administration; however, the pellets should not be crushed or chewed. Give 0.1 to 0.2 mg/kg up to 15 mg IM/SC or slow IV q 4 h. Titrate dose as high as necessary to relieve cancer or nonmalignant pain where chronic opioids are necessary. [Generic only: Tabs, immediate-release 15, 30 mg ($). Oral soln 10 mg/5 mL, 20 mg/5 mL, 20 mg/mL (concentrate). Rectal supps 5, 10, 20, 30 mg. Generic/Trade: Controlled-release tabs (MS Contin) 15, 30, 60, 100, 200 mg ($$$$). Controlled-release caps (Kadian) 10, 20, 30, 50, 60, 80, 100 mg ($$$$$). Extended-release caps (Avinza) 30, 45, 60, 75, 90, 120 mg. Trade only: Controlled-release caps (Kadian) 40, 200 mg.] ▶LK ♀ C ▶+ ⊚ll varies by therapy ■

OXYCODONE (*Roxicodone, OxyContin, Percolone, OxyIR, OxyFAST, Oxecta, ✦Endocodone, Supeudol, OxyNEO*) Immediate-release preparations: 5 mg PO q 4 to 6 h prn. Controlled-release (OxyContin): 10 to 40 mg PO q 12 h (no supporting data for shorter dosing intervals for controlled-release tabs). Titrate dose as high as necessary to relieve cancer or nonmalignant pain where chronic opioids are necessary. Do not break, chew, or crush controlled-release preparations or Oxecta. [Generic only: Immediate-release: Tabs 5, 10, 20 mg. Caps 5 mg. Oral soln 5 mg/5 mL. Generic/Trade: Tab 15, 30 mg. Oral concentrate 20 mg/mL. Trade only: Immediate-release abuse-deterrent tabs (Oxecta): 5, 7.5 mg. Controlled-release tabs 10, 15, 20, 30, 40, 60, 80 mg ($$$$$).] ▶L ♀B ▶— ⊚ll varies by therapy ■

OXYMORPHONE (*Opana, Opana ER*) 10 to 20 mg PO q 4 to 6 h (immediate-release) or 5 mg q 12 h (extended-release) in opioid-naive patients, 1 h before or 2 h after meals. 1 to 1.5 mg IM/SC q 4 to 6 h prn. 0.5 mg IV q 4 to 6 h prn, increase dose until pain adequately controlled. [Generic/Trade: Immediate-release (IR) tabs 5, 10 mg. Extended-release tabs (ER) 5, 7.5, 10, 15, 20, 30, 40 mg. Trade only: Injection 1 mg/mL.] ▸L ♀C ▸? ⊚II $$$$$ ■

Opioid Analgesic Combinations

NOTE: *Refer to individual components for further information. May cause drowsiness and/or sedation, which may be enhanced by alcohol and other CNS depressants. Opioids, carisoprodol, and butalbital may be habit forming. Avoid exceeding 4 g/day of acetaminophen in combination products. Caution people who drink 3 or more alcoholic drinks/ day to limit acetaminophen use to 2.5 g/day due to additive liver toxicity. Opioids commonly cause constipation; concurrent laxatives are recommended. All opioids are pregnancy class D if used for prolonged periods or in high doses at term.*

ANEXSIA (**hydrocodone + acetaminophen**) Multiple strengths; write specific product on Rx. 1 tab PO q 4 to 6 h prn. [Generic only: Tabs 5/325, 7.5/325, 10/325 mg hydrocodone/mg acetaminophen, scored.] ▸LK ♀C ▸– ⊚II $

CAPITAL WITH CODEINE SUSPENSION (**acetaminophen + codeine**) 15 mL PO q 4 h prn. Give 5 mL q 4 to 6 h prn for age 3 to 6 yo, give 10 mL PO q 4 to 6 h prn for age 7 to 12 yo, use adult dose for age older than 12 yo. [Generic only: Soln 120 mg/5 mL, 12 mg/5 mL (APAP/Codeine). Trade only: Susp 120 mg/5 mL, 12 mg/5 mL (APAP/Codeine).] ▸LK ♀C ▸? ⊚V $

COMBUNOX (**oxycodone + ibuprofen**) 1 tab PO q 6 h prn for no more than 7 days. Max 4 tabs per day. [Generic only: Tabs 5 mg oxycodone/400 mg ibuprofen.] ▸L ♀C (D in 3rd trimester) ▸? ⊚II $$$

EMPIRIN WITH CODEINE (acetylsalicylic acid + codeine, ✚*292 tab*) Multiple strengths; write specific product on Rx. 1 to 2 tabs PO q 4 h prn. [Generic/Trade: No US formulation available. Tabs 325/30, 325/60 mg aspirin/mg codeine] ▶LK ♀D ▶– ⊝III $

FIORICET WITH CODEINE (acetaminophen + butalbital + caffeine + codeine) 1 to 2 caps PO q 4 h prn. Max 6 caps per day. [Generic/Trade: Caps 325 mg acetaminophen/50 mg butalbital/40 mg caffeine/30 mg codeine.] ▶LK ♀C ▶– ⊝III $$$

FIORINAL WITH CODEINE (acetylsalicylic acid + butalbital + caffeine + codeine, ✚*Fiorinal C-1/4, Fiorinal C-1/2, Trianal C-1/4, Trianal C-1/2*) 1 to 2 caps PO q 4 h prn. Max 6 caps/24 h. [Generic/Trade: Caps 325 mg aspirin/50 mg butalbital/40 mg caffeine/30 mg codeine.] ▶LK ♀D ▶– ⊝III $$$

IBUDONE REPREXAIN (hydrocodone + ibuprofen) 1 tab PO q 4 to 6 h prn, max dose 5 tabs/day. [Generic/Trade: Tabs 2.5/200, 5/200, 10/200 mg hydrocodone/ibuprofen.] ▶LK ♀– ▶? ⊝II $$

LORCET (hydrocodone + acetaminophen) 1 to 2 caps (5/325) PO q 4 to 6 h prn, max dose 8 caps/day. 1 tab PO q 4 to 6 h prn (7.5/325 and 10/325), max dose 6 tabs/day. [Gene] ▶LK ♀C ▶– ⊝II $$

LORTAB (hydrocodone + acetaminophen) 1 to 2 tabs (2.5/325 and 5/325) PO q 4 to 6 h prn, max dose 8 tabs/day. 1 tab (7.5/325 and 10/325 PO) q 4 to 6 h prn, max dose 5 tabs/day. [Generic/Trade: Lortab 5/325 (scored), Lortab 7.5/325 (trade scored), Lortab 10/325 mg hydrocodone/mg acetaminophen. Generic only: Tabs 2.5/325 mg.] ▶LK ♀C ▶– ⊝II $

MERSYNDOL WITH CODEINE (acetaminophen + codeine + doxylamine) Canada only. 1 to 2 tabs PO q 4 to 6 h prn. Max 12 tabs per day. [Canada trade only: OTC tab 325 mg acetaminophen/8 mg codeine phosphate/5 mg doxylamine.] ▶LK ♀C ▶? $

NORCO (hydrocodone + acetaminophen) 1 to 2 tabs PO q 4 to 6 h prn (5/325), max dose 12 tabs/day. 1 tab (7.5/325 and 10/325) PO q 4 to 6 h prn, max dose 8 and 6 tabs/day respectively. [Generic/Trade: Tabs 5/325, 7.5/325, 10/325 mg hydrocodone/acetaminophen, scored. Generic only: Soln 7.5/325 mg per 15 mL.] ▶L ♀C ▶? ⊝II $$

PERCOCET (oxycodone + acetaminophen, **✦***Percocet-Demi*, *Oxycocet, Endocet*) Multiple strengths; write specific product on Rx. 1 to 2 tabs PO q 4 to 6 h prn (2.5/325 and 5/325 mg). 1 tab PO q 4 to 6 h prn (7.5/325 and 10/325 mg). [Generic/Trade: Oxycodone/acetaminophen tabs 2.5/325, 5/325, 7.5/325, 10/325 mg. Trade only: (Primlev) tabs 2.5/300, 5/300, 7.5/300, 10/300 mg. Generic only: 10/325 mg.] ▶L ♀C ▶– ⊚II $

PERCODAN (oxycodone + acetylsalicylic acid, **✦***Oxycodan*) 1 tab PO q 6 h prn. [Generic/Trade: Tabs 4.88/325 mg oxycodone/ aspirin (trade scored).] ▶LK ♀D ▶– ⊚II $$

ROXICET (oxycodone + acetaminophen) Multiple strengths; write specific product on Rx. 1 tab PO q 6 h prn. Soln: 5 mL PO q 6 h prn. [Generic/Trade: Tabs 5/325 mg. Caps/caplets 5/325 mg. Soln 5/325 per 5 mL, mg oxycodone/acetaminophen.] ▶L ♀C ▶– ⊚II $

SOMA COMPOUND WITH CODEINE (carisoprodol + acetylsalicylic acid + codeine) Moderate to severe musculoskeletal pain: 1 to 2 tabs PO four times per day prn. [Generic only: Tabs 200 mg carisoprodol/ 325 mg aspirin/16 mg codeine.] ▶L ♀D ▶– ⊚III $$$$

SYNALGOS-DC (dihydrocodeine + acetylsalicylic acid + caffeine) 2 caps PO q 4 h prn. [Generic/Trade: Caps 16 mg dihydrocodeine/356.4 mg aspirin/30 mg caffeine.] ▶L ♀C ▶– ⊚III $$$

TYLENOL WITH CODEINE (codeine + acetaminophen, **✦***Tylenol #1, Tylenol #2, Tylenol #3, Tylenol #4, Atasol 8, Atasol 15, Atasol 30*) Multiple strengths; write specific product on Rx. Give 1 to 2 tabs PO q 4 h prn. Elixir: give 5 mL q 4 to 6 h prn for age 3 to 6 yo; give 10 mL q 4 to 6 h prn for age 7 to 12 yo. [Generic only: Tabs Tylenol #2 (15/300). Tylenol with Codeine Elixir/Susp/Soln 12/120 per 5 mL, mg codeine/mg acetaminophen. Generic/Trade: Tabs Tylenol #3 (30/300), Tylenol #4 (60/300).] ▶LK ♀C ▶? ⊚III $

TYLOX (oxycodone + acetaminophen) 1 cap PO q 6 h prn. [Trade only: Caps 5 mg oxycodone/325 mg acetaminophen.] ▶L ♀C ▶– ⊚II $

***VICODIN* (hydrocodone + acetaminophen)** 5/300 mg (max dose 8 tabs/day) and 7.5/300 mg (max dose of 6 tabs/day): 1 to 2 tabs PO q 4 to 6 h prn. 10/300 mg: 1 tab PO q 4 to 6 h prn (max of 6 tabs/day). [Generic/Trade: Tabs Vicodin (5/300), Vicodin ES (7.5/300), Vicodin HP (10/300), mg hydrocodone/mg acetaminophen, scored.] ▶LK ♀C ▶? ⊚ll $$$

***VICOPROFEN* (hydrocodone + ibuprofen)** 1 tab PO q 4 to 6 h prn, max dose 5 tabs/day. [Generic/Trade: Tabs 7.5/200 mg hydrocodone/ibuprofen. Generic only: Tabs 2.5/200, 5/200, 10/200 mg.] ▶LK ♀– ▶– ⊚ll $$

***XODOL* (hydrocodone + acetaminophen)** 1 tab PO q 4 to 6 h prn, max 6 doses/day. [Generic/Trade: Tabs 5/300, 7.5/300, 10/300 mg hydrocodone/acetaminophen.] ▶LK ♀C ▶– ⊚ll $$$

Opioid Antagonists

NALOXONE (*Narcan, Evzio*) Adult opioid overdose: 0.4 to 2 mg q 2 to 3 min prn. Adult post-op reversal: 0.1 to 0.2 mg q 2 to 3 min prn. Peds opioid overdose: 0.01 mg/kg IV; may give 0.1 mg/kg if inadequate response. Peds post-op reversal: 0.005 to 0.01 mg q 2 to 3 min prn. May use IM/SC/ET if IV not available. Nasal spray dosage form: give 4 mg (1 spray) every 2-3 minutes until patient responds or medical assistance arrives. [Trade only: solution for injection: 0.4 mg/mL or 1 mg/mL 10 mL multiple-dose vials. Ampules for injection: 0.02 mg/mL 2 mL ampule (box of 10), 0.4 mg/mL 1 mL ampule (box of 10), 1 mg/mL 2 mL ampule (box of 10). Nasal spray: 4 mg/0.1 mL, two blister packages of one dose each. Autoinjector (Evzio): 0.4 mg/injection, carton of 2.] ▶LK ♀B ▶ $

Other Analgesics

ACETAMINOPHEN (*Tylenol, Panadol, Tempra, Ofirmev, paracetamol, ✦Abenol, Atasol, Pediatrix*) 325 to 650 mg PO/PR q 4 to 6 h prn. Max dose 4 g/day, possibly changing to 3 g/day in near future. Adults and adolescents wt less than 50 kg, give

(cont.)

15 mg/kg IV q 6 h or 12.5 mg/kg IV q 4 h. Max dose 75 mg/kg/day. Adults and adolescents wt 50 kg or greater, give 1000 mg IV q 6 h or 650 mg IV q 4 h. Max dose 4 g/day. OA: 2 extended-release caplets (ie, 1300 mg) PO q 8 h around the clock. Peds: 10 to 15 mg/kg/dose PO/PR q 4 to 6 h prn. Children age 2 to 12 yo, give 15 mg/kg IV q 6 h or 12.5 mg/kg q 4 h. Max dose 75 mg/kg/day. [OTC: Tabs 325, 500, 650 mg. Chewable tabs 80 mg. Orally disintegrating tabs 80, 160 mg. Caps/gelcaps 500 mg. Extended-release caplets 650 mg. Liquid 160 mg/5 mL, 500 mg/15 mL. Supps 80, 120, 325, 650 mg.] ▸LK ♀B ▶+ $

MIDOL TEEN FORMULA (**acetaminophen+pamabrom**) 2 caps PO q 4 to 6 h. [Generic/Trade OTC: Caps 325 mg acetaminophen/25 mg pamabrom (diuretic).] ▸LK ♀B ▶+ $

TAPENTADOL (*Nucynta, Nucynta ER*) Moderate to severe acute pain: Immediate-release: 50 to 100 mg PO q 4 to 6 h prn, max 600 mg/day. Moderate to severe chronic pain: Extended-release: 50 to 250 mg PO twice daily. Adjust dose in elderly, renal and hepatic dysfunction. Avoid in opioid-dependent patients. Seizures may occur with concurrent antidepressants or seizure disorder. [Trade only: Immediate-release ($$$$): Tabs 50, 75, 100 mg. Extended-release ($$$$$): Tabs 50, 100, 150, 200, 250 mg.] ▸LK ♀C ▶– ⊝II $$$$

TRAMADOL (*Ultram, Ultram ER, Ryzolt, ConZip, Rybix ODT, ✦Zytram XL, Tridural, Ralivia, Durela*) Moderate to moderately severe pain: 50 to 100 mg PO q 4 to 6 h prn, max 400 mg/day. Chronic pain, extended-release: 100 to 300 mg PO daily. Adjust dose in elderly, renal, and hepatic dysfunction. Avoid in opioid-dependent patients. Seizures may occur with concurrent serotonergic agents or seizure disorder. [Generic/Trade: Tabs, immediate-release 50 mg. Extended-release tabs 100, 200, 300 mg. Trade only: (ConZip) Extended-release caps 100, 150, 200, 300 mg. (Rybix) ODT 50 mg.] ▸KL ♀C ▶– ⊝IV $$$

ANESTHESIA

Anesthetics and Sedatives

DEXMEDETOMIDINE (*Precedex*) ICU sedation less than 24 h: Load 1 mcg/kg over 10 min followed by infusion 0.6 mcg/kg/h (ranges from 0.2 to 1.0 mcg/kg/h) titrated to desired sedation endpoint. Beware of bradycardia and hypotension. Reduce dose in impaired hepatic function and geriatric patients. ▶LK ♀C ▶? $$$$$

ETOMIDATE (*Amidate*) Induction: Give 0.3 mg/kg IV. ▶L ♀C ▶? $

KETAMINE (*Ketalar*) Dissociative sedation: 1 to 2 mg/kg IV over 1-2 min (sedation lasting 10-20 min) repeat 0.5 mg/kg doses every 5 to 15 in PRN; 4 to 5 mg/kg IM (sedation lasting 15-30 min) repeat 2-4 mg/kg IM every 10 to 15 min PRN. Anesthesia induction: Adult: 1 to 2 mg/kg IV over 1 to 2 min (produces 5 to 10 min dissociative state) or 6.5 to 13 mg/kg IM (produces 10 to 20 min dissociative state). Concurrent administration of atropine no longer recommended. Consider prohylactic ondansetron to reduce vomiting and prophylactic midazolam to reduce recovery reactions. Peds: Age older than 3 mo: 1 to 2 mg/kg IV over 1 to 2 min or 4 to 5 mg/kg IM. Analgesia adjunct subdissociative dose: 0.01 to 0.5mg/kg in conjunction with opioid analgesia. [Generic/Trade: 10, 50, 100 mg/mL.] ▶L ♀C ▶? ©III $ ■

METHOHEXITAL (*Brevital*) Anesthesia induction: 1 to 2.0 mg/kg IV, duration 5 min, followed by 0.25-1 mg/kg IV every 4-7 min prn. ▶L ♀B ▶? ©IV $$

MIDAZOLAM (*Versed*) Adult sedation/anxiolysis: 5 mg or 0.07 mg/kg IM; or 1 mg IV slowly q 2 to 3 min up to 5 mg. Peds: 0.25 to 1 mg/kg to max of 20 mg PO, or 0.1 to 0.15 mg/kg IM. IV route (6 mo to 5 yo): initial dose 0.05 to 0.1 mg/kg IV, then titrated to max 0.6 mg/kg. IV route (6 to 12 yo): initial dose 0.025 to 0.05 mg/kg IV, then titrated to max 0.4 mg/kg. Monitor for respiratory depression. [Generic only: Injection 1 mg/mL, 5 mg/mL. Oral liquid 2 mg/mL.] ▶LK ♀D ▶– ©IV $

PROPOFOL (*Diprivan*)   Induction: 40 mg IV q 10 sec until induction (2 to 2.5 mg/kg). ICU ventilator sedation: Infusion 5 to 50 mcg/kg/min. Deep sedation: 1 mg/kg IV over 20 to 30 seconds. Repeat 0.5 mg/kg IV prn. ▶L ♀B ▶– $

Local Anesthetics

NOTE: *Risk of chondrolysis in patients receiving intra-articular infusions of local anesthetics following arthroscopic and other surgical procedures.*

ARTICAINE (*Septocaine, Zorcaine*)   4% injection (includes epinephrine) up to 7 mg/kg total dose   [4% (includes epinephrine 1:100,000).] ▶LK ♀C ▶? $

BUPIVACAINE (*Marcaine, Sensorcaine*)   Up to 2.5 mg/kg without epinephrine and up 3.0 mg/kg with epinephrine [0.25%, 0.5%, 0.75%, all with or without epinephrine]. ▶LK ♀C ▶? $ ■

EMLA (prilocaine—topical + lidocaine—topical)   Topical anesthesia: Apply 2.5 g cream or 1 disc to region at least 1 h before procedure. Cover with occlusive dressing. [Generic/Trade: Cream (2.5% lidocaine + 2.5% prilocaine) 5, 30 g.] ▶LK ♀B ▶? $$

LIDOCAINE—LOCAL ANESTHETIC (*Xylocaine*)   Without epinephrine: Max dose 4.5 mg/kg not to exceed 300 mg. With epinephrine: Max dose 7 mg/kg not to exceed 500 mg. Dose for regional block varies by region. [0.5, 1, 1.5, 2%. With epi: 0.5, 1, 1.5, 2%.] ▶LK ♀B ▶? $

MEPIVACAINE (*Carbocaine, Polocaine*)   Onset 3 to 5 min, duration 45 to 90 min. Amide group. Max local dose 5 to 6 mg/kg. [1, 1.5, 2, 3%.] ▶LK ♀C ▶? $

PRILOCAINE (*Citanest*)   Contraindicated if younger than 6 to 9 mo. If younger than 5 yo, max local dose is 3 to 4 mg/kg (with or without epinephrine). If 5 yo or older, max local dose is 5 mg/kg without epinephrine and 7 mg/kg with epinephrine. [4%, 4% with epinephrine.] ▶LK ♀B ▶? $

Neuromuscular Blockade Reversal Agents

NEOSTIGMINE (*Bloxiverz*) 0.03 to 0.07 mg/kg slow IV (preceded by atropine or glycopyrrolate). Max 0.07 mg/kg or 5 mg, whichever is less. ▶L ♀C ▶? $$$$

SUGAMMEDEX (*Bridion*) Rapid reversal of rocuronium (within 3 minutes): 16 mg/kg reverses a single dose of 1.2 mg/kg of rocuronium. Reversal of rocuronium and vecuronium: 4 mg/kg is recommended if spontaneous recovery of the twitch response has reached 1 to 2 post-tetanic counts (PTC) and there are no twitch responses to train-of-four (TOF) stimulation. 2 mg/kg is recommended if spontaneous recovery has reached the reappearance of the second twitch in response to TOF stimulation. ▶ renal excretion of unchanged drug ♀ 0/0/0 no data on pregnant women but no evidence of teratogenicity in animals; reduced efficacy of hormonal contraceptives for one week after administration ▶? $$$$$

Neuromuscular Blockers

CISATRACURIUM (*Nimbex*) Paralysis: 0.15 to 0.2 mg/kg IV. Peds: 0.1 mg/kg. Duration 30 to 60 min. ▶Plasma ♀B ▶? $

ROCURONIUM (*Zemuron*) Rapid-sequence intubation: 0.6 to 1.2 mg/kg IV. Paralysis: 0.6 mg/kg IV. Duration 30 min. ▶L ♀B ▶? $$

SUCCINYLCHOLINE (*Anectine, Quelicin*) Rapid sequence intubation paralysis: 1 to 2 mg/kg IV or up to 3–4 mg/kg IM (maximum 150 mg). Paralysis: 0.6 to 1.1 mg/kg IV or up to 3–4 mg/kg IM (maximum 150 mg). Peds: 2 mg/kg IV. ▶Plasma ♀C ▶? $

VECURONIUM (*Norcuron*) Paralysis: 0.08 to 0.1 mg/kg IV. Duration 15 to 30 min. ▶LK ♀C ▶? $

ANESTHESIA

ANTIMICROBIALS

ACUTE BACTERIAL SINUSITIS IN ADULTS AND CHILDREN[a] IDSA TREATMENT RECOMMENDATIONS

Initial therapy: mild to moderate infection and no risk factors for resistance

Adults: Treat for 5 to 7 days with: 1) Amoxicillin-clavulanate 500 mg/125 mg PO three times per day or 875 mg/125 mg PO two times per day for 5 to 7 days 2) Doxycycline 100 mg PO two times per day or 200 mg PO once daily	Peds: Amoxicillin-clavulanate[a] 45 mg/kg/day PO two times per day for 10 to 14 days

Initial therapy: severe infection, risk factors for resistance,[b] or high endemic rate of invasive, penicillin-nonsusceptible *S. pneumoniae* (≥10%)

Adults: Treat for 5 to 7 days with: 1) Amoxicillin-clavulanate[c] 2000 mg/125 mg PO two times per day 2) Doxycycline 100 mg PO two times per day or 200 mg PO once daily	Peds: Amoxicillin-clavulanate[a, c] 90 mg/kg/day PO two times per day for 10 to 14 days

(cont.)

ACUTE BACTERIAL SINUSITIS IN ADULTS AND CHILDREN[a] IDSA TREATMENT RECOMMENDATIONS (*continued*)

Beta-lactam allergy
Adults: Treat for 5 to 7 days with: 1) Doxycycline 100 mg PO two times per day or 200 mg PO once daily 2) Levofloxacin[d] 500 mg PO once daily 3) Moxifloxacin[d] 400 mg PO once daily	Peds, type 1 hypersensitivity: Levofloxacin[d] 10 to 20 mg/kg/day PO divided q 12 to 24 h for 10 to 14 days Peds, not type 1 hypersensitivity: Clindamycin[e] 30 to 40 mg/kg/day PO three times per day plus cefixime 8 mg/kg/day PO two times per day or cefpodoxime 10 mg/kg/day PO two times per day for 10 to 14 days

(cont.)

(cont.)

Risk factors for antibiotic resistance[b] or failed first-line therapy

Adults: Treat for 5 to 7 days with: 1) Amoxicillin-clavulanate[c] 2000 mg/125 mg PO two times per day 2) Levofloxacin[d] 500 mg PO once daily 3) Moxifloxacin[d] 400 mg PO once daily	Peds: Treat for 10 to 14 days with: 1) Amoxicillin-clavulanate[c] 90 mg/kg/day PO two times per day 2) Clindamycin[e] 30 to 40 mg/kg/day PO three times per day plus cefixime 8 mg/kg/day PO two times per day or cefpodoxime 10 mg/kg/day PO two times per day 3) Levofloxacin[d] 10 to 20 mg/kg/day PO q 12 to 24 h

ACUTE BACTERIAL SINUSITIS IN ADULTS AND CHILDREN[a] IDSA TREATMENT RECOMMENDATIONS (continued)

Severe infection requiring hospitalization
Adults: 1) Ampicillin-sulbactam 1.5 to 3 g IV q 6 h 2) Levofloxacin[d] 500 mg PO/IV once daily 3) Moxifloxacin[d] 400 mg PO/IV once daily 4) Ceftriaxone 1 to 2 g IV q 12 to 24 h 5) Cefotaxime 2 g IV q 4 to 6 h
Peds: 1) Ampicillin-sulbactam 200 to 400 mg/kg/day IV q 6 h 2) Cefotaxime 50 mg/kg/day IV q 12 h 3) Ceftriaxone 100 to 200 mg/kg/day IV q 6 h 4) Levofloxacin[d] 10 to 20 mg/kg/day IV q 12 to 24 h

Adapted from *Clin Infect Dis* 2012;54(8):e72–e112. Available online at: http://www.idsociety.org.

[a] AAP (*Pediatrics* 2013;132:e262–e280; pediatrics.aappublications.org) recommends amoxicillin 1st-line for uncomplicated acute sinusitis in children if antimicrobial resistance is not suspected. It recommends amoxicillin 45 mg/kg/day PO divided two times per day for mild-moderate sinusitis in children 2 yo or older who do not attend daycare and have not received an antibiotic in the past month. It recommends amoxicillin 80 to 90 mg/kg/day (max

(cont.)

4 g/day) divided two times per day in communities with a high prevalence of nonsusceptible *S. pneumoniae* (at least 10%). Amoxicillin-clavulanate 80 to 90 mg/kg/day (max 4 g/day) PO divided two times per day is an option for moderate-severe sinusitis, and for children younger than 2 yo, attending daycare, or who received an antibiotic in the past month.

[b]Risk factors for antibiotic resistance include attendance at daycare, age younger than 2 yo or older than 65 yo, recent hospitalization, antibiotic use within the past month, or patients who are immunocompromised.

[c]High-dose amoxicillin-clavulanate is recommended for geographic regions with high endemic rates (atleast 10%) of invasive penicillin-nonsusceptible *S. pneumoniae*, severe infection (eg, evidence of systemic toxicity with fever of 39° C or higher, and threat of suppurative complications), or risk factors for antibiotic resistance. Use the 14:1 formulation that provides amoxicillin 90 mg/kg/day and clavulanate 6.4 mg/kg/day. If the 14:1 is not available, use the 7:1 formulation with additional amoxicillin. Do not increase the dose of the 4:1 or 7:1 formulation in order to achieve a higher dose of amoxicillin; an excessive clavulanate dose increases the risk of diarrhea.

[d]As of May 2016, FDA advises that, for patients with other treatment options, the risk of serious adverse events exceeds the benefit of treating acute sinusitis with a fluoroquinolone. Therefore, fluoroquinolones should be reserved for patients with acute sinusitis who do not have other treatment options.

[e]Clindamycin resistance in *S. pneumoniae* is common in some areas of the United States.

Anthrax: CDC and AAP Preferred Regimens

Adults[a]	Children, 1 month of age and older[b]
Post-exposure prophylaxis.[c] Treat for 60 days with:	
Ciprofloxacin 500 mg PO q 12 h OR Doxycycline 100 mg PO q 12 h	Ciprofloxacin 30 mg/kg/day PO divided q 12 h (max 500 mg/dose) OR Doxycycline[g] 4.4 mg/kg/day PO divided q 12 h for wt <45 kg (max 100 mg/dose); 100 mg PO divided q 12 h for wt >45 kg

(cont.)

(cont.)

Cutaneous anthrax without systemic involvement.[c,d] Treat naturally-acquired disease for 7 to 10 days; treat bioterrorism-related disease for 60 days with:	
Ciprofloxacin 500 mg PO q 12 h OR Doxycycline 100 mg PO q 12 h OR Levofloxacin 750 mg PO q 24 h OR Moxifloxacin 400 mg PO q 24 h	Ciprofloxacin 30 mg/kg/day PO divided q 12 h (max 500 mg/dose)

Anthrax: CDC and AAP Preferred Regimens (*continued*)

Adults[a]	Children, 1 month of age and older[b]
Systemic anthrax[d] without meningitis. Treat for at least 2 weeks and until clinically stable with:[e]	
Ciprofloxacin 400 mg IV q 8 h[c] PLUS Clindamycin 900 mg IV q 8 h OR Linezolid 600 mg IV q 12 h	Ciprofloxacin 30 mg/kg/day IV divided q 8 h (max 400 mg/dose)[c] PLUS Clindamycin 40 mg/kg/day IV divided q 8 h (max 900 mg/dose)

(cont.)

(cont.)

Systemic anthrax[d] with possible/confirmed meningitis. Treat for 2 to 3 weeks and until clinically stable with:[e]	
Ciprofloxacin 400 mg IV q 8 h PLUS Meropenem 2 g IV q 8 h[c] PLUS Linezolid 600 mg IV q 12 h[f]	Ciprofloxacin 30 mg/kg/day IV divided q 8 h (max 400 mg/dose) PLUS Meropenem 120 mg/kg/day divided q 8 h (max 2 g/dose)[e] PLUS Linezolid 30 mg/kg/day divided q 8 h for age less than 12 yo; divide q 12 h for age 12 fyo and older (max 600 mg/dose)

Adapted from *Emerg Infect Dis* [Internet]. 2014 Feb. http://dx.doi.org/10.3201/eid2002. 130687 and *Pediatrics* 2014;133(5):e1411 at http://pediatrics.aappublications.org/content/early/2014/04/22/ peds. 2014–0563.

Anthrax: CDC and AAP Preferred Regimens (*continued*)

a For women who are pregnant or breastfeeding, refer to *Emerg Infect Dis* [Internet]. 2014 Feb. http://dx.doi.org/10.3201/eid2002.130611.

b Refer to AAP report cited above for dosage regimens to treat infants younger than 1 mo.

c Alternatives for penicillin-susceptible strains. Post-exposure prophylaxis or cutaneous anthrax. Adults: amoxicillin 1000 mg PO q 8 h OR penicillin 500 mg PO q 6 h. Children: amoxicillin 75 mg/kg/day PO divided q 8 h (max 1 g/dose) OR penicillin 50 to 75 mg/kg/day divided q 6 to 8 h. Systemic anthrax. Adults: penicillin G 4 million units IV q 4h OR ampicillin 3 g IV q 6 h. Children: penicillin G 400,000 units/kg/day IV divided q 4 h (max 4 million units/dose).

d Systemic anthrax is inhalation, injection, or GI anthrax; cutaneous anthrax with systemic involvement, extensive edema, or head or neck lesions; or meningitis. In addition to antibiotics, patients with suspected systemic anthrax should receive an antitoxin from the US Strategic National Stockpile. Three antitoxins bind the protective antigen on *B. anthracis* lethal and edema toxins. Obiltoxaximab (Anthim) and raxibacumab are monoclonal antibodies; anthrax immune globulin intravenous (AIGIV; Anthrasil) is human IgG polyclonal antibodies. Recommendations for prioritizing antitoxin use are available at: www.cdc.gov/mmwr/pdf/rr/rr6404.pdf.

e For patients exposed to aerosolized spores, provide prophylaxis to complete 60 days of treatment from the onset of illness.

f Linezolid can cause myelosuppression; monitor CBC weekly esp. in patients with myelosuppression and for courses longer than 2 weeks.

g In children younger than 8 yo, the benefit of preventing anthrax outweighs the risk of permanent tooth staining with doxycycline.

C. difficile Infection (CDI) in Adults: IDSA/SHEA and ACG Treatment Recommendations

Clinical signs	Treatment
Initial episode: mild to moderate	
IDSA: WBC ≤15,000 AND serum creatinine <1.5 times premorbid level ACG: Diarrhea with signs or symptoms not meeting severe or complicated criteria	Metronidazole 500 mg PO q 8 h for 10 to 14 days[a] ACG: If no response to metronidazole in 5 to 7 days, consider vancomycin. If unable to take metronidazole, use vancomycin 125 mg PO q 6 h for 10 days.
Initial episode: severe	
IDSA: WBC ≥15,000 OR serum creatinine ≥1.5 times premorbid level ACG: Serum albumin <3 g/dL plus either: • WBC ≥15,000 • Abdominal tenderness	Vancomycin 125 mg PO q 6 h for 10 to 14 days

(cont.)

C. difficile Infection (CDI) in Adults: IDSA/SHEA and ACG Treatment Recommendations (continued)

Clinical signs	Treatment
Initial episode: severe and complicated	
IDSA: Hypotension or shock, ileus, megacolon ACG: Any of the following attributable to CDI: • ICU admission for CDI • Hypotension ± required use of vasopressors • Fever ≥38.5°C • Ileus or significant abdominal distention • Mental status changes • WBC ≥35,000 or <2000 • Serum lactate >2.2 mmol/L • End organ failure	Vancomycin 500 mg PO/NG q 6 h plus metronidazole 500 mg IV q 8 h IDSA: Consider adding vancomycin 500 mg/100 mL[c] normal saline retention enema q 6 h if complete ileus. ACG: Add vancomycin 500 mg/500 mL[c] normal saline enema q 6 h if complicated CDI with ileus or toxic colon and/or significant abdominal distention.

(cont.)

(cont.)

First recurrent episode	
	Same as initial episode, stratified by severity. IDSA: Use vancomycin if WBC ≥15,000 or serum creatinine is increasing.

Second recurrent episode	
	Vancomycin taper and/or pulsed regimen[d]

Adapted from: *Infect Control Hosp Epidemiol* 2010;31:431. Available online at: http://www.idsociety.org.
Am J Gastroenterol 2013;108:478–98. Available online at: http://gi.org.

[a] ACG recommends 10 days of therapy because that is what clinical trials evaluated.

C. difficile Infection (CDI) in Adults: IDSA/SHEA and ACG Treatment Recommendations

[b] IDSA: Consider colectomy for severe CDI. ACG: Consult surgeon for complicated CDI. Consider surgery for any of the following attributed to CDI: hypotension requiring vasopressors; clinical signs of sepsis and organ dysfunction; mental status changes; WBC ≥50,000; lactate ≥5 mmol/L; or failure to improve after 5 days on medical therapy.

[c] IDSA recommends diluting vancomycin in 100 mL for administration as enema. ACG recommends diluting vancomycin in a larger volume (500 mL) in order to ensure delivery to ascending and transverse colon.

[d] IDSA taper example: Vancomycin 125 mg PO QID for 10 to 14 days, then 125 mg two times per day for 7 days, then 125 mg once daily for 7 days, then 125 mg every 2 or 3 days for 2 to 8 weeks. ACG proposed pulse regimen: Vancomycin 125 mg PO q 6 h for 10 days, then 125 mg once every 3 days for 10 doses. Note: If there is a third recurrence after a pulsed vancomycin regimen, ACG recommends considering fecal microbiota transplant.

PROPHYLAXIS FOR BACTERIAL ENDOCARDITIS*

Limited to dental or respiratory tract procedures in patients at highest risk. All regimens are single dose administered 30–60 minutes prior to procedure.

Standard regimen	Amoxicillin 2 g PO
Unable to take oral meds	Ampicillin 2 g IM/IV; or cefazolin† or ceftriaxone† 1 g IM/IV
Allergic to penicillin	Clindamycin 600 mg PO; or cephalexin† 2 g PO; or azithromycin or clarithromycin 500 mg PO
Allergic to penicillin and unable to take oral meds	Clindamycin 600 mg IM/IV; or cefazolin† or ceftriaxone† 1 g IM/IV
Pediatric drug doses	Pediatric dose should not exceed adult dose. Amoxicillin 50 mg/kg, ampicillin 50 mg/kg, azithromycin 15 mg/kg, cephalexin† 50 mg/kg, cefazolin† 50 mg/kg, ceftriaxone† 50 mg/kg, clarithromycin 15 mg/kg, clindamycin 20 mg/kg.

*For additional details of the 2007 AHA guidelines, see http://www.heart.org.
†Avoid cephalosporins if prior penicillin-associated anaphylaxis, angioedema, or urticaria.

ACUTE OTITIS MEDIA (AOM) IN CHILDREN: AMERICAN ACADEMY OF PEDIATICS

Initial Treatment (immediate or delayed[a])	
First-line	Alternative for Penicillin Allergy[d]
Amoxicillin 80 to 90 mg/kg/day PO divided 2 times per day[b] or Amoxicillin-clavulanate[c] 90 mg/kg/day PO divided 2 times per day[b]	Cefdinir 14 mg/kg/day PO divided 1 or 2 times per day[b] or Cefuroxime 30 mg/kg/day PO divided 2 times per day[b] or Cefpodoxime 10 mg/kg/day PO divided 2 times per day[b] or Ceftriaxone 50 mg IM/IV once daily for 1 or 3 days

(cont.)

(cont.)

Treatment After First Antibiotic Failure

If initial treatment was amoxicillin, use amoxicillin–clavulanate[c] 90 mg/kg/day PO divided 2 times per day.[b]

If initial treatment was amoxicillin–clavulanate or oral 3rd generation cephalosporin, use ceftriaxone 50 mg IM/IV once daily for 3 days.

Consider clindamycin 30 to 40 mg/kg/day PO divided 3 times per day ± 3rd generation cephalosporin if penicillin-resistant *S. pneumoniae* suspected.[b]

Treatment After Second Antibiotic Failure

Clindamycin 30 to 40 mg/kg/day PO divided 3 times per day + 3rd generation cephalosporin.[b]

Consider tympanocentesis and consult infectious diseases specialist if multidrug-resistant bacteria detected.

Adapted from *Pediatrics* 2013;131:e964–e999. Available online at: http://pediatrics.aappublications.org.

ACUTE OTITIS MEDIA (AOM) IN CHILDREN: AMERICAN ACADEMY OF PEDIATICS (*continued*)

[a]This applies to uncomplicated AOM in children age 6 mo to 12 yo. Immediate treatment is recommended for children with otorrhea or severe symptoms (moderate to severe pain, pain for ≥48 h, or temperature ≥39°C), and bilateral AOM in children age 6 to 23 mo. Observation for 48 to 72 h before antibiotic therapy is an option for children age 6 to 23 mo with unilateral AOM and mild symptoms (mild pain for <48 h and temperature <39°C), or children 2 yo and older with unilateral/bilateral AOM and mild symptoms. Observation must have mechanism to follow-up and start an antibiotic if symptoms do not improve within 48 to 72 hours. Do not use observation if follow-up is unsure.

[b]Treat for 10 days if age <2 yo or any age with severe symptoms, 7 days for age 2 to 5 yo with mild to moderate symptoms, and 5 to 7 days for age 6 yo or older with mild to moderate symptoms.

[c] Consider in patients who have received amoxicillin in the past 30 days or who have the otitis-conjunctivitis syndrome. Use the 14:1 formulation of amoxicillin-clavulanate that provides amoxicillin 90 mg/kg/day and clavulanate 6.4 mg/kg/day. If the 14:1 formulation is not available, give the 7:1 formulation with additional amoxicillin. Do not increase the dose of a 4:1 or 7:1 formulation to achieve a higher dose of amoxicillin; an excessive clavulanate dose increases the risk of diarrhea.

(cont.)

d Cefdinir, cefuroxime, cefpodoxime, and ceftriaxone are highly unlikely to cross-react with penicillin. Excluding patients with a history of a severe reaction, the reaction rate in patients who have not undergone penicillin skin testing is estimated at 0.1%. A drug allergy practice parameter (Ann Allergy Asthma Immunol 2010;105:259–73; available at http://www.allergyparameters.org) recommends that a cephalosporin can be given to patients who do not have a history of a severe and/or recent allergic reaction to penicillin. Options for patients with a history of an IgE-mediated reaction to penicillin include substitution of a non-beta-lactam antibiotic, or penicillin or cephalosporin skin testing to evaluate the risk of cephalosporin administration.

OVERVIEW OF BACTERIAL PATHOGENS (Selected)

By bacterial class

Gram-Positive Aerobic Cocci: Staphylococci. Coagulase-positive: *S. aureus*. Coagulase-negative: *S. epidermidis, S. lugdunensis, S. saprophyticus.* Streptococci. Alpha-hemolytic: *S. pneumoniae* (pneumococcus), Viridans group. Other: *S. anginosus* group. Beta-hemolytic: *S. pyogenes* (Group A), *S. agalactiae* (Group B). Enterococcus: *E. facium, E. faecalis.*

Gram-Positive Anaerobic Cocci: *Peptostreptococcus.*

Gram-Positive Aerobic/Facultative Anaerobic Bacilli: *Arcanobacterium, Bacillus, Corynebacterium diphtheriae, C. jeikeium, Erysipelothrix rhusiopathiae, Listeria monocytogenes, Nocardia.*

Gram-Positive Anaerobic Bacilli: *Actinomyces, Clostridium botulinum, C. difficile, C. perfringens, C. tetani, Lactobacillus, Propionibacterium acnes.*

Gram-Negative Aerobic Diplococci: *Moraxella catarrhalis, Neisseria gonorrhoeae, N. meningitides.*

Gram-Negative Aerobic Coccobacilli: *Haemophilus ducreyi, H. influenzae.*

(cont.)

Gram-Negative Aerobic Bacilli: *Acinetobacter, Bartonella, Bordetella pertussis, Brucella, Burkholderia cepacia, Campylobacter, Francisella tularensis, Helicobacter pylori, Legionella pneumophila, Pseudomonas aeruginosa, Stenotrophomonas maltophilia, Vibriocholerae, V. parahaemolyticus, V. vulnificus.*

Gram-Negative Facultative Anaerobic Bacilli: *Aeromonas hydrophila, Capnocytophaga, Eikenella corrodens, Kingella kingae, Pasteurella multocida,* Enterobacteriaceae: *Citrobacter, Escherichia coli, Enterobacter, Hafnia, Klebsiella pneumoniae, K. granulomatis, Morganella morganii, Proteus mirabilis, P. vulgaris, Providencia, Salmonella, Serratia, Shigella, Yersinia.*

Gram-Negative Anaerobic Bacilli: *Bacteroides fragilis, Fusobacterium, Prevotella.*

Intracellular Bacteria: *Anaplasma, Chlamydia pneumoniae, C. psittaci, C. trachomatis, Coxiella burnetii, Ehrlichia, Mycoplasma genitalium, M. pneumoniae, Rickettsia prowazekii, R. rickettsii, R. typhi, Ureaplasma urealyticum.*

Spirochetes: *Borrelia burgdorferi, B. miyamotoi, Leptospira, Treponema pallidum.*

Mycobacteria: *M. avium complex, M. kansasii, M. leprae, M. tuberculosis.*

OVERVIEW OF BACTERIAL PATHOGENS (Selected) (*continued*)

By bacterial name
Acinetobacter **Gram-negative aerobic bacilli**
Actinomyces **Gram-positive anaerobic bacilli**
Aeromonas hydrophila **Gram-negative facultative anaerobic bacilli**
Anaplasma **Intracellular bacteria**
Arcanobacterium **Gram-positive aerobic/facultative anaerobic bacilli**
Bacillus **Gram-positive aerobic/facultative anaerobic bacilli**
Bacteroides fragilis **Gram-negative anaerobic bacilli**
Bartonella **Gram-negative aerobic bacilli**
Bordetella pertussis **Gram-negative aerobic bacilli**
Borrelia burgdorferi **Spirochete**
Borrelia miyamotoi **Spirochete**
Brucella **Gram-negative aerobic bacilli**
Burkholderia cepacia **Gram-negative aerobic bacilli**
Campylobacter **Gram-negative aerobic bacilli**

(cont.)

Capnocytophaga **Gram-negative facultative anaerobic bacilli**

Chlamydia pneumoniae **Intracellular bacteria**

Chlamydia psittaci **Intracellular bacteria**

Chlamydia trachomatis **Intracellular bacteria**

Citrobacter **Gram-negative facultative anaerobic bacilli**

Clostridium botulinum **Gram-positive anaerobic bacilli**

Clostridium difficile **Gram-positive anaerobic bacilli**

Clostridium perfringens **Gram-positive anaerobic bacilli**

Clostridium tetani **Gram-positive anaerobic bacilli**

Corynebacterium diphtheriae **Gram-positive aerobic/facultative anaerobic bacilli**

Corynebacterium jeikeium **Gram-positive aerobic/facultative anaerobic bacilli**

Coxiella burnetii **Intracellular bacteria**

Ehrlichia **Intracellular bacteria**

Eikenella corrodens **Gram-negative facultative anaerobic bacilli**

Enterobacter **Gram-negative facultative anaerobic bacilli**

Enterobacteriaceae **Gram-negative facultative anaerobic bacilli**

Enterococcus facium **Gram-positive aerobic cocci**

OVERVIEW OF BACTERIAL PATHOGENS (Selected) (*continued*)

By bacterial name (*continued*)

Enterococcus faecalis **Gram-positive aerobic cocci**

Erysipelothrix rhusiopathiae **Gram-positive aerobic/facultative anaerobic bacilli**

Escherichia coli **Gram-negative facultative anaerobic bacilli**

Francisella tularensis **Gram-negative aerobic bacilli**

Fusobacterium **Gram-negative anaerobic bacilli**

Haemophilus ducreyi **Gram-negative aerobic coccobacilli**

Haemophilus influenzae **Gram-negative aerobic coccobacilli**

Hafnia **Gram-negative facultative anaerobic bacilli**

Helicobacter pylori **Gram-negative aerobic bacilli**

Kingella kingae **Gram-negative facultative anaerobic bacilli**

Klebsiella granulomatis **Gram-negative facultative anaerobic bacilli**

Klebsiella pneumoniae **Gram-negative facultative anaerobic bacilli**

Lactobacillus **Gram-positive anaerobic bacilli**

Legionella pneumophila **Gram-negative aerobic bacilli**

(cont.)

Leptospira **Spirochete**
Listeria monocytogenes **Gram-positive aerobic/facultative anaerobic bacilli**
Moraxella catarrhalis **Gram-negative aerobic diplococci**
Morganella morganii **Gram-negative facultative anaerobic bacilli**
Mycobacterium avium complex **Mycobacteria**
Mycobacterium kansasii **Mycobacteria**
Mycobacterium leprae **Mycobacteria**
Mycobacterium tuberculosis **Mycobacteria**
Mycoplasma pneumoniae **Intracellular bacteria**
Mycoplasma genitalium **Intracellular bacteria**
Neisseria gonorrhoeae **Gram-negative aerobic diplococci**
Neisseria meningitidis **Gram-negative aerobic diplococci**
Nocardia **Gram-positive aerobic/facultative anaerobic bacilli**
Pasteurella multocida **Gram-negative facultative anaerobic bacilli**
Peptostreptococcus **Gram-positive anaerobic cocci**
Pneumococcus (Streptococcus pneumoniae) **Gram-positive aerobic cocci**

OVERVIEW OF BACTERIAL PATHOGENS (Selected) (*continued*)

By bacterial name (*continued*)
Prevotella Gram-negative anaerobic bacilli
Propionibacterium acnes Gram-positive anaerobic bacilli
Proteus mirabilis Gram-negative facultative anaerobic bacilli
Proteus vularis Gram-negative facultative anaerobic bacilli
Providencia Gram-negative facultative anaerobic bacilli
Pseudomonas aeruginosa Gram-negative aerobic bacilli
Rickettsia prowazekii Intracellular bacteria
Rickettsia rickettsii Intracellular bacteria
Rickettsia typhi Intracellular bacteria
Salmonella Gram-negative facultative anaerobic bacilli
Serratia Gram-negative facultative anaerobic bacilli
Shigella Gram-negative facultative anaerobic bacilli
Staphylococcus aureus (coagulase-positive) Gram-positive aerobic cocci
Staphylococcus epidermidis (coagulase-negative) Gram-positive aerobic cocci

(cont.)

Staphylococcus lugdunensis (coagulase-negative) **Gram-positive aerobic cocci**

Staphylococcus saprophyticus (coagulase-negative) **Gram-positive aerobic cocci**

Stenotrophomonas maltophilia **Gram-negative aerobic bacilli**

Streptococcus agalactiae (Group B; beta-hemolytic) **Gram-positive aerobic cocci**

Streptococcus anginosus group **Gram-positive aerobic cocci**

Streptococcus pneumoniae (pneumococcus; alpha-hemolytic) **Gram-positive aerobic cocci**

Streptococcus pyogenes (Group A; beta-hemolytic) **Gram-positive aerobic cocci**

Treponema pallidum **Spirochete**

Ureaplasma urealyticum **Intracellular bacteria**

Vibrio cholerae **Gram-negative aerobic bacilli**

Vibrio parahaemolyticus **Gram-negative aerobic bacilli**

Vibrio vulnificus **Gram-negative aerobic bacilli**

Viridans group *Streptococcus* (alpha-hemolytic) **Gram-positive aerobic cocci**

Yersinia **Gram-negative facultative anaerobic bacilli**

SEXUALLY TRANSMITTED DISEASES & VAGINITIS*

Bacterial vaginosis	(1) metronidazole 5 g of 0.75% gel intravaginally daily for 5 days OR 500 mg PO two times per day for 7 days; (2) clindamycin 5 g of 2% cream intravaginally at bedtime for 7 days. Alternative: (1) tinidazole 2 g PO once daily for 2 days OR 1 g PO once daily for 5 days; (2) clindamycin 300 mg PO two times per day for 7 days. Treat all symptomatic pregnant women.
Candidal vaginitis	(1) Intravaginal butoconazole, clotrimazole, miconazole, terconazole, or tioconazole; (2) fluconazole 150 mg PO single dose.
Cervicitis	Treat based on NAAT results for chlamydia and gonorrhea. Presumptively treat at-risk women (age <25 yo; sex partner is new, has other partners, or has STD), esp if follow-up not ensured or NAAT not available. Presumptive regimen: (1) azithromycin 1 g PO single dose; (2) doxycycline 100 mg PO two times per day for 7 days. Presumptively treat for gonorrhea if at-risk or high community prevalence.

(cont.)

Chancroid	(1) azithromycin 1 g PO single dose; (2) ceftriaxone 250 mg IM single dose; (3) ciprofloxacin 500 mg PO two times per day for 3 days; (4) erythromycin base 500 mg PO three times per day for 7 days.
Chlamydia	(1) azithromycin 1 g PO single dose; (2) doxycycline 100 mg PO two times per day for 7 days. Alternative: (1) erythromycin base 500 mg PO four times per day for 7 days; (2) levofloxacin 500 mg PO once daily for 7 days. In pregnancy: azithromycin 1 g PO single dose. Alternative: (1) amoxicillin 500 mg PO three times per day for 7 days. (2) erythromycin base 500 mg PO four times per day for 7 days or 250 mg PO four times per day for 14 days. Repeat NAAT 3 to 4 weeks after treatment in pregnant women.
Lymphogranuloma venereum *(Chlamydia trachomatis)*	(1) doxycycline 100 mg PO two times per day for 21 days. Alternative: erythromycin base 500 mg PO four times per day for 21 days.

(cont.)

SEXUALLY TRANSMITTED DISEASES & VAGINITIS* (continued)

Epididymitis, acute	Chlamydia and gonorrhea likely: ceftriaxone 250 mg IM single dose + doxycycline 100 mg PO two times per day for 10 days. Chlamydia-gonorrhea and enteric organisms likely: ceftriaxone 250 mg IM single dose + levofloxacin 500 mg PO once daily for 10 days. Enteric organisms likely: levofloxacin 500 mg PO once daily for 10 days.
Genital herpes, first episode	(1) acyclovir 400 mg PO three times per day for 7 to 10 days; (2) famciclovir 250 mg PO three times per day for 7 to 10 days; (3) valacyclovir 1 g PO two times per day for 7 to 10 days.
Genital herpes, recurrent	(1) acyclovir 400 mg PO three times per day for 5 days; (2) acyclovir 800 mg PO three times per day for 2 days or two times per day for 5 days; (3) famciclovir 125 mg PO two times per day for 5 days; (4) famciclovir 1 g PO two times per day for 1 day; (5) famciclovir 500 mg PO 1st dose, then 250 mg PO two times per day for 2 days; (6) valacyclovir 500 mg PO two times per day for 3 days; (7) valacyclovir 1 g PO daily for 5 days.

(cont.)

Genital herpes, suppressive therapy	(1) acyclovir 400 mg PO two times per day; (2) famciclovir 250 mg PO two times per day; (3) valacyclovir 500 or 1000 mg PO daily. Valacyclovir 500 mg PO daily reduces transmission in patients with 9 or fewer recurrences per year, but other valacyclovir/acyclovir regimens may be more effective for suppression in patients who have 10 or more recurrences per year. Pregnant women with recurrent genital herpes: Start at 36 weeks gestation with (1) acyclovir 400 mg PO three times per day; (2) valacyclovir 500 mg PO two times per day.
Genital herpes, recurrent in HIV infection	(1) acyclovir 400 mg PO three times per day for 5 to 10 days; (2) famciclovir 500 mg PO two times per day for 5 to 10 days; (3) valacyclovir 1 g PO two times per day for 5 to 10 days.
Genital herpes, suppressive therapy in HIV infection	(1) acyclovir 400 to 800 mg PO two or three times per day; (2) famciclovir 500 mg PO two times per day; (3) valacyclovir 500 mg PO two times per day.

(cont.)

SEXUALLY TRANSMITTED DISEASES & VAGINITIS* *(continued)*

Genital warts	External anogenital, patient-applied: (1) imiquimod 3.75% or 5% cream; (2) podofilox 0.5% soln or gel; (3) sinecatechins 15% ointment. External anogenital, provider-administered: (1) cryotherapy with liquid nitrogen or cryoprobe; (2) surgical removal; (3) trichloroacetic or bichloroacetic acid 80% to 90% soln. Urethral meatus: (1) cryotherapy with liquid nitrogen; (2) surgical removal. Vaginal, cervical, or intra-anal: (1) cryotherapy with liquid nitrogen; (2) surgical removal; (3) trichloroacetic or bichloroacetic acid 80% to 90% soln.
Gonorrhea[a]	Ceftriaxone 250 mg IM single dose + azithromycin 1 g PO single dose. For cervix, urethra, and rectum if ceftriaxone is unavailable: cefixime 400 mg PO single dose + azithromycin 1 g PO single dose.[a] Ceftriaxone-allergic: consult infectious disease expert and consider (1) gemifloxacin 320 mg PO single dose + azithromycin 2 g PO single dose; (2) gentamicin 240 mg IM single dose + azithromycin 2 g PO single dose.

(cont.)

(cont.)

Gonorrhea, disseminated	Arthritis/arthritis-dermatitis syndrome: ceftriaxone 1 g IM/IV q 24 h + azithromycin 1 g PO single dose. After substantial improvement, can switch to PO drug based on antimicrobial susceptibility to complete at least 7 days of treatment. Alternative: cefotaxime 1 g IV q 8 h OR ceftizoxime 1 g IV q 8 h + azithromycin 1 g PO single dose. Meningitis, endocarditis: ceftriaxone 1 to 2 g IV q 12 to 24 h + azithromycin 1 g PO single dose. Treat IM/IV for at least 10 to 14 days for meningitis, and at least 4 weeks for endocarditis.

SEXUALLY TRANSMITTED DISEASES & VAGINITIS* *(continued)*

Granuloma inguinale	Azithromycin 1 g PO once weekly or 500 mg PO once daily for at least 3 weeks and until lesions completely healed. See STD guideline for alternative treatment regimens.
Non-gonococcal urethritis (NGU)	(1) azithromycin 1 g PO single dose; (2) doxycycline 100 mg PO two times per day for 7 days. Alternative: (1) erythromycin base 500 mg PO four times per day for 7 days; (2) levofloxacin 500 mg PO once per day for 7 days. Persistant/recurrent: (1) azithromycin 1 g PO single dose for men who initially received doxycycline; (2) moxifloxacin 400 mg PO once daily for 7 days if azithromycin failed; (3) metronidazole or tinidazole 2 g PO single dose for heterosexual men in areas of high *T vaginalis* prevalence.

(cont.)

(cont.)

ANTIMICROBIALS

Pelvic inflammatory disease (PID)	Parenteral: (1) cefotetan 2 g IV q 12 h + doxycycline 100 mg IV/PO q 12 h OR cefoxitin 2 g IV q 6 h + doxycycline 100 mg IV/PO q 12 h. After 24 to 48 h of improvement, switch to PO doxycycline to complete 14 days. (2) clindamycin 900 mg IV q 8 h + gentamicin IM/IV 2 mg/kg loading dose, then 1.5 mg/kg q 8 h (can substitute 3 to 5 mg/kg once-daily dosing). After 24 to 48 h of improvement, switch to clindamycin 450 mg PO four times per day or doxycycline 100 mg PO two times per day to complete 14 days. For tubo-ovarian abscess, add clindamycin 450 mg PO four times per day or metronidazole 500 mg PO two times per day to doxycycline to provide anaerobic activity. IM/oral regimen: ceftriaxone 250 mg IM single dose + doxycycline 100 mg PO two times per day ± metronidazole 500 mg PO two times per day for 14 days. Metronidazole is added to provide anaerobic coverage and treat bacterial vaginosis.

SEXUALLY TRANSMITTED DISEASES & VAGINITIS* *(continued)*

Proctitis	Ceftriaxone 250 mg IM single dose + doxycycline 100 mg PO two times per day for 7 days.
Pubic lice	(1) permethrin 1% cream rinse (2) pyrethrins with piperonyl butoxide. Apply to affected areas and wash off after 10 minutes. Alternatives: (1) malathion 0.5% lotion; apply to affected areas and wash off after 8 to 12 h (can be used if treatment failure may be due to resistance); (2) ivermectin 250 mcg/kg PO taken with food; repeat in 2 weeks.

(cont.)

(cont.)

Scabies	(1) permethrin 5% cream applied to body from neck down and washed off after 8 to 14 h; (2) ivermectin 200 mcg/kg PO taken with food; repeat in 2 weeks. Use permethrin for infants and children. Alternative: lindane 1% 1 oz of lotion or 30 g of cream applied to body from neck down and thoroughly washed off after 8 h; not for age less than 10 yo. Crusted scabies: 5% benzyl benzoate or 5% permethrin cream, full-body application daily for 7 days then twice weekly until discharge or cure + ivermectin 200 mcg/kg PO on days 1, 2, 8, 9, and 15. Consider additional doses on days 22 and 29 if severe.
Sexual assault prophylaxis	Ceftriaxone 250 mg IM single dose + metronidazole or tinidazole 2 g PO single dose + azithromycin 1 g PO single dose. Consider HBV and HPV vaccination and HIV prophylaxis when appropriate.

SEXUALLY TRANSMITTED DISEASES & VAGINITIS* (continued)

Syphilis, primary, secondary, or early latent, ie, duration less than 1 year	Benzathine penicillin 2.4 million units IM single dose. Penicillinallergic: doxycycline 100 mg PO two times per day for 14 days if primary or secondary syphilis and 28 days if early latent syphilis. Use skin testing and penicillin desensitization protocol if medication compliance or follow-up cannot be ensured.
Syphilis, late latent or unknown duration	Benzathine penicillin 2.4 million units IM q week for 3 doses. Penicillin-allergic: doxycycline 100 mg PO two times per day for 4 weeks.
Syphilis, tertiary	Benzathine penicillin 2.4 million units IM q week for 3 doses. This regimen is for patients with normal CSF exam; use neurosyphilis regimen if CSF abnormalities. Consult infectious disease specialist for management of penicillin-allergic patients.

(cont.)

Syphilis, neuro and ocular	(1) penicillin G 18 to 24 million units/day continuous IV infusion or 3 to 4 million units IV q 4 h for 10 to 14 days; (2) if compliance can be ensured, consider procaine penicillin 2.4 million units IM daily + probenecid 500 mg PO four times per day, both for 10 to 14 days. Penicillin-allergic: (1) ceftriaxone 2 g IM/IV once daily for 10 to 14 days; (2) skin testing and penicillin desensitization protocol.
Syphilis in pregnancy	Treat with penicillin regimen for stage of syphilis as noted above. For primary, secondary, or early latent syphilis, consider a second dose of benzathine penicillin 2.4 million units IM one week after initial dose. Use skin-testing and penicillin desensitization protocol if penicillin-allergic.

SEXUALLY TRANSMITTED DISEASES & VAGINITIS* *(continued)*

Trichomoniasis	Metronidazole or tinidazole 2 g PO single dose. Use metronidazole if pregnant. Persistent/recurrent: metronidazole 500 mg PO two times per day for 7 days. Treatment-failure: metronidazole or tinidazole 2 g PO two times per day for 7 days. HIV-infected women: metronidazole 500 mg PO two times per day for 7 days.

* MMWR 2015;64(No. RR-3): 1-137 or www.cdc.gov/std/tg2015/default.htm. Treat sexual partners for all except herpes, candida, and bacterial vaginosis. Refer to the STD guideline for additional alternative regimens.

a For suspected cephalosporin treatment failure, consult infectious disease specialist, an STD/HIV Prevention Training Center clinical expert (www.nnptc.org), or local/state health department STD program or CDC (phone 404-639-8659). Report suspected treatment failure to health department within 24 hours of diagnosis. When reinfection is likely, retreat with ceftriaxone 250 mg IM + azithromycin 1 g PO. For suspected treatment failure after cefixime-azithromycin regimen: Treat with ceftriaxone 250 mg IM single dose + azithromycin 2 g PO single dose. Obtain test-of-cure 7 to 14 days later, preferably with culture (and susceptibility testing of *N. gonorrhoeae* if isolated) and simultaneous NAAT.

NAAT = nucleic acid amplification test.

Aminoglycosides

NOTE: *See also Dermatology and Ophthalmology. Can cause nephrotoxicity, ototoxicity.*

AMIKACIN Adults: 15 mg/kg/day (up to 1500 mg/day) IM/IV divided q 8 to12 h or 15 mg/kg IV q 24 h. Peds, age 1 mo and older: 15 to 22.5 mg/kg/day divided q 8 to 12 h or 15 to 20 mg/kg IV q 24 h. Conventional dosing: Peak 20 to 35 mcg/mL, trough less than 5 mcg/mL. Once daily dosing: Peak 35 to 60 mcg/mL (if obtained), trough less than 4 mcg/mL. ▶K ♀D ▶? $$ ■

GENTAMICIN Adults: 3 to 5 mg/kg/day IM/IV divided q 8 h or 5 to 7 mg/kg IV q 24 h. Peds, age 1 mo and older: 2 to 2.5 mg/kg IM/IV q 8 h or 5 to 7.5 mg/kg IV q 24 h. Conventional dosing: Peak 5 to 10 mcg/mL, trough less than 2 mcg/mL. Once daily dosing: Peak 15 to 20 mcg/mL (if obtained), trough less than 1 mcg/mL. ▶K ♀D ▶+ $$ ■

STREPTOMYCIN Combo therapy for TB: 15 mg/kg (up to 1 g) IM daily; 10 mg/kg (up to 750 mg) for age 60 yo or older. Peds: 20 to 40 mg/kg (up to 1 g) IM daily; ATS recommends 15 to 20 mg/kg IM once daily. ▶K ♀D ▶+ $$$$$ ■

TOBRAMYCIN (*Bethkis, Kitabis Pak, Tobi*) Adults: 3 to 5 mg/kg/day IM/IV divided q 8 h or 5 to 7 mg/kg IV q 24 h. Peds, age 1 mo and older: 2 to 2.5 mg/kg q 8 h or 5 to 7.5 mg/kg IV q 24 h. Conventional dosing: Peak 5 to 10 mcg/mL, trough less than 2 mcg/mL. Once daily dosing: Peak 15 to 20 mcg/mL, trough less than 1 mcg/mL. Cystic fibrosis, age 6 yo to adult: 300 mg nebulized or 4 caps inhaled (Tobi Podhaler) two times per day 28 days on, then 28 days off. [Generic/Trade (Tobi): 300 mg/5 mL ampules for nebulizer. Trade only: Bethkis 300 mg/4 mL ampules for nebulizer. Tobi Podhaler 28 mg caps for inhalation. Kitabis Pak 300 mg/5 mL ampules copackaged with nebulizer.] ▶K ♀D ▶+ $$ ■

Antifungal Agents—Azoles

CLOTRIMAZOLE Oral troches five times per day for 14 days. [Generic only: Oral troches 10 mg.] ▶L ♀C ▶? $$$$

FLUCONAZOLE (*Diflucan*, ✶*CanesOral*) Vaginal candidiasis: 150 mg PO single dose ($). Other dosing regimens IV/PO. Oropharyngeal candidiasis: 100 to 200 mg daily for 7 to 14 days. Esophageal candidiasis: 200 to 400 mg daily for 14 to 21 days. Candidemia: 800 mg on 1st day, then 400 mg daily. Cryptococcal meningitis (IDSA regimen): Amphotericin B preferably in combo with flucytosine for at least 2 weeks (induction), then fluconazole 400 mg PO once daily for 8 weeks (consolidation), then chronic suppression with fluconazole 200 mg PO once daily until immune system reconstitution. Peds: Oropharyngeal candidiasis: 6 mg/kg on 1st day, then 3 mg/kg daily for 7 to 14 days. Esophageal candidiasis: 12 mg/kg on 1st day, then 6 mg/kg daily for 14 to 21 days. Systemic candidiasis; cryptococcal meningitis in AIDS: 12 mg/kg on 1st day, then 6 to 12 mg/kg daily. Many drug interactions. [Generic/Trade: Tabs 50, 100, 150, 200 mg. 150 mg tab in single-dose blister pack. Susp 10, 40 mg/mL (35 mL).] ▶K ♀C for single-dose treatment of vaginal candidiasis, D for all other indications. Possible increased risk of miscarriage; 400 to 800 mg/day linked to birth abnormalities. ▶+ $$$$

ISAVUCONAZONIUM (*Cresemba*, *isavuconazole*) Invasive aspergillosis, mucormycosis: Loading dose of 372 mg isavuconazonium IV/PO q 8 h for 6 doses, then 372 mg IV/PO once daily starting 12 to 24 h after last loading dose. Infuse IV doses over at least 1 h with in-line filter. Isavuconazonium is prodrug of isavuconazole; 372 mg isavuconazonium = 200 mg isavuconazole. P-glycoprotein and moderate CYP3A4 inhibitor. [Trade only: Caps 186 mg (100 mg isavuconazole).] ▶L glucuronidation ♀C ▶– $$$$$

ITRACONAZOLE (*Onmel*, *Sporanox*) Oral caps for onychomycosis "pulse dosing": 200 mg PO two times per day for 1st week of

(cont.)

month for 2 months (fingernails) or 3 to 4 months (toenails). Standard regimen, toenail onychomycosis: 200 mg PO daily with full meal for 12 weeks. Fluconazole-refractory oropharyngeal or esophageal candidiasis: Oral soln 200 mg PO daily for 14 to 21 days. Strong CYP3A4 and P-glycoprotein inhibitor; contraindicated with many drugs due to drug interactions. Negative inotrope; not for onychomycosis if ventricular dysfunction. [Trade only: Tabs 200 mg (Onmel). Oral soln 10 mg/mL (Sporanox-150 mL). Generic/Trade: Caps 100 mg.] ▶L ♀C ▶– $$$$$ ∎

MICONAZOLE—BUCCAL (*Oravig*) Oropharyngeal candidiasis, age 16 yo and older: Apply 50 mg buccal tab to gums once daily for 14 days. Increased INR with warfarin. CYP3A4 inhibitor. [Trade only: Buccal tabs 50 mg.] ▶L ♀C ▶? $$$$$

POSACONAZOLE (*Noxafil*, ✦*Posanol*) Prevention of invasive *Aspergillus* or *Candida* infection, Susp, age 13 yo and older: 200 mg (5 mL) PO three times per day with meals. Delayed-release tabs, age 13 yo and older: Load with 300 mg PO two times per day on 1st day, then 300 mg PO once daily taken with food. Injection, age 18 yo and older: Load with 300 mg IV two times per day on 1st day, then 300 mg IV once daily. Can infuse 1st dose over 30 minutes by peripheral line; infuse additional doses over 90 minutes by central venous line or peripherally-inserted central catheter. Susp for oropharyngeal candidiasis, age 13 yo or older: 100 mg (2.5 mL) PO two times on day 1, then 100 mg PO once daily for 13 days. Susp for oropharyngeal candidiasis resistant to itraconazole/fluconazole, age 13 yo or older: 400 mg (10 mL) PO two times per day. Take susp with full meal or liquid nutritional supplement. Susp and delayed-release tabs not interchangeable. Strong CYP3A4 inhibitor. [Trade only: Delayed-release tabs 100 mg. Oral susp 40 mg/mL (105 mL).] ▶Glucuronidation ♀C ▶– $$$$$

VORICONAZOLE (*Vfend*) Invasive aspergillosis, systemic *Candida* infections, adults and age 12 yo and older with wt 50 kg or greater: 6 mg/kg IV q 12 h for 2 doses, then 3 to 4 mg/kg IV

(cont.)

q 12 h (use 4 mg/kg for aspergillosis). Esophageal candidiasis or maintenance therapy of aspergillosis/candidiasis: 200 mg PO two times per day. For wt less than 40 kg, reduce to 100 mg PO two times per day. Dosage adjustment for efavirenz: Voriconazole 400 mg PO two times per day with efavirenz 300 mg PO once daily (use caps). Invasive aspergillosis, systemic *Candida* infections, age 2 to 11 yo and age 12 to 14 yo with wt less than 50 kg: 9 mg/kg IV q 12 h for 2 doses, then 8 mg/kg IV q 12 h. After 1 week and clinical improvement, convert to 9 mg/kg (max 350 mg) PO q 12 h. Therapeutic drug monitoring recommended due to variable pharmacokinetics in children. Take tabs or susp 1 h before or after meals. Strong CYP3A4 inhibitor. Many drug interactions. [Generic/Trade: Tabs 50, 200 mg (contains lactose). Susp 40 mg/mL (75 mL).] ▶L ♀D ▶? $$$$$

Antifungal Agents—Echinocandins

ANIDULAFUNGIN (*Eraxis*) Candidemia: 200 mg IV load on day 1, then 100 mg IV once daily. Esophageal candidiasis: 100 mg IV load on day 1, then 50 mg IV once daily. Max infusion rate of 1.1 mg/min to prevent histamine reactions. ▶Degraded chemically ♀B ▶? $$$$$

CASPOFUNGIN (*Cancidas*) Infuse over 1 h. Aspergillosis, candidemia, empiric therapy in febrile neutropenia: Load with 70 mg IV on day 1, then 50 mg once daily. Esophageal candidiasis: 50 mg IV once daily. Peds, age 3 mo and older: Load with 70 mg/m^2 IV on day 1, then 50 mg/m^2 once daily (max of 70 mg/day). ▶KL ♀C ▶? $$$$$

MICAFUNGIN (*Mycamine*) Esophageal candidiasis, age 4 mo and older: 3 mg/kg IV once daily for wt 30 kg or less; 2.5 mg/kg IV up to 150 mg once daily for wt greater than 30 kg. Candidemia, acute disseminated candidiasis, *Candida* peritonitis/abscess, age 4 mo and older: 2 mg/kg up to 100 mg IV once daily. Prevention of candidal infections in bone marrow

(cont.)

transplant patients, age 4 mo and older: 1 mg/kg up to 50 mg IV once daily. Infuse over 1 h to reduce histamine reactions. Flush IV line with NS before infusing micafungin. ▶L, feces ♀C ▶? $$$$$

Antifungal Agents—Polyenes

AMPHOTERICIN B DEOXYCHOLATE Test dose 0.1 mg/kg up to 1 mg slow IV. Wait 2 to 4 h, and if tolerated then begin 0.25 mg/kg IV daily and advance to 0.5 to 1.5 mg/kg/day depending on fungal type. ▶Tissues ♀B ▶? $$$$$ ■

AMPHOTERICIN B LIPID FORMULATIONS (*Abelcet, AmBisome*) Abelcet: 5 mg/kg/day IV at 2.5 mg/kg/h. AmBisome: 3 to 5 mg/kg/day IV over 2 h. ▶? ♀B ▶? $$$$$

Antifungal Agents—Other

FLUCYTOSINE (*Ancobon*) 50 to 150 mg/kg/day PO divided four times per day. Myelosuppression. [Generic/Trade: Caps 250, 500 mg.] ▶K ♀C Contraindicated in first trimester. ▶− $$$$$ ■

GRISEOFULVIN Tinea capitis: 500 mg PO daily in adults; 10 to 20 mg/kg (up to 1 g) PO daily in peds. Treat for 4 to 6 weeks, continuing for 2 weeks past symptom resolution. [Generic only: Susp 125 mg/5 mL (120 mL). Tabs 500 mg.] ▶Skin ♀ X/?/?. Contraindicated in pregnancy. ▶? $$$$$

NYSTATIN Thrush: 4 to 6 mL susp PO, swish and swallow four times per day. Infants: 2 mL/dose with 1 mL in each cheek four times per day. Non-esophageal mucus membrane gastrointestinal candidiasis: 1 to 2 tabs PO three times per day. [Generic only: Susp 100,000 units/mL (60, 480 mL). Film-coated tabs 500,000 units.] ▶Not absorbed ♀C ▶+ $

TERBINAFINE (*Lamisil*) Onychomycosis: 250 mg PO daily for 6 weeks (fingernails) or 12 weeks (toenails).Tinea capitis, age 4 yo or older: Give PO once daily with food for 6 weeks: 125 mg for wt less than 25 kg, 187.5 mg for wt 25 to 35 kg, 250 mg for

(cont.)

wt more than 35 kg. Treat *T tonsurans* for 2 to 4 weeks, *M canis* for 4 to 6 weeks. [Generic/Trade: Tabs 250 mg. No pediatric formulation, but pharmacists can compound a suspension.] ▶LK ♀B ▶− $$$$$

Antimalarials

NOTE: *For help treating malaria or getting antimalarials, see www.cdc.gov/malaria or call the "malaria hotline" at CDC. Call 770-488-7788 or 855-856-4713 toll-free Monday-Friday 9 am to 5 pm EST; after hours call 770-488-7100 and ask for the Malaria Branch clinician. Pediatric doses of antimalarials should never exceed adult doses.*

CHLOROQUINE (*Aralen*) Malaria prophylaxis, chloroquine-sensitive areas: 8 mg/kg up to 500 mg PO q week starting 1 to 2 weeks before exposure to 4 weeks after exposure. Chloroquine resistance is widespread. Can prolong QT interval and cause torsades. [Generic only: Tabs 250 mg. Generic/Trade: Tabs 500 mg (500 mg phosphate equivalent to 300 mg base).] ▶KL ♀C but +. ▶+ $ ■

COARTEM (**artemether + lumefantrine**) Uncomplicated malaria: Take PO with food two times per day for 3 days. On day 1, give 2nd dose 8 h after 1st dose. Dose based on wt: 1 tab for 5 to 14 kg; 2 tabs for 15 to 24 kg; 3 tabs for 25 to 34 kg; 4 tabs for 35 kg or greater. Repeat dose if vomiting occurs within 1 to 2 h. Can prolong QT interval. [Trade only: Tabs, artemether 20 mg + lumefantrine 120 mg. Call 1-855-COARTEM for availability.] ▶L ♀C ▶? $$$$

MALARONE (**atovaquone + proguanil**) Prevention of malaria: Give the following dose PO once daily from 1 to 2 days before exposure until 7 days after. Dose based on wt: ½ ped tab for 5 to 8 kg; ¾ ped tab for 9 to 10 kg; 1 ped tab for 11 to 20 kg; 2 ped tabs for 21 to 30 kg; 3 ped tabs for 31 to 40 kg; 1 adult tab for all patients wt greater than 40 kg. Treatment

(cont.)

of malaria: Give the following dose PO once daily for 3 days. Dose based on wt: 2 ped tabs for 5 to 8 kg; 3 ped tabs for 9 to 10 kg; 1 adult tab for 11 to 20 kg; 2 adult tabs for 21 to 30 kg; 3 adult tabs for 31 to 40 kg; 4 adult tabs for all patients wt greater than 40 kg. Take with food or milky drink. [Generic/Trade: Adult tabs atovaquone 250 mg + proguanil 100 mg. Pediatric tabs 62.5 mg + 25 mg.] ▶ Feces; LK ♀C ▶? $$$$$

MEFLOQUINE Malaria prophylaxis for chloroquine-resistant areas: 250 mg PO once a week from at least 2 weeks before exposure to 4 weeks after. Malaria treatment: 1250 mg PO single dose. Peds malaria prophylaxis: Give PO once a week starting at least 2 weeks before exposure to 4 weeks after at a dose of: 5 mg/kg (prepared by pharmacist) for wt 9 kg or less; ¼ tab for wt greater than 9 to 19 kg; ½ tab for wt greater than 19 to 30 kg; ¾ tab for wt greater than 30 to 45 kg; 1 tab for wt greater than 45 kg. Peds malaria treatment: 20 to 25 mg/kg PO single dose or divided into 2 doses given 6 to 8 h apart. Take on full stomach. Neuropsychiatric adverse events. [Generic only: Tabs 250 mg.] ▶L ♀B ▶? $$ ■

PRIMAQUINE Prevention of relapse, *P. vivax/ovale* malaria: 0.5 mg/kg (up to 30 mg) base PO daily for 14 days. Do not use unless normal G6PD level. [Generic only: Tabs 26.3 mg (equiv to 15 mg base).] ▶L ♀– ▶– $$$ ■

QUININE (*Qualaquin*) Malaria: 648 mg PO three times per day. Peds: 25 to 30 mg/kg/day (up to 2 g/day) PO divided q 8 h. Treat for 3 days (Africa/South America) or 7 days (Southeast Asia). Also give 7-day course of doxycycline, tetracycline, or clindamycin. Nocturnal leg cramps: 325 mg PO at bedtime. Per FDA, risk of life-threatening adverse events exceeds potential benefit for leg cramps. These include cinchonism; hemolysis with G6PD deficiency; hypersensitivity; thrombocytopenia; HUS/TTP; QT interval prolongation; many drug interactions. [Generic/Trade: Caps 324 mg.] ▶L ♀C ▶+? $$$$$ ■

Antimycobacterial Agents

NOTE: *Treat active mycobacterial infection with at least 2 drugs. See guidelines at www.thoracic.org/statements/ and www.aidsinfo.nih.gov.*

DAPSONE (*Aczone*) Pneumocystis pneumonia prophylaxis: 100 mg PO daily. Pneumocystis pneumonia treatment: 100 mg PO daily with trimethoprim 5 mg/kg PO three times per day for 21 days. Leprosy: See www.hrsa.gov/hansensdisease/ for regimens. Acne (Aczone; $$$$$): Apply 5% topically two times per day; apply 7.5% once daily. [Generic only: Tabs 25, 100 mg. Trade only (Aczone): Topical gel 5% and 7.5% in 30, 60, 90 g.] ▶LK ♀C ▶– $$$$

ETHAMBUTOL (*Myambutol*, ✷*Etibi*) TB: 15 to 20 mg/kg PO daily. Dose with whole tabs based on estimated lean body weight: Give 800 mg PO daily for wt 40 to 55 kg, 1200 mg for wt 56 to 75 kg, 1600 mg for wt 76 to 90 kg. Peds: 15 to 20 mg/kg (up to 1 g) PO daily. [Generic/Trade: Tabs 100, 400 mg.] ▶LK ♀C but + ▶+ $$$$

ISONIAZID (*INH*, ✷*Isotamine*) Adults: 5 mg/kg (up to 300 mg) PO daily. Peds: 10 to 15 mg/kg (up to 300 mg) PO daily. Hepatotoxicity. Give pyridoxine 25 to 50 mg daily to patients at risk for neuropathy. [Generic only: Tabs 100, 300 mg. Syrup 50 mg/5 mL.] ▶LK ♀C but + ▶+ $ ■

PYRAZINAMIDE (*PZA*, ✷*Tebrazid*) TB: 20 to 25 mg/kg (up to 2000 mg) PO daily. Dose with whole tabs based on estimated lean body weight: Give PO daily 1000 mg for 40 to 55 kg, 1500 mg for 56 to 75 kg, 2000 mg for 76 to 90 kg. Peds: 15 to 30 mg/kg (up to 2000 mg) PO daily. Hepatotoxicity. [Generic only: Tabs 500 mg.] ▶LK ♀C ▶? $$$$ ■

RIFABUTIN (*Mycobutin*) Mycobacterium avium complex disease, TB: 300 mg PO daily or 150 mg PO two times per day. Dosage reduction required with HIV protease inhibitors. [Generic/Trade: Caps 150 mg.] ▶L ♀B ▶? $$$$$ ■

RIFAMATE (isoniazid + rifampin) TB, age 15 yo and older: 2 caps PO daily on empty stomach. [Trade only: Caps isoniazid 150 mg + rifampin 300 mg.] ▶LK ♀C but + ▶+ $$$$$ ■

RIFAMPIN (*Rifadin, ★Rofact*) TB: 10 mg/kg (up to 600 mg) PO/IV daily. Peds: 10 to 20 mg/kg (up to 600 mg) PO/IV daily. *Neisseria meningitidis* carriers: 600 mg PO two times per day for 2 days. Peds: Age younger than 1 mo: 5 mg/kg PO two times per day for 2 days. Age 1 mo or older: 10 mg/kg (up to 600 mg) PO two times per day for 2 days. IV and PO doses are the same. Take oral doses on empty stomach. Strong enzyme inducer; many drug interactions. [Generic/Trade: Caps 150, 300 mg. Pharmacists can make oral susp.] ▶L ♀C but + ▶+ $$$$ ■

RIFAPENTINE (*Priftin, RPT*) Active pulmonary TB, age 12 yo and older: 600 mg PO two times per week for 2 months, then once weekly for 4 months. Use for continuation therapy only in selected HIV-negative patients. Latent TB, age 2 yo and older: Give with isoniazid both PO once weekly for 12 weeks. Use wt-based rifapentine dose of 300 mg for 10 to 14 kg; 450 mg for 14.1 to 25 kg; 600 mg for 25.1 to 32 kg; 750 mg for 32.1 to 50 kg; 900 mg for wt greater than 50 kg. Take with food. Intended for directly observed therapy. [Trade only: Tabs 150 mg.] ▶esterases, feces ♀C ▶? $$$$

RIFATER (isoniazid + rifampin + pyrazinamide) TB, initial 2 months of treatment, age 15 yo and older: Take on empty stomach PO daily at a dose of 4 tabs for wt less than 45 kg; 5 tabs for wt 45 to 54 kg, 6 tabs for wt 55 kg or greater. [Trade only: Tabs isoniazid 50 mg + rifampin 120 mg + pyrazinamide 300 mg.] ▶LK ♀C ▶? $$$$$ ■

Antiparasitics

ALBENDAZOLE (*Albenza*) Hydatid disease, neurocysticercosis: 15 mg/kg/day (up to 800 mg/day) PO divided in two doses for wt less than 60 kg; 400 mg PO two times per day for wt 60 kg or greater. [Trade only: Tabs 200 mg.] ▶L ♀C ▶? $$$$$

ANTIMICROBIALS

ATOVAQUONE (*Mepron*) Pneumocystis pneumonia, age 13 yo and older. Treatment: 750 mg PO two times per day for 21 days. Prevention: 1500 mg PO daily. Take with meals. [Generic/Trade: Susp 750 mg/5 mL (210 mL). Trade only: Foil pouch 750 mg/5 mL (5 mL).] ▶feces ♀C ▶? $$$$$

IVERMECTIN (*Stromectol*) Scabies: 200 mcg/kg PO on day 1 (3 mg for wt 15 to 24 kg, 6 mg for 25 to 35 kg, 9 mg for 36 to 50 kg, 12 mg for 51 to 65 kg, 15 mg for 66 to 79 kg); repeat dose in 7 to 14 days. Peds head lice: 200 or 400 mcg/kg PO on days 1 and 8. Single PO dose of 200 mcg/kg for strongyloidiasis, 150 mcg/kg for onchocerciasis. Not for children less than 15 kg. Take on empty stomach with water. [Generic/Trade: Tabs 3 mg.] ▶L ♀C ▶+ $$

MEBENDAZOLE (*Emverm*) Pinworm: 100 mg PO once; repeat in 2 weeks. Roundworm, whipworm, hookworm: 100 mg PO two times per day for 3 days. [Trade only: Chewable tabs 100 mg.] ▶L ♀C ▶? $$$$$

NITAZOXANIDE (*Alinia*) Cryptosporidial or giardial diarrhea: Give PO two times per day with food for 3 days. Dose is 100 mg for age 1 to 3 yo; 200 mg for age 4 to 11 yo; 500 mg for adults and children 12 yo and older. Use susp if younger than 12 yo. [Trade only: Oral susp 100 mg/5 mL (60 mL). Tabs 500 mg.] ▶L ♀?/?/? ▶? $$$$

PAROMOMYCIN Intestinal amebiasis: 25 to 35 mg/kg/day PO divided three times per day with or after meals. [Generic only: Caps 250 mg.] ▶Not absorbed ♀C ▶? $$$$$

PENTAMIDINE (*Pentam, NebuPent*) Pneumocystis pneumonia, treatment: 4 mg/kg IM/IV daily for 21 days. Pneumocystis pneumonia, prevention: 300 mg nebulized q 4 weeks. [Trade only: Aerosol 300 mg.] ▶K ♀C ▶– $$$$

PRAZIQUANTEL (*Biltricide*) Schistosomiasis: 20 mg/kg PO q 4 to 6 h for 3 doses. [Trade only: Tabs 600 mg.] ▶LK ♀B ▶– $$$$

PYRANTEL (*Pinworm, Pin-X, ✦Combantrin*) Pinworm, roundworm: 11 mg/kg (up to 1 g) PO single dose. Repeat in 2 weeks for pinworm. [OTC Trade only (Pin-X): Susp 144 mg/mL

(cont.)

(equivalent to 50 mg/mL of pyrantel base) 30, 60 mL. Tabs 720.5 mg (equivalent to 250 mg of pyrantel base).] ▶Not absorbed ♀C ▶? $

PYRIMETHAMINE (*Daraprim*) CNS toxoplasmosis in adults with AIDS. Acute therapy: For wt less than 60 kg give pyrimethamine 200 mg PO for first dose, then 50 mg PO once daily with sulfadiazine 1000 mg PO q 6 h and leucovorin 10 to 25 mg PO once daily (up to 50 mg once daily or two times per day). For wt 60 kg or greater give pyrimethamine 200 mg PO for first dose, then 75 mg PO once daily with sulfadiazine 1500 mg PO q 6 h and leucovorin 10 to 25 mg PO once daily (up to 50 mg once daily or two times per day). Treat for at least 6 weeks. Chronic maintenance therapy: Pyrimethamine 25 to 50 mg PO once daily with sulfadiazine 2000 to 4000 mg/day PO divided two to four times per day and leucovorin 10 to 25 mg PO once daily. [Trade only: Tabs 25 mg.] ▶L ♀C ▶+ $$$$$

TINIDAZOLE (*Tindamax*) Adults: 2 g PO daily for 1 day for trichomoniasis or giardiasis, 3 days for amebiasis. Bacterial vaginosis: 2 g PO once daily for 2 days or 1 g PO once daily for 5 days. See STD table. Peds, age older than 3 yo: 50 mg/kg (up to 2 g) PO daily for 1 day for giardiasis, 3 days for amebiasis. Take with food. [Generic/Trade: Tabs 250, 500 mg. Pharmacists can compound oral susp.] ▶KL ♀C ▶? $$ ■

Antiviral Agents—Anti-CMV

CIDOFOVIR CMV retinitis in AIDS: 5 mg/kg IV once a week for 2 weeks, then 5 mg/kg every other week. Severe nephrotoxicity. ▶K ♀C ▶– $$$$$ ■

FOSCARNET (*Foscavir*) CMV retinitis: 60 mg/kg IV (over 1 h) q 8 h or 90 mg/kg IV (over 1.5 to 2 h) q 12 h for 2 to 3 weeks, then 90 to 120 mg/kg IV daily over 2 h. HSV infection: 40 mg/kg (over 1 h) q 8 to 12 h. Nephrotoxicity, seizures. ▶K ♀C ▶? $$$$$ ■

GANCICLOVIR (*Cytovene*) CMV retinitis: Induction 5 mg/kg IV q 12 h for 14 to 21 days. Maintenance 6 mg/kg IV daily for 5 days per week. Myelosuppression; potential carcinogen and teratogen; may impair fertility. ▶K ♀C ▶– $$$$$ ■

VALGANCICLOVIR (*Valcyte*) CMV retinitis: 900 mg PO two times per day for 21 days, then 900 mg PO daily. Prevention of CMV disease in high-risk transplant patients: 900 mg PO daily given within 10 days post-transplant until 100 days post-transplant for heart or kidney/pancreas or 200 days for kidney transplant. See prescribing information for peds dose. Give with food. Myelosuppression; potential carcinogen and teratogen; may impair fertility. [Generic/Trade: Tabs 450 mg. Oral soln 50 mg/mL.] ▶K ♀C ▶– $$$$$ ■

Antiviral Agents—Anti-Hepatitis B

ENTECAVIR (*Baraclude*) Chronic hepatitis B, 16 yo and older: 0.5 mg PO once daily if treatment-naive; give 1 mg if lamivudine- or telbivudine-resistant, history of viremia despite lamivudine treatment, decompensated liver disease, or HIV coinfected. Peds. Chronic hepatitis B, treatment-naïve , age 2 to 15 yo: Give oral soln PO once daily at a dose of 3 mL for 10 to 11 kg; 4 mL for greater than 11 to 14 kg; 5 mL for greater than 14 to 17 kg; 6 mL for greater than 17 to 20 kg; 7 mL for greater than 20 to 23 kg; 8 mL for greater than 23 to 26 kg; 9 mL for greater than 26 to 30 kg; 10 mL or 0.5 mg tab for greater than 30 kg. Lamivudine-experienced , age 2 to 15 yo: Give oral soln PO once daily at a dose of 6 mL for 10 to 11 kg; 8 mL for greater than 11 to 14 kg; 10 mL for greater than 14 to 17 kg; 12 mL for greater than 17 to 20 kg; 14 mL for greater than 20 to 23 kg; 16 mL for greater than 23 to 26 kg; 18 mL for greater than 26 to 30 kg; 20 mL or 1 mg tab for greater than 30 kg. Take on empty stomach. [Generic/Trade: Tabs 0.5, 1 mg. Trade only: Oral soln 0.05 mg/mL (210 mL).] ▶K ♀C ▶– $$$$$ ■

Antiviral Agents—Anti-Hepatitis C

NOTE: *Treatment recommendations for HCV infection can change rapidly; refer to www.hcvguidelines.org for current guidance.*

Hepatitis C Direct-Acting Antiviral Agents

NS5B RNA Polymerase Inhibitors "buvirs"	NS3/4A Protease Inhibitors "previrs"	NS5A Protein Inhibitors "asvirs"
dasabuvir (in *Viekira Pak/XR*) sofosbuvir* (in *Harvoni*)	grazoprevir (in *Zepatier*) paritaprevir (in *Technivie, Viekira Pak/XR*) simeprevir*	daclatasvir* elbasvir (in *Zepatier*) ledipasvir (in *Harvoni*) ombitasvir (in *Technivie, Viekira Pak/XR*) velpatasvir (in *Epclusa*)

*Available as single-drug product, but HCV drugs are not intended for monotherapy.

DACLATASVIR (*Daklinza*) Chronic hepatitis C, genotype 1, 2, or 3, with no cirrhosis: 60 mg PO once daily + sofosbuvir 400 mg PO once daily for 12 weeks. Increase daclatasvir to 90 mg/day for moderate CYP3A4 inducers such as efavirenz or etravirine; avoid strong CYP3A4 inducers. Reduce to 30 mg/day for strong CYP3A4 inhibitors such as ritonavir-boosted atazanavir (see cytochrome P450 table). Cost of daclatasvir is $25,200/month. [Trade only: Tabs 30, 60 mg.] ▶L ♀?/?/? ▶? $$$$$

EPCLUSA (*sofosbuvir + velpatasvir*) Chronic hepatitis C, all genotypes, no cirrhosis or compensated cirrhosis (Child-Pugh A): 1 tab PO once daily for 12 weeks. Also for decompensated cirrhosis in combo with ribavirin. Cost of Epclusa is $29,900/month. [Trade only: Tabs velpatasvir 100 mg + sofosbuvir 400 mg.] ▶LK ♀?/?/?. Regimens with ribavirin: X/X/X ▶? $$$$$

***HARVONI* (ledipasvir + sofosbuvir)** Chronic hepatitis C . Harvoni dose is 1 tab PO once daily without regard to meals. Genotype 1, treatment-naïve ± compensated cirrhosis: Harvoni alone for 12 weeks. Can consider 8 weeks if pre-treatment HCV RNA <6 million international units/mL and no cirrhosis, HIV infection, African-American, or known IL28B polymorphism CT or TT. Genotype 4, 5, 6, treatment-naïve, ± compensated cirrhosis: Harvoni alone for 12 weeks. Also FDA-approved for genotype 1, 4, 5, 6, treatment-experienced patients; genotype 1 and 4 post-liver transplant; genotype 1 with decompensated cirrhosis . Warn patients that OTC antacids, H2 blockers, and proton pump inhibitors can reduce Harvoni levels. Cost of Harvoni is $33,750/month. [Trade only: Tabs ledipasvir 90 mg + sofosbuvir 400 mg.] ▶Bile, LK ♀?/?/? ▶? $$$$$

RIBAVIRIN—ORAL (*Rebetol, Copegus, Ribasphere*) Combination therapy of chronic hepatitis C in adults: Daily dose of 1000 mg/day PO for wt less than 75 kg, 1200 mg/day PO for wt 75 kg or greater. Divide daily dose of ribavirin two times per day and give with food. Chronic hepatitis C, peds: Rebetol, age 3 yo and older: 15 mg/kg/day PO divided two times per day with peginterferon alfa-2b (PegIntron). Copegus, age 5 yo and older: 15 mg/kg/day PO divided two times per day with peginterferon alfa-2a (Pegasys). Can cause hemolytic anemia; dosage adjustments required based on Hb. Teratogenic: Female patients and female partners of male patients must avoid pregnancy by using 2 effective forms of birth control during and for 6 months after stopping ribavirin. [Generic/Trade: Caps 200 mg, Tabs 200 mg. Generic only: Tabs 400, 600 mg. Trade only (Rebetol): Oral soln 40 mg/mL (100 mL).] ▶Cellular, K ♀X ▶– $$$$$ ■

SIMEPREVIR (*Olysio, SMV, ✦Galexos*) Chronic hepatitis C: Simeprevir dose for use only in combination regimens is 150 mg PO once daily with food. Genotype 1, treatment-naive and -experienced, no cirrhosis (guideline-recommended regimen): Simeprevir 150 mg + sofosbuvir 400 mg both PO once daily for 12 weeks. Genotype 1, treatment-naive and -experienced,

(cont.)

compensated cirrhosis, without Q80K polymorphism for genotype 1a (guideline alternative regimen): Simeprevir + sofosbuvir ± wt-based ribavirin (1000 mg/day PO for wt less than75 kg; 1200 mg/day PO for 75 kg or greater) for 24 weeks. HCV guideline no longer recommends FDA-approved regimen of simeprevir + wt-based ribavirin + peginterferon alfa. Cost of simeprevir is $26,500/month. [Trade only: Caps 150 mg.] ▶L bile ♀?/?/?. Regimens with ribavirin: X/X/X ▶— $$$$$

SOFOSBUVIR (*Sovaldi, SOF*) Chronic hepatitis C: Dose of sofosbuvir for use only in combination regimens is 400 mg PO once daily without regard to food. HCV guideline no longer recommends FDA-approved 12-week regimen of sofosbuvir + peginterferon + ribavirin for genotype 1. See daclasvir entry for daclatasvir-sofosbuvir regimens. See simeprevir entry for simeprevir-sofosbuvir regimens. Cost of sofosbuvir is $28,000/month. [Trade only: Tabs 400 mg.] ▶LK ♀B Regimens with ribavirin: X ▶? $$$$$

TECHNIVIE **(ombitasvir-paritaprevir-ritonavir)** Chronic hepatitis C, genotype 4: 2 tabs PO once daily with breakfast for 12 weeks. Intended for use with ribavirin (1000 mg/day for wt less than 75 kg and 1200 mg/day for wt 75 kg or greater PO divided two times per day with food) in patients without cirrhosis. Many drug interactions. Ribavirin is teratogenic; female patients and female partners of male patients must avoid pregnancy by using 2 forms of birth control during and for 6 months after stopping ribavirin. Cost of Technivie is $30,600/month. [Trade only: Tabs ombitasvir 12.5 mg + paritaprevir 75 mg + ritonavir 50 mg.] ▶L ♀X ▶— $$$$$

VIEKIRA PAK **(ombitasvir + paritaprevir + ritonavir + dasabuvir, *Viekira XR*, ✦*Holkira Pak*)** Chronic hepatitis C. Viekira Pak regimen is 2 tabs of ombitasvir-paritaprevir-ritonavir PO once each morning + 1 tab dasabuvir (250 mg) PO two times per day with a meal. Viekira XR regimen is 3 tabs of dasabuvir-ombitasvir-paritaprevir-ritonavir PO once daily with a meal. Genotype 1a, no cirrhosis: Viekira Pak/XR + ribavirin

(cont.)

for 12 weeks. Genotype 1a, compensated cirrhosis (Child-Pugh A): Viekira Pak/XR + ribavirin for 24 weeks. HCV guideline considers this an alternative regimen only for patients who can be monitored closely during the first 4 weeks for changes in liver function. Genotype 1b, ± compensated cirrhosis (Child-Pugh A): Viekira Pak/XR alone for 12 weeks. Ribavirin dose is 1000 mg/day for wt less than 75 kg and 1200 mg/day for wt 75 kg or greater PO divided two times per day with food. Many drug interactions. Viekira XR: Do not split, crush, or chew tabs; do not drink alcohol within 4 hours after a dose. Cost of Viekira Pak or Viekira XR is $33,327/month. [Viekira Pak. Trade only: Tabs ombitasvir 12.5 mg + paritaprevir 75 mg + ritonavir 50 mg plus separate tabs dasabuvir 250 mg. Viekira XR. Trade only: Extended-release tabs: dasabuvir 200 mg + ombitasvir 8.33 mg + paritaprevir 50 mg + ritonavir 33.33 mg.] ▶L feces ♀?/?/? ▶? $$$$$

ZEPATIER (elbasvir + grasoprevir) Chronic hepatitis C. Zapatier dose is 1 tab PO once daily without regard to meals. Treatment duration and need for ribavirin varies by genotype, NS5A resistance polymorphisms, and treatment experience. Test genotype 1a for NS5A resistance. Genotype 1a, treatment-naive: Zapatier alone for 12 weeks if no resistance; Zapatier + wt-based ribavirin for 16 weeks if baseline resistance. Ribavirin dose is 800 mg/day for wt less than 66 kg; 1000 mg/day for 66 to 80 kg; 1200 mg/day for 81 to 105 kg; 1400 mg/day for greater than 105 kg; give PO divided two times per day with food. Genotype 1b and 4, treatment-naive: Zapatier alone for 12 weeks. Also for treatment-experienced genotype 1a, 1b, and 4. Cost of Zepatier is $21,800/month. [Trade only: Tabs elbasvir 50 mg + grazoprevir 100 mg.] ▶L ♀?/?/? Regimens with ribavirin: X/X/X ▶? $$$$$

Antiviral Agents—Anti-Herpetic

ACYCLOVIR (Zovirax, Sitavig) Genital herpes: 400 mg PO three times per day for 7 to 10 days for 1st episode, or for 5 days
(cont.)

for recurrent episodes. Chronic suppression of genital herpes: 400 mg PO two times per day; in HIV infection use 400 to 800 mg PO two to three times per day. See STD table. Zoster: 800 mg PO five times per day for 7 to 10 days. Chickenpox, age 2 yo to adult: 20 mg/kg (up to 800 mg) PO four times per day for 5 days. Adult IV: 5 to 10 mg/kg IV q 8 h, each dose over 1 h. Herpes simplex encephalitis: 10 to 15 mg/kg IV q 8 h for age 3 mo to 12 yo; 10 mg/kg IV q 8 h for age 12 yo or older. Treat for 14 to 21 days. Neonatal herpes: 20 mg/kg IV q 8 h for 21 days for disseminated/CNS disease, for 14 days for skin/mucous membrane infections. Suppressive therapy after neonatal herpes, birth to 7 mo: 300 mg/m^2 PO three times per day for 6 months. Sitavig for recurrent herpes labialis in immunocompetent adults: Within 1 h of prodromal symptom onset, apply buccal tab once to upper gum above incisor on the side of mouth affected by herpes; then press slightly on upper lip for 30 seconds. [Generic/Trade: Caps 200 mg. Tabs 400, 800 mg. Susp 200 mg/5 mL. Trade only: Buccal tab (Sitavig-$$$$$) 50 mg.] ▶K ♀B ▶+ $

FAMCICLOVIR (*Famvir*) First episode genital herpes: 250 mg PO three times per day for 7 to 10 days. Recurrent genital herpes: 1000 mg PO two times per day for 2 days; give 500 mg two times per day for 7 days if HIV-infected. Chronic suppression of genital herpes: 250 mg PO two times per day; 500 mg PO two times per day if HIV-infected. See STD table. Recurrent herpes labialis: 1500 mg PO single dose; 500 mg two times per day for 7 days if HIV-infected. Zoster: 500 mg PO three times per day for 7 days. [Generic/Trade: Tabs 125, 250, 500 mg.] ▶K ♀B ▶? $$

VALACYCLOVIR (*Valtrex*) First episode genital herpes: 1 g PO two times per day for 10 days. Recurrent genital herpes: 500 mg PO two times per day for 3 days; if HIV-infected, give 1 g PO two times per day for 5 to 10 days. Chronic suppression of genital herpes: 500 to 1000 mg PO daily; if HIV-infected, give 500 mg PO two times per day. Reduction of genital herpes transmission in immunocompetent patients with no more than

(cont.)

ANTIMICROBIALS

9 recurrences per year: 500 mg PO daily for source partner, in conjunction with safer sex practices. See STD table. Herpes labialis, age 12 yo or older: 2 g PO q 12 h for 2 doses. Zoster: 1000 mg PO three times per day for 7 days. Chickenpox, age 2 to 18 yo: 20 mg/kg (max of 1 g) PO three times per day for 5 days. [Generic/Trade: Tabs 500, 1000 mg.] ▶K ♀B ▶+ $$$$

Antiviral Agents—Anti-HIV—CCR5 Antagonists

MARAVIROC (*Selzentry, MVC, ✦Celsentri*) 150 mg PO two times per day with strong CYP3A4 inhibitors (clarithromycin, itraconazole, ketoconazole, most HIV protease inhibitors); 300 mg PO two times per day with drugs that are not strong CYP3A4 inducers/inhibitors (NRTIs, tipranavir-ritonavir, nevirapine, raltegravir; rifabutin without a strong CYP3A4 inhibitor or inducer); 600 mg PO two times per day with strong CYP3A4 inducers (efavirenz, etravirine, rifampin, carbamazepine, phenobarbital, phenytoin). Tropism test before treatment; not for dual/mixed or CXCR4-tropic HIV infection. Hepatotoxicity with allergic features. [Trade only: Tabs 150, 300 mg.] ▶LK ♀B ▶– $$$$$ ∎

Antiviral Agents—Anti-HIV—Combinations

***ATRIPLA* (efavirenz + emtricitabine + tenofovir disoproxil fumarate)** HIV infection, alone or in combination with other antiretrovirals: 1 tab PO once daily on empty stomach, preferably at bedtime. [Trade only: Tabs efavirenz 600 mg + emtricitabine 200 mg + tenofovir disoproxil fumarate 300 mg.] ▶KL ♀D ▶– $$$$$ ∎

***COMBIVIR* (lamivudine + zidovudine)** Combination therapy of HIV infection: 1 tab PO two times per day for wt 30 kg or greater. [Generic/Trade: Tabs lamivudine 150 mg + zidovudine 300 mg.] ▶LK ♀C ▶– $$$$$ ∎

***COMPLERA* (emtricitabine + rilpivirine + tenofovir disoproxil fumarate)** HIV infection, treatment-naive with baseline HIV RNA up to 100,000 copies/mL, adults and age 12 yo and older: 1 tab PO once daily with food. When coadministered with

(cont.)

rifabutin, give 1 tab Complera plus 25 mg rilpivirine PO once daily with a meal. Also used to replace a stable regimen in certain virologically-suppressed patients; monitor HIV RNA for virologic failure/rebound after switching to Complera. [Trade only: Tabs emtricitabine 200 mg + rilpivirine 25 mg + tenofovir disoproxil fumarate 300 mg.] ▶KL ♀B▶— $$$$$ ■

DESCOVY (emtricitabine + tenofovir alafenamide) Combination therapy for HIV infection, age 12 yo and older and wt 35 kg and greater: 1 tab PO once daily with other antiretroviral drugs. [Trade only (emtricitabine/tenofovir disoproxil fumarate): Tabs emtricitabine 200 mg + tenofovir alafenamide 25 mg.] ▶K ♀?/?/? R▶— $$$$$ ■

EPZICOM (abacavir + lamivudine, ★*Kivexa*) Combination therapy of HIV infection, adults and children with wt 25 kg or greater: 1 tab PO daily. [Trade only: Tabs abacavir 600 mg + lamivudine 300 mg.] ▶LK ♀C▶— $$$$$ ■

GENVOYA (elvitegravir + cobicistat + emtricitabine + tenofovir alafenamide) HIV infection, age 12 yo and older: 1 tab PO once daily with food. Not for use with other antiretroviral drugs. Many drug interactions. [Trade only: Tabs elvitegravir 150 mg + cobicistat 150 mg + emtricitabine 200 mg + tenofovir alafenamide 10 mg.] ▶KL ♀B R▶— $$$$$ ■

ODEFSEY (emtricitabine + rilpivirine + tenofovir alafenamide) HIV infection, treatment-naive with baseline HIV RNA up to 100,000 copies/mL, adults and age 12 yo and older: 1 tab PO once daily with food. Also used to replace a stable regimen in certain virologically-suppressed patients; monitor HIV RNA for virologic failure/rebound after switching to Odefsey. [Trade only: Tabs emtricitabine 200 mg + rilpivirine 25 mg + tenofovir alafenamide 25 mg.] ▶LK ♀?/?/? R▶— $$$$$ ■

STRIBILD (elvitegravir + cobicistat + emtricitabine + tenofovir disoproxil fumarate) HIV infection: 1 tab PO once daily with food. Not for use with other antiretroviral drugs. Many drug interactions. [Trade only: Tabs elvitegravir 150 mg + cobicistat 150 mg + emtricitabine 200 mg + tenofovir disoproxil fumarate 300 mg.] ▶KL ♀B▶— $$$$$ ■

***TRIUMEQ* (abacavir + dolutegravir + lamivudine)** HIV infection, alone or in combination with other drugs: 1 tab PO once daily. Coadministration with carbamazepine, efavirenz, fosamprenavir-ritonavir, tipranavir-ritonavir, or rifampin: Add dolutegravir 50 mg PO at least 12 hours after dose of Triumeq. Do not use Triumeq alone in patients with INSTI resistance substitutions or suspected INSTI resistance. [Trade only: Tabs abacavir 600 mg + dolutegravir 50 mg + lamivudine 300 mg.] ▶LK ♀C ▶– $$$$$ ■

***TRIZIVIR* (abacavir + lamivudine + zidovudine)** HIV infection, alone (not a preferred regimen) or in combination with other agents: 1 tab PO two times per day. [Generic/Trade: Tabs abacavir 300 mg + lamivudine 150 mg + zidovudine 300 mg.] ▶LK ♀C ▶– $$$$$ ■

***TRUVADA* (emtricitabine + tenofovir disoproxil fumarate)** Combination therapy for HIV infection, adults and peds with wt 17 kg or greater: Give 1 tab PO once daily at a dose of 100/150 mg for wt 17 to less than 22 kg; 133/200 mg for 22 to less than 28 kg; 167/250 mg for 28 to less than 35 kg; 200/300 mg for adults and peds with wt 35 kg or greater. Pre-exposure prophylaxis (PrEP) of HIV in adults at high risk for sexually acquired HIV or injection-drug users: 1 tab 200/300 mg PO once daily. Screen for HIV q 3 months in PrEP patients. [Trade only (emtricitabine/tenofovir disoproxil fumarate): Tabs 200/300 mg, 167/250 mg, 133/200 mg, 100/150 mg.] ▶K ♀B ▶– $$$$$ ■

Antiviral Agents—Anti-HIV—Integrase Strand Transfer Inhibitor

DOLUTEGRAVIR (*Tivicay, DTG*) Combination therapy of HIV, integrase strand inhibitor (INSTI)-naïve, adults or peds with wt 30 kg or greater: 35 mg PO once daily (25 mg tab + 10 mg tab) for wt 30 to less than 40 kg; 50 mg PO once daily for adults and peds wt 40 kg or greater. Adjust dosing interval to two times per

(cont.)

day for coadministration of certain CYP3A4 or UGT1A inducers (carbamazepine, efavirenz, fosamprenavir-ritonavir, rifampin, tipranavir-ritonavir). INSTI-experienced with INSTI resistance substitutions or suspected INSTI resistance, adults only: 50 mg PO two times per day. [Trade only: Tabs 10, 25, 50 mg.] ▶glucuronidation ♀?/?/? R ▶– $$$$$

ELVITEGRAVIR (*Vitekta, EVG*) Combination therapy for HIV infection: Give with ritonavir-boosted protease inhibitor regimens listed here plus antiretroviral drug. Elvitegravir 85 mg + atazanavir-ritonavir 300 mg-100 mg all PO once daily. Elvitegravir 85 mg PO once daily + lopinavir-ritonavir 400 mg-100 mg PO two times per day. Elvitegravir 150 mg PO once daily + darunavir-ritonavir 600 mg-100 mg PO two times per day. Elvitegravir 150 mg PO once daily + fosamprenavir-ritonavir 700 mg-100 mg PO two times per day. Elvitegravir 150 mg PO once daily + tipranavir-ritonavir 500 mg-200 mg PO two times per day. Take with food. [Trade only: Film-coated tabs 85, 150 mg.] ▶L glucuronidation ♀B ▶– $$$$$

RALTEGRAVIR (*Isentress, RAL*) Combination therapy of HIV infection. Adults: 400 mg PO two times per day. Increase to 800 mg PO two times per day if given with rifampin. Peds. Film-coated tabs, wt 25 kg or greater: 400 mg PO two times per day. Chew tabs, 11 kg or greater: Give PO two times per day at a dose of 75 mg for wt 11 to less than 14 kg; 100 mg for 14 to less than 20 kg; 150 mg for 20 to less than 28 kg; 200 mg for 28 to less than 40 kg; 300 mg for 40 kg or greater. Oral susp, age 4 weeks and older and wt 3 to 20 kg: Give PO two times per day at a dose of 20 mg for 3 to less than 4 kg; 30 mg for 4 to less than 6 kg; 40 mg for 6 to less than 8 kg; 60 mg for 8 to less than 11 kg; 80 mg for 11 to less than 14 kg; 100 mg for 14 to less than 20 kg. Do not substitute chew tab or susp for film-coated tabs. Give all formulations without regard to meals. [Trade only: Film-coated tabs 400 mg. Chewable tabs (contain phenylalanine): 25, 100 mg. Single-use packets of powder for oral susp: 100 mg/5 mL.] ▶glucuronidation ♀C ▶– $$$$$

ANTIMICROBIALS

Antiviral Agents—Anti-HIV—Non-Nucleoside Reverse Transcriptase Inhibitors

EFAVIRENZ (*Sustiva, EFV*) Combination therapy of HIV, adults and children wt 40 kg or greater: 600 mg PO once daily on an empty stomach, preferably at bedtime. With voriconazole: Use voriconazole 400 mg PO two times per day and efavirenz 300 mg PO once daily. With rifampin: Increase efavirenz to 800 mg PO once daily if wt is 50 kg or greater. Peds, age 3 mo or older and wt 3.5 to 40 kg: Consider antihistamine prophylaxis to prevent rash before starting. Give PO once daily at a dose of 100 mg for 3.5 to less than 5 kg; 150 mg for 5 to less than 7.5 kg; 200 mg for 7.5 to less than 15 kg; 250 mg for 15 to less than 20 kg; 300 mg for 20 to less than 25 kg; 350 mg for 25 to less than 32.5 kg; 400 mg for 32.5 to less than 40 kg. Take on empty stomach, preferably at bedtime. Can sprinkle capsule contents on 1 to 2 teaspoons of food with no additional food for 2 h. [Trade only: Caps 50, 200 mg. Tabs 600 mg.] ▶L ♀X/O/O. Risk of neural tube defects in 1st 8 weeks; may use later. R. R ▶─ $$$$$

ETRAVIRINE (*Intelence, ETR*) Combination therapy for treatment-resistant HIV. Adults: 200 mg PO two times per day after meals. Peds, age 6 yo and older: Give PO two times per day after meals at a dose of 100 mg for 16 to less than 20 kg; 125 mg for 20 to less than 25 kg; 150 mg per dose for 25 to less than 30 kg; 200 mg for 30 kg or greater. [Trade only: Tabs 25, 100, 200 mg.] ▶L ♀B ▶─ $$$$$

NEVIRAPINE (*Viramune, Viramune XR, NVP*) Combination therapy for HIV: 200 mg PO daily for 14 days initially. If tolerated, increase to 200 mg PO two times per day or Viramune XR 400 mg PO once daily. Patients maintained on immediate-release tabs can switch directly to Viramune XR. Peds, age 15 days or older: 150 mg/m^2 PO once daily for 14 days, then 150 mg/m^2 two times per day (max dose 200 mg two times per day). Viramune XR, age 6 yo and older: 200 mg PO once daily

(cont.)

for BSA 0.58 to 0.83 m^2; 300 mg PO once daily for BSA 0.84 to 1.16 m^2; 400 mg PO once daily for BSA 1.17 m^2 or greater. To reduce risk of rash, give immediate-release nevirapine 150 mg/m^2 once daily (max 200 mg/day) for at least 14 days before conversion to Viramune XR. Patients already taking twice-daily immediate-release nevirapine can switch directly to Viramune XR. Severe skin reactions and hepatotoxicity. [Generic/Trade: Tabs 200 mg. Susp 50 mg/5 mL (240 mL). Extended-release tabs 100, 400 mg.] ▶LK ♀C ▷— $$$$$ ■

RILPIVIRINE (*Edurant, RPV*) Combination therapy of HIV infection, treatment-naive with HIV RNA ≤100,000 copies/mL, age 12 yo and older: 25 mg PO once daily with a meal. Dosage adjustment for rifabutin: Rilpivirine 50 mg PO once daily with a meal. [Trade only: Tabs 25 mg.] ▶L ♀B ▷— $$$$$

Antiviral Agents—Anti-HIV—Nucleoside/Nucleotide Reverse Transcriptase Inhibitors

ABACAVIR (*Ziagen, ABC*) Combination therapy for HIV. Adult and peds with wt 25 kg or greater: 300 mg PO two times per day or 600 mg PO daily. Peds: Oral soln, age 3 mo or older: 16 mg/kg (up to 600 mg/day) PO divided one or two times per day. Do not start therapy with once-daily dose of oral soln; can convert from twice- to once-daily dose of oral soln after 6 months with undetectable viral load and stable CD4 count. Peds, tabs: 150 mg PO two times per day or 300 mg PO once daily for wt 14 to less than 20 kg; 150 mg PO q am and 300 mg PO q pm or 450 mg PO once daily for wt 20 to less than 25 kg. Potentially fatal hypersensitivity. HLA-B*5701 predisposes to hypersensitivity; screen before starting and avoid if positive test. Never rechallenge with abacavir after suspected reaction. [Generic/Trade: Tabs 300 mg scored. Trade only: Soln 20 mg/mL (240 mL).] ▶L ♀C ▷— $$$$$ ■

DIDANOSINE (*Videx, Videx EC, DDI*) Combination therapy for HIV. Videx EC: Give 200 mg PO once daily for wt 20 to 24 kg; 250 mg PO once daily for wt 25 to 59 kg; 400 mg PO once daily for wt

(cont.)

60 kg or greater. Dosage reduction of Videx EC with tenofovir in adults: 200 mg for wt less than 60 kg; 250 mg for wt 60 kg or greater. Dosage reduction unclear with tenofovir if CrCl <60 mL/min. Buffered powder, peds: 100 mg/m^2 PO two times per day for age 2 weeks to 8 mo; 120 mg/m^2 PO two times per day for age older than 8 mo (do not exceed adult dose). Take on an empty stomach. [Generic/Trade: Delayed-release caps (Videx EC): 125, 200, 250, 400 mg. Trade only: Pediatric powder for oral soln (buffered with antacid) 10 mg/mL.] ▶LK ♀B ▶– $$$$$ ■

EMTRICITABINE (*Emtriva, FTC*) Combination therapy for HIV. Adults: 200 mg cap or 240 mg oral soln PO once daily. Peds, oral soln: 3 mg/kg PO once daily for age 3 mo or younger; 6 mg/kg PO once daily (up to 240 mg) for age older than 3 mo. Can give 200 mg cap PO once daily if wt greater than 33 kg. [Trade only: Caps 200 mg. Oral soln 10 mg/mL (170 mL).] ▶K ♀B ▶– $$$$$ ■

LAMIVUDINE (*Epivir, Epivir-HBV, 3TC, ✦Heptovir*) Epivir for HIV infection. Adults and peds with wt of 25 kg or greater: 150 mg PO two times per day or 300 mg PO daily. Peds, 3 mo and older: 8 mg/kg (up to 300 mg/day) PO divided one or two times per day. Epivir tabs, wt 14 kg or greater (preferred over oral soln for children who can swallow tabs): 75 mg two times per day or 150 mg once daily for wt 14 to less than 20 kg; 75 mg q am and 150 mg q pm or 225 mg once daily for wt 20 to less than 25 kg. Generally avoid once-daily dosing of oral soln in infants and young children; soln may suppress HIV less than tabs due to lower absorption. Epivir-HBV for hepatitis B: Adults: 100 mg PO daily. Peds: 3 mg/kg (up to 100 mg) PO daily. [Generic/Trade: Tabs 100, 150 (scored), 300 mg. Oral soln 10 mg/mL. Trade only (Epivir-HBV, Heptovir): Oral soln 5 mg/mL.] ▶K ♀ +/+/+ R ▶– $$$$$ ■

TENOFOVIR DISOPROXIL FUMARATE (*Viread, TDF*) Combination therapy for HIV. Adults and adolescents: 300 mg PO daily. Peds, 2 yo and older: 8 mg/kg PO once daily (max 300 mg/day) as oral powder. Tabs for peds, wt 17 kg or greater: Give PO once

(cont.)

daily at dose of 150 mg for wt 17 to less than 22 kg; 200 mg for wt 22 to less than 28 kg; 250 mg for wt 28 to less than 35 kg; 300 mg for wt 35 kg or greater. Chronic hepatitis B, adults and peds age 12 yo and older and wt 35 kg or greater: 300 mg PO daily (7.5 scoops of power for those who cannot swallow tabs) without regard to meals. Mix powder with soft food (not liquid) and use immediately. [Trade only: Tabs 150, 200, 250, 300 mg. Oral powder 40 mg tenofovir disoproxil fumarate/1 g scoop of powder, 60 g bottle.] ▶K ♀B ▶– $$$$$ ■

ZIDOVUDINE (*Retrovir, AZT, ZDV*) Combination therapy of HIV infection: 600 mg/day PO divided two or three times per day for wt 30 kg or greater. Peds dose based on wt: Give 24 mg/kg/day PO divided two or three times per day for wt 4 to 8 kg, 18 mg/kg/day PO divided two or three times per day for wt 9 to 29 kg. [Generic/Trade: Caps 100 mg. Syrup 50 mg/5 mL (240 mL). Generic only: Tabs 300 mg.] ▶LK ♀C ▶– $$$$$ ■

Antiviral Agents—Anti-HIV—Protease Inhibitors and Boosters

NOTE: *Many serious drug interactions: Always check before prescribing. Protease inhibitors and cobicistat inhibit CYP3A4. Contraindicated with alfuzosin, dronedarone, ergot alkaloids, lovastatin, pimozide, rifampin, rifapentine, salmeterol, high-dose sildenafil for pulmonary hypertension, simeprevir, simvastatin, St. John's wort, triazolam. Midazolam contraindicated in labeling; but can use single dose IV cautiously with monitoring for procedural sedation. Monitor INR with warfarin. Avoid inhaled/nasal budesonide/fluticasone with ritonavir/cobicistat if possible; increased corticosteroid levels can cause Cushing's syndrome/adrenal suppression. Other protease inhibitors may increase budesonide/fluticasone levels; find alternatives for long-term use. Reduce colchicine dose; do not coadminister colchicine and protease inhibitors in patients with renal or hepatic dysfunction. Adjust dose of bosentan or tadalafil for*

(cont.)

pulmonary hypertension. Reduce quetiapine dose to 1/6 of original dose if protease inhibitor or cobicistat is added; use lowest initial quetiapine dose if it is added to protease inhibitor or cobicistat. Erectile dysfunction: Single dose of sildenafil 25 mg q 48 h, tadalafil 5 mg (not more than 10 mg) q 72 h, or vardenafil initially 2.5 mg q 72 h. Protease inhibitor class adverse effects include spontaneous bleeding in hemophiliacs, hyperglycemia, hyperlipidemia, immune reconstitution syndrome, and fat redistribution. Coinfection with hepatitis C or other liver disease increases the risk of hepatotoxicity with protease inhibitors; monitor LFTs at least twice in 1st month of therapy, then q 3 months.

ATAZANAVIR (*Reyataz, ATV*) Combination therapy of HIV. Adults, therapy-naive: 300 mg + ritonavir 100 mg PO both once daily. With efavirenz, therapy-naive: 400 mg + ritonavir 100 mg PO both once daily. Do not give atazanavir with efavirenz in therapy-experienced patients. Adults, therapy-experienced: 300 mg + ritonavir 100 mg PO both once daily. Peds: Oral powder, age 3 mo and older and wt 5 kg to less than 25 kg: 200 mg atazanavir powder (4 packets) with 80 mg ritonavir oral soln PO once daily for wt 5 kg to less than 15 kg; 250 mg atazanavir powder (5 packets) with 80 mg ritonavir oral soln PO once daily for wt 15 to less than 25 kg. Mix powder with food or beverage and give ritonavir immediately after. Oral capsules, age 6 yo or older: Atazanavir-ritonavir PO once daily 150/100 mg for wt 15 to less than 20 kg; 200/100 mg for wt 20 to less than 40 kg; 300/100 mg for 40 kg or greater. Give atazanavir with food. Give atazanavir 2 h before or 1 h after buffered didanosine. Do not give to infants less than 3 mo due to risk of kernicterus. [Trade only: Caps 150, 200, 300 mg. Powder packets (contain phenylalanine) 50 mg.] ▶L ♀ O/0/0 Ritonavir-boosted atazanavir is a preferred protease inhibitor in ARV-naive pregnant women; maternal hyperbilirubinemia. R ▶– $$$$$

COBICISTAT (*Tybost, COBI*) Combination therapy for HIV: Cobicistat 150 mg + atazanavir 300 mg both PO once daily OR cobicistat 150 mg + darunavir 800 mg both PO once daily. Take cobicistat with food at the same time as atazanavir or darunavir. Dosage adjustment of cobicistat-atazanavir for efavirenz, treatment-naive patients: Cobicistat 150 mg + atazanavir 400 mg both PO once daily with food + efavirenz 600 mg PO once daily on an empty stomach, preferably at bedtime. Do not use cobicistat-atazanavir with efavirenz in treatment-experienced patients. Cobicistat is a strong CYP3A4 inhibitor that boosts atazanavir and darunavir levels (no antiviral activity). Many drug interactions. Not interchangeable with ritonavir; do not assume interactions are the same. [Trade only: Film-coated tabs 150 mg.] ▶L ♀B ▶– $$$$$

DARUNAVIR (*Prezista, DRV*) Combination therapy of HIV. Therapy-naive or -experienced adults with no darunavir resistance substitutions: 800 mg + ritonavir 100 mg both PO once daily. Therapy-experienced adults with at least 1 darunavir resistance substitution: 600 mg + ritonavir 100 mg both PO two times per day. Dose in pregnancy: 600 mg + ritonavir 100 mg PO two times per day. Peds: Treatment-naïve or treatment-experienced without resistance substitutions, age 3 yo or older: Give darunavir + ritonavir both PO once daily according to wt: Darunavir 35 mg/kg + ritonavir 7 mg/kg for wt 10 to less than 15 kg; darunavir 600 mg + ritonavir 100 mg for wt 15 to less than 30 kg; darunavir 675 mg + ritonavir 100 mg for wt 30 to less than 40 kg; darunavir 800 mg + ritonavir 100 mg for wt 40 kg or greater. Treatment-experienced with at least 1 resistance substitution, age 3 yo or older: Give darunavir + ritonavir both PO two times per day according to wt: Darunavir 20 mg/kg + ritonavir 7 mg/kg for wt 10 to less than 15 kg; darunavir 375 mg + ritonavir 48 mg for wt 15 to less than 30 kg; darunavir 450 mg + ritonavir 60 mg for wt 30 to less than 40 kg; darunavir 600 mg + ritonavir 100 mg for wt 40 kg or greater. Take with food. [Trade only:

(cont.)

ANTIMICROBIALS

Tabs 75, 150, 600, 800 mg. Susp 100 mg/mL (200 mL).] ▶L ♀ 0/0/0. Darunavir-ritonavir is a preferred protease inhibitor regimen for ARV-naive pregnant women. R. ▶– $$$$$

EVOTAZ (atazanavir + cobicistat) Combination therapy of HIV, adults: 1 tab PO once daily with food. [Trade only: Tabs atazanavir 300 mg + cobicistat 150 mg.] ▶L ♀B ▶– $$$$$

FOSAMPRENAVIR (*Lexiva, FPV, ✦Telzir*) Combination therapy of HIV. Protease inhibitor–experienced adults: 700 mg + ritonavir 100 mg PO both two times per day. Peds: Fosamprenavir-ritonavir for protease inhibitor–experienced patients, 6 mo or older: Give PO two times per day according to wt: Fosamprenavir 45 mg/kg plus ritonavir 7 mg/kg for wt less than 11 kg; fosamprenavir 30 mg/kg plus ritonavir 3 mg/kg for wt 11 to less than 15 kg; fosamprenavir 23 mg/kg plus ritonavir 3 mg/kg for wt 15 to less than 20 kg; fosamprenavir 18 mg/kg plus ritonavir 3 mg/kg for wt 20 kg or greater. Do not exceed adult dose of fosamprenavir 700 mg plus ritonavir 100 mg both PO two times per day. For fosamprenavir-ritonavir, can use fosamprenavir tabs if wt 39 kg or greater and ritonavir caps if wt 33 kg or greater. Do not use once-daily dosing of fosamprenavir in children. Take tabs without regard to meals. Adults should take susp without food; children should take with food. [Trade only: Tabs 700 mg. Susp 50 mg/mL.] ▶L ♀C ▶– $$$$$

KALETRA (lopinavir + ritonavir, *LPV/r*) Combination therapy of HIV. Adults: 400/100 mg PO two times per day (tabs or oral soln). Can use 800/200 mg PO once daily in patients with less than 3 lopinavir resistance–associated substitutions. Coadministration with efavirenz, nevirapine, fosamprenavir, or nelfinavir: 500/125 mg tabs (use two 200/50 mg + one 100/25 mg tab) or 533/133 mg oral soln (6.5 mL) PO two times per day. Peds: Infants, age 14 days to 6 mo: Lopinavir 16 mg/kg PO two times per day. Peds age 6 mo to 12 yo: Lopinavir 12 mg/kg PO two times per day for wt less than 15 kg, use 10 mg/kg PO two times per day for wt 15 to 40 kg. Coadministration with efavirenz, nevirapine, fosamprenavir, or nelfinavir: Lopinavir

(cont.)

13 mg/kg PO two times per day for wt less than 15 kg, 11 mg/kg PO two times per day for wt 15 to 45 kg. Do not exceed adult dose in children. No once-daily dosing for pediatric or pregnant patients; coadministration with carbamazepine, phenobarbital, phenytoin, efavirenz, nevirapine, fosamprenavir, or nelfinavir; or in patients with 3 or more lopinavir resistance–associated substitutions. Give tabs without regard to meals; give oral soln with food. [Trade only (lopinavir-ritonavir): Tabs 200/50 mg, 100/25 mg. Oral soln 80/20 mg/mL (160 mL).] ▶L ♀C ▶– $$$$$

PREZCOBIX (darunavir + cobicistat) Combination therapy of HIV, adults: 1 tab PO once daily with food. Genotypic testing recommended at baseline, especially for treatment-experienced patients. [Trade only: Tabs darunavir 800 mg + cobicistat 150 mg.] ▶L ♀C ▶– $$$$$

RITONAVIR (Norvir, RTV) Adult doses of 100 to 400 mg/day PO are used to boost levels of other protease inhibitors. See specific protease inhibitor entries for adult and pediatric boosting doses of ritonavir. Take ritonavir with food. [Trade only: Caps 100 mg, tabs 100 mg. Oral soln 80 mg/mL (240 mL).] ▶L ♀B ▶– $$$$$ ■

SAQUINAVIR (Invirase, SQV) Combination therapy for HIV infection: Regimens must contain ritonavir. Saquinavir 1000 mg + ritonavir 100 mg both PO two times per day, taken together within 2 h after meals. [Trade only: Caps 200 mg. Tabs 500 mg.] ▶L ♀B ▶– $$$$$

TIPRANAVIR (Aptivus, TPV) Combination therapy for HIV infection, Treatment-experienced patients with resistance to multiple protease inhibitors: 500 mg boosted by ritonavir 200 mg PO two times per day with food. Peds: 14 mg/kg with 6 mg/kg ritonavir PO two times per day; do not exceed adult dose. Hepatotoxicity. [Trade only: Caps 250 mg. Oral soln 100 mg/mL (95 mL in unit-of-use amber glass bottle).] ▶Feces ♀C ▶– $$$$$ ■

Antiviral Agents—Anti-Influenza

NOTE: See table for recommendations to prevent and treat influenza with antiviral drugs.

ANTIVIRAL DRUGS FOR INFLUENZA

ANTIVIRAL DRUGS FOR INFLUENZA	Treatment[a] (Duration of 5 days for oseltamivir/zanamivir)	Prevention[b] (Duration of 7 to 10 days post-exposure)
OSELTAMIVIR (*Tamiflu*)		
Adults and adolescents age 13 years and older		
	75 mg PO bid	75 mg PO once daily
Children, 1 year of age and older[c]		
Body weight ≤15 kg	30 mg PO bid	30 mg PO once daily
Body weight >15 to 23 kg	45 mg PO bid	45 mg PO once daily
Body weight >23 to 40 kg	60 mg PO bid	60 mg PO once daily
Body weight >40 kg	75 mg PO bid	75 mg PO once daily

(cont.)

Infants, newborn to 11 months of age[c]		
Age 3 to 11 months old[d]	3 mg/kg/dose PO bid	3 mg/kg/dose PO once daily
Age younger than 3 months old[e]	3 mg/kg/dose PO bid	Not for routine prophylaxis in infants <3 months old

ZANAMIVIR (*Relenza*)[f]

Adults and children (7 years and older for treatment, 5 years and older for prophylaxis)

	10 mg (two 5-mg inhalations) bid	10 mg (two 5-mg inhalations) once daily

PERAMIVIR (*Rapivab*)

Adults with uncomplicated influenza[g]

600 mg IV over 15 to 30 minutes as single dose		

ANTIMICROBIALS

(cont.)

ANTIVIRAL DRUGS FOR INFLUENZA (*continued*)

Adapted from http://www.cdc.gov/flu/professionals/antivirals/summary-clinicians.htm. bid = two times per day

[a]Treatment: Start antivirals as soon as possible (ideally within 2 days of symptom onset); do not wait for lab test confirmation. Starting later may help severe/complicated/hospitalized patients. Consider treating longer if patients remain severely ill after 5 days of treatment, especially if immunosuppressed. Treat patients at high risk of influenza complications: age younger than 2 yo or at least 65 yo; chronic pulmonary, cardiovascular (except hypertension only), renal, hepatic, hematologic, metabolic, neurologic/ neurodevelopment disorders; immunosuppressed or HIV; pregnant or within 2 weeks postpartum; child or adolescent on long-term aspirin; native American/ Alaskan native; morbid obesity; resident of nursing home or chronic care facility.

[b]Prevention: Treat for 10 days after household exposure, and for 7 days after most recent known exposure in other situations. For long-term care facilities and hospitals, treat for a minimum of 14 days and up to 7 days after the most recent case was identified.

[c]If Tamiflu suspension is unavailable, pharmacists can compound 6 mg/mL suspension from package insert recipe. Capsule contents of 30, 45, and 75 mg capsules can be mixed with sweetened liquid. Unit of measure is mL for 10 mL Tamiflu suspension oral dispenser; make sure units of measure in dosing instructions match dosing device provided. Tamiflu is FDA-approved for treatment of influenza in infants 2 weeks of age and older and prevention of influenza in children 1 yo and older.

(cont.)

(cont.)

[d]AAP (pediatrics.aappublications.org/content/early/2016/09/01/peds.2016-2527.full-text.pdf) recommends that infants age 9 to 11 mo receive oseltamivir 3.5 mg/kg/dose PO twice daily for treatment and once daily for prevention. This is based on pharmacokinetic data that suggests a higher dose is needed for adequate oseltamivir exposure in this age group. There is no data to suggest the higher dose is more effective or causes more adverse effects than the usual dose.

[e]This dose is not intended for premature infants who may have increased oseltamivir exposure due to immature renal function.

[f]Zanamivir should not be used by patients with underlying pulmonary disease. Do not use Relenza in a nebulizer or ventilator; lactose in the formulation may clog the device.

[g]IV peramivir is FDA-approved for uncomplicated influenza in adults. Per CDC, there is insufficient data to evaluate the efficacy of IV peramivir for influenza in hospitalized patients. CDC recommends PO/NG oseltamivir for influenza in hospitalized patients. In patients who cannot tolerate or absorb PO/NG oseltamivir (due to gastric stasis, malabsorption, or GI bleeding), consider IV peramivir (Age 6 yo and older: 10 mg/kg up to 600 mg IV once daily for at least 5 days) or investigational IV zanamivir. In oseltamivir-resistant influenza, consider IV zanamivir. Contact gsksclinicalsupportHD@gsk.com, or call 1-877-626-8019 or 1-866-341-9160 (24 h/day) for availability of IV zanamivir.

AMANTADINE Parkinsonism: 100 mg PO two times per day. Max 300 to 400 mg/day divided three to four times per day. Prevention/treatment of influenza A: 5 mg/kg/day up to 150 mg/day PO divided two times per day for age 1 to 9 yo and any child wt less than 40 kg. Give 100 mg PO two times per day for adults and children age 10 yo or older; reduce to 100 mg PO daily if age 65 yo or older. The CDC generally recommends against amantadine/rimantadine for treatment/prevention of influenza A in the United States due to high levels of resistance. [Generic only: Caps 100 mg. Tabs 100 mg. Syrup 50 mg/5 mL (480 mL).] ▶K ♀C ▶? $$$$

OSELTAMIVIR (*Tamiflu*) Influenza A/B: For treatment, give each dose two times per day for 5 days starting within 2 days of symptom onset. For prevention, give each dose once daily for 10 days starting within 2 days of exposure. For adults each dose is 75 mg. For peds, age 1 yo or older, each dose is 30 mg for wt 15 kg or less; 45 mg for wt 16 to 23 kg; 60 mg for wt 24 to 40 kg; and 75 mg for wt greater than 40 kg or age 13 yo or older. Influenza treatment in infants age 2 weeks old to 1 yo: 3 mg/kg/dose PO two times per day for 5 days. Influenza prophylaxis in infants 3 to 11 mo: 3 mg/kg PO once daily. Due to limited data, prophylaxis is not recommended for infants younger than 3 mo unless the situation is critical. Can take with food to improve tolerability. [Trade only: Caps 30, 45, 75 mg. Susp 6 mg/mL (60 mL) with 10 mL dosing device (contains sorbitol). Pharmacist can also compound susp (6 mg/mL).] ▶LK ♀C, but + ▶? $$$$

PERAMIVIR (*Rapivab*) Influenza, uncomplicated in adults: 600 mg IV single dose infused over 15 to 30 minutes. ▶K ♀C ▶? $$$$$

RIMANTADINE (*Flumadine*) Treatment or prevention of influenza A in adults: 100 mg PO two times per day. Reduce dose to 100 mg PO once daily for age older than 65 yo. Peds influenza A prophylaxis: 5 mg/kg (up to 150 mg/day) PO once daily for age 1 to 9 yo. Use adult dose for age 10 yo or older. The CDC generally recommends against amantadine/rimantadine for

(cont.)

treatment/prevention of influenza A in the United States due to high levels of resistance. [Generic/Trade: Tabs 100 mg. Pharmacist can compound susp.] ▶LK ♀C ▶– $$

ZANAMIVIR (*Relenza*) Influenza A/B treatment: 2 puffs two times per day for 5 days for adults and children 7 yo or older. Influenza A/B prevention: 2 puffs once daily for 10 days for adults and children 5 yo or older starting within 2 days of exposure. Do not use if chronic airway disease. [Trade only: Rotadisk inhaler 5 mg/puff (20 puffs).] ▶K ♀C ▶? $$$

Antiviral Agents—Other

INTERFERON ALFA-2B (*Intron A*) Chronic hepatitis B: 5 million units/day or 10 million units three times per week SC/IM for 16 weeks if HBeAg+, for 48 weeks if HBeAg–. [Trade only: Powder/soln for injection 10, 18, 50 million units/vial. Soln for injection 18, 25 million units/multidose vial.] ▶K ♀C ▶?+ $$$$$ ■

PALIVIZUMAB (*Synagis*) Prevention of respiratory syncytial virus pulmonary disease in high-risk infants: 15 mg/kg IM once monthly for a max of 5 doses per RSV season. ▶L ♀C ▶? $$$$$

PEGINTERFERON ALFA-2A (*Pegasys*) Chronic hepatitis C: Regimens of sofosbuvir or simeprevir plus peginterferon are not recommended. Refer to www.hcvguidelines.org for info on remaining indication, genotypes 2, 3, 5, or 6, with GFR 30 mL/min or less and urgency to treat before kidney transplantation. Hepatitis B: 180 mcg SC in abdomen or thigh once a week for 48 weeks. Peds. Chronic hepatitis C, age 5 yo or older: 180 mcg/1.73 m^2 (max dose of 180 mcg) SC once weekly with PO ribavirin for 24 weeks (genotype 2 or 3) or 48 weeks (genotype 1 or 4). May cause or worsen severe autoimmune, neuropsychiatric, ischemic, and infectious diseases. Frequent clinical and lab monitoring. [Trade only: 180 mcg/1 mL soln in single-use vial, 180 mcg/0.5 mL prefilled syringe, 180 mcg/0.5 mL, 135 mcg/0.5 mL auto-injector.] ▶LK ♀C ▶– $$$$$ ■

RIBAVIRIN—INHALED (*Virazole*) Severe respiratory syncytial virus infection in children: Aerosol 12 to 18 h/day for 3 to 7 days.

(cont.)

ANTIMICROBIALS

Beware of sudden pulmonary deterioration; drug precipitation can cause ventilator dysfunction. Minimize exposure to healthcare workers, especially pregnant women. ▶Lung ♀X ▶– $$$$$ ■

Carbapenems

NOTE: *Carbapenems can dramatically reduce valproic acid levels; use another antibiotic (preferred) or add a supplemental anticonvulsant.*

DORIPENEM (*Doribax*) Complicated intra-abdominal infection, complicated UTI/pyelonephritis: 500 mg IV q 8 h infused over 1 h. Not indicated for ventilator-associated bacterial pneumonia due to higher mortality rate. ▶K ♀B ▶? $$$$$

ERTAPENEM (*Invanz*) 1 g IV/IM q 24 h. Prophylaxis, colorectal surgery: 1 g IV 1 h before incision. Peds, younger than 13 yo: 15 mg/kg IV/IM q 12 h (up to 1 g/day). Infuse IV over 30 min. ▶K ♀B ▶? $$$$$

MEROPENEM (*Merrem IV*) Complicated skin infection, 3 mo and older: 10 mg/kg up to 500 mg IV q 8 h; use 500 mg IV for adults and peds with wt greater than 50 kg. Complicated skin infection caused by *P. aeruginosa*, 3 mo and older: 20 mg/kg IV q 8 h up to 1 g IV q 8 h; use 1 g IV q 8 h for adults and peds with wt greater than 50 kg. Complicated intra-abdominal infection. Age 3 mo and older: 20 mg/kg up to 1 g IV q 8 h; use 1 g IV q 8 h for adults and peds with wt greater than 50 kg. Age 2 weeks to less than 3 mo: 20 mg/kg IV q 8 h if gestational age less than 32 weeks; 30 mg/kg IV q 8 h if gestational age 32 weeks and older. Age less than 2 weeks: 20 mg/kg IV q 12 h if gestational age less than 32 weeks; 20 mg/kg IV q 8 h if gestational age 32 weeks and older. Peds meningitis, 3 mo and older: 40 mg/kg IV q 8 h; 2 g IV q 8 h for wt greater than 50 kg. Anthrax: See table. ▶K ♀B ▶? $$$$$

PRIMAXIN (imipenem-cilastatin) 250 to 1000 mg IV q 6 to 8 h. Peds, age older than 3 mo: 15 to 25 mg/kg IV q 6 h. Seizures (especially if given with ganciclovir, elderly with renal dysfunction, or cerebrovascular or seizure disorder). ▶K ♀C ▶? $$$$$

Cephalosporins—1st Generation

CEFADROXIL 1 to 2 g/day PO once daily or divided two times per day. Peds: 30 mg/kg/day divided two times per day. Group A streptococcal pharyngitis: 30 mg/kg/day to max of 1 g/day PO divided once or twice daily for 10 days. [Generic only: Tabs 1 g. Caps 500 mg. Susp 250, 500 mg/5 mL.] ▶K ♀B ▶+ $$$

CEFAZOLIN 0.5 to 1.5 g IM/IV q 6 to 8 h. Peds: 25 to 50 mg/kg/day divided q 6 to 8 h (up to 100 mg/kg/day for severe infections). ▶K ♀B ▶+ $$

CEPHALEXIN (*Keflex*) 250 to 500 mg PO four times per day. Peds: 25 to 50 mg/kg/day. Group A streptococcal pharyngitis: 20 mg/kg/dose to max of 500 mg/dose PO two times per day for 10 days. Not for otitis media, sinusitis. [Generic/Trade (Keflex $$$$$): Caps 250, 500, 750 mg. Generic only: Tabs 250, 500 mg. Susp 125, 250 mg/5 mL.] ▶K ♀B ▶? $$

CEPHALOSPORINS: GENERAL ANTIMICROBIAL SPECTRUM

1st generation	Gram-positive (including *S. aureus*); basic Gram-negative coverage
2nd generation	diminished *S. aureus*, improved Gram-negative coverage compared to 1st generation; some with anaerobic coverage
3rd generation	further diminished *S. aureus*, further improved Gram-negative coverage compared to 1st and 2nd generation; some with pseudomonal coverage and diminished Gram-positive coverage
4th generation	same as 3rd generation plus coverage against *Pseudomonas*
5th generation	Gram-negative coverage similar to 3rd generation; also active against *S. aureus* (including MRSA) and *S. pneumoniae*

Cephalosporins—2nd Generation

CEFACLOR (✢Ceclor) Usual adult dose: 250 to 500 mg PO three times per day. Extended-release tabs for acute exacerbation of chronic bronchitis ($$$$$): 500 mg PO two times per day for 7 days. Peds: 20 to 40 mg/kg/day PO divided three times per day. Group A streptococcal pharyngitis (2nd line to penicillin): 20 mg/kg/day PO divided two times per day for 10 days. Serum sickness—like reactions with repeated use. [Generic only: Caps 250, 500 mg. Susp 125, 250, 375 mg per 5 mL. Extended-release tabs: 500 mg.] ▸K ♀B ▸+ $$$$

CEFOXITIN 1 to 2 g IM/IV q 6 to 8 h. Peds: 80 to 160 mg/kg/day IV divided q 4 to 8 h. ▸K ♀B ▸+ $$$$

CEFPROZIL 250 to 500 mg PO two times per day. Peds: Otitis media: 15 mg/kg/dose PO two times per day. Group A streptococcal pharyngitis (2nd line to penicillin): 7.5 mg/kg/dose PO two times per day for 10 days. [Generic only: Tabs 250, 500 mg. Susp 125, 250 mg/5 mL.] ▸K ♀B ▸+ $$$$

CEFUROXIME (Zinacef, Ceftin) Adults: 750 to 1500 mg IM/IV q 8 h. 250 to 500 mg PO two times per day. Peds: 50 to 100 mg/kg/day IV divided q 6 to 8 h; not for meningitis; 20 to 30 mg/kg/day susp PO divided two times per day. [Generic/Trade (Ceftin $$$$$): Tabs 500 mg. Susp 125, 250 mg/5 mL. Generic only: Tabs 250 mg.] ▸K ♀B ▸? $$$$

Cephalosporins—3rd Generation

CEFDINIR (Omnicef) 14 mg/kg/day up to 600 mg/day PO once daily or divided two times per day. See otitis media table. [Generic only: Caps 300 mg. Susp 125, 250 mg/5 mL.] ▸K ♀B ▸? $$$$

CEFDITOREN (Spectracef) 200 to 400 mg PO two times per day with food. [Generic/Trade: Tabs 200, 400 mg.] ▸K ♀B ▸? $$$$$

CEFIXIME (Suprax) 400 mg PO once daily. Gonorrhea (not pharyngeal): 400 mg PO single dose + azithromycin 1 g PO single dose. CDC now considers cefixime an alternative for when

(cont.)

ceftriaxone cannot be used. See STD table. Peds: 8 mg/kg/day once daily or divided two times per day. Use only susp/chew tabs for otitis media (better blood levels). See acute sinusitis table. [Generic/Trade: Susp 100, 200 mg/5 mL. Trade only: Susp 500 mg/5 mL. Chewable tabs 100, 200 mg. Caps 400 mg.] ▶K/Bile ♀B▶? $$$$$

CEFOTAXIME (*Claforan*) Usual dose: 1 to 2 g IM/IV q 6 to 8 h. Peds: 50 to 180 mg/kg/day IM/IV divided q 4 to 6 h. AAP dose for pneumococcal meningitis: 225 to 300 mg/kg/day IV divided q 6 to 8 h. ▶KL ♀B▶+ $$$$

CEFPODOXIME 100 to 400 mg PO two times per day. Peds: 10 mg/kg/day divided two times per day. See acute sinusitis and otitis media tables. [Generic: Tabs 100, 200 mg. Susp 50, 100 mg/5 mL.] ▶K ♀B▶? $$$$

CEFTAZIDIME (*Fortaz, Tazicef*) 1 g IM/IV or 2 g IV q 8 to 12 h. Peds: 30 to 50 mg/kg IV q 8 h. ▶K ♀B▶+ $$$$

CEFTIBUTEN (*Cedax*) Group A streptococcal pharyngitis, acute exacerbation of chronic bronchitis, otitis media not due to *S. pneumoniae*: 400 mg PO once daily. Peds: 9 mg/kg (up to 400 mg) PO once daily. Treat pharyngitis for 10 days. See otitis media table. [Generic/Trade: Caps 400 mg. Susp 180 mg/5 mL. Trade only: Susp 90 mg/5 mL.] ▶K ♀B▶? $$$$$

CEFTRIAXONE (*Rocephin*) 1 to 2 g IM/IV q 24 h. Meningitis: 2 g IV q 12 h. Gonorrhea: 250 mg IM plus azithromycin 1 g PO both single dose. See STD table. Peds: 50 to 75 mg/kg/day (up to 2 g/day) divided q 12 to 24 h. Peds meningitis: 100 mg/kg/day (up to 4 g/day) IV divided q 12 to 24 h. Otitis media: 50 mg/kg up to 1 g IM single-dose or once daily for 3 days. May dilute in 1% lidocaine for IM. See acute sinusitis and otitis media tables. Contraindicated in neonates who require or may require IV calcium (including in TPN) due to risk of fatal lung/kidney precipitation of ceftriaxone-calcium. In other patients, do not give ceftriaxone and calcium-containing IV solns simultaneously; sequential administration is acceptable if lines are flushed with a compatible fluid between infusions. ▶K/Bile ♀B▶+ $

ANTIMICROBIALS

Cephalosporins—4th Generation

AVYCAZ (ceftazidime-avibactam) Complicated intra-abdominal infection (in combination with metronidazole), complicated UTI, pyelonephritis: 2.5 g IV q 8 h infused over 2 h. Avycaz 2.5 g = 2 g ceftazidime + 0.5 g avibactam. ▶K ♀?/?/? ▶? $$$$

CEFEPIME (*Maxipime*) 0.5 to 2 g IM/IV q 12 h. Peds: 50 mg/kg IV q 8 to 12 h. ▶K♀B▶? $$$$

ZERBAXA (ceftolozane-tazobactam) Complicated intra-abdominal infections (in combination with metronidazole), complicated UTI, pyelonephritis: 1.5 g IV q 8 h infused over 1 h. Zerbaxa 1.5 g = 1 g ceftolozane + 0.5 g tazobactam. ▶K ♀B ▶? $$$$$

Cephalosporins—5th Generation

CEFTAROLINE (*Teflaro*) Community-acquired pneumonia, skin infections. Adults: 600 mg IV q 12 h. Treat pneumonia for 5 to 7 days, skin infections for 5 to 14 days. Peds. Age 2 mo to less than 2 yo: 8 mg/kg IV q 8 h. Age 2 yo and older: 12 mg/kg IV q 8 h for wt 33 kg or less; 400 mg IV q 8 h or 600 mg IV q 12 h for wt greater than 33 kg. Treat peds for 5 to 14 days. Infuse over 5 to 60 minutes. ▶K♀B▶? $$$$$

Glycopeptides

DALBAVANCIN (*Dalvance*) Gram-positive skin infections, including MRSA: Single dose of 1500 mg IV infused over 30 min or 1000 mg followed 1 week later by 500 mg. Rapid infusion can cause "red man" syndrome. ▶K ♀?/?/? ▶? $$$$$

ORITAVANCIN (*Orbactiv*) Gram-positive skin infections, including MRSA: 1200 mg IV single dose infused over 3 h. Do not give IV heparin for 120 h after oritavancin dose. Increases warfarin exposure; INR inaccurate for 12 h after oritavancin dose. ▶K feces ♀C ▶? $$$$$

TELAVANCIN (*Vibativ*) Complicated skin infections including MRSA, hospital-acquired/ventilator-associated *S. aureus*

(cont.)

pneumonia (not 1st-line), adults: 10 mg/kg IV once daily for 7 to 14 days (skin infections) or 7 to 21 days (pneumonia). Infuse over 1 h. May be teratogenic; get serum pregnancy test before use in women of childbearing potential. Nephrotoxic; monitor renal function. Not for CrCl of 50 mL/min or less unless potential benefit exceeds risk. ▶K ♀C ▶? $$$$$ ■

VANCOMYCIN (*Vancocin*) Usual adult dose: 15 to 20 mg/kg IV q 8 to 12 h; consider loading dose of 25 to 30 mg/kg for severe infection. Infuse over 1 h; infuse over 1.5 to 2 h if dose greater than 1 g; slow infusion rate to reduce risk of Red Man syndrome. Peds: 10 to 15 mg/kg IV q 6 h. *C. difficile* diarrhea: 40 mg/kg/day PO up to 2 g/day divided four times per day for at least 10 days. IV administration ineffective for this indication. Dose depends on severity and complications, see table for management of *C. difficile* infection in adults. [Generic/Trade: Caps 125, 250 mg. Pharmacist can compound oral liquid from IV formulation.] ▶K ♀C ▶? $$$$$

Macrolides

AZITHROMYCIN (*Zithromax, Zmax*) Usual dose: 10 mg/kg (up to 500 mg) PO on day 1, then 5 mg/kg (up to 250 mg) daily for 4 days. Usual IV dose for adults:500 mg IV once daily. Azithromycin is a poor option for otitis media and sinusitis due to pneumococcal and *H. influenzae* resistance; see otitis media and sinusitis treatment tables for alternatives. Otitis media: 30 mg/kg PO single dose or 10 mg/kg PO daily for 3 days. Peds sinusitis: 10 mg/kg PO daily for 3 days. Group A streptococcal pharyngitis (2nd-line to penicillin): 12 mg/kg (up to 500 mg) PO daily for 5 days. Adult acute sinusitis or exacerbation of chronic bronchitis: 500 mg PO daily for 3 days. Zmax for community-acquired pneumonia, acute sinusitis: 60 mg/kg (up to 2 g) PO single dose on empty stomach; give adult dose of 2 g for wt 34 kg or greater.

(cont.)

Chlamydia (including pregnancy), chancroid: 1 g PO single dose. See STD table. Prevention of disseminated *Mycobacterium avium* complex disease: 1200 mg PO once a week. Pertussis treatment/post-exposure prophylaxis: 10 mg/kg PO once daily for 5 days for infants age younger than 6 mo; 10 mg/kg (max 500 mg) PO on day 1, then 5 mg/kg (max 250 mg) PO once daily for 4 days for children 6 mo and older; 500 mg PO on day 1, then 250 mg PO daily for 4 days for adolescents and adults. [Generic/Trade: Tabs 250, 500, 600 mg. Susp 100, 200 mg/5 mL. Packet 1000 mg. Z-Pak: #6, 250 mg tab. Tri-Pak: #3, 500 mg tab. Trade only: Extended-release oral susp (Zmax): 2 g in 60 mL single-dose bottle.] ▶L ♀B ▶? $$

CLARITHROMYCIN (*Biaxin*) Usual dose: Adult: 250 to 500 mg PO two times per day. Peds: 7.5 mg/kg PO two times per day. *H. pylori*: See table in GI section. See table for prophylaxis of bacterial endocarditis. *Mycobacterium avium* complex disease prevention: 7.5 mg/kg up to 500 mg PO two times per day. [Generic/Trade: Tabs 250, 500 mg. Extended-release tabs 500 mg. Susp 125, 250 mg/5 mL.] ▶KL ♀C ▶? $$$

ERYTHROMYCIN BASE (*Ery-Tab, PCE, ✦Eryc*) Adult: 250 to 500 mg PO four times per day, 333 mg PO three times per day, or 500 mg PO two times per day. Peds: 30 to 50 mg/kg/day PO divided four times per day. [Generic only: Tabs 250, 500 mg. Delayed-release caps 250 mg. Trade only: Delayed-release tabs (Ery-Tab, PCE) 250, 333, 500 mg.] ▶L ♀B ▶+ $$$$

ERYTHROMYCIN ETHYL SUCCINATE (*EES, EryPed*) Adult: 400 mg PO four times per day. Peds: 30 to 50 mg/kg/day PO divided four times per day. [Generic/Trade: Tabs 400 mg. Trade only: Susp 200, 400 mg/5 mL.] ▶L ♀B ▶+ $

ERYTHROMYCIN LACTOBIONATE (*Erythrocin IV*) Adult: 15 to 20 mg/kg/day (max 4 g) IV divided q 6 h. Peds: 15 to 50 mg/kg/day IV divided q 6 h. ▶L ♀B ▶+ $$$$$

FIDAXOMICIN (*Dificid*) *C. difficile*–associated diarrhea: 200 mg PO two times per day for 10 days. [Trade only: 200 mg tabs.] ▶minimal absorption ♀B ▶? $$$$$

PENICILLINS — GENERAL ANTIMICROBIAL SPECTRUM

1st generation	Most streptococci; oral anaerobic coverage
2nd generation	Most streptococci; *S. aureus* (but not MRSA)
3rd generation	Most streptococci; basic Gram-negative coverage
4th generation	*Pseudomonas*

Penicillins—1st Generation—Natural

BENZATHINE PENICILLIN (*Bicillin L-A*) Usual dose: 1.2 million units IM for adults and peds wt greater than 27 kg; 600,000 units IM for peds wt 27 kg or less. Give single dose for group A streptococcal pharyngitis. Give IM q month for secondary prevention of rheumatic fever (q 3 weeks for high-risk patients). See STD table for treatment of syphilis in adults. Dose lasts 2 to 4 weeks. [Trade only: For IM use, 600,000 units/mL; 1, 2, 4 mL syringes.] ▸K ♀B ▸? $$$ ■

BICILLIN C-R **(procaine penicillin + benzathine penicillin)** Scarlet fever; erysipelas; upper respiratory, skin, and soft-tissue infections due to group A strep: 600,000 units IM for wt less than 13.6 kg; 900,000 to 1.2 million units IM for wt 13.6 to 27 kg; 2.4 million units IM for wt greater than 27 kg. Pneumococcal infections other than meningitis: 600,000 units IM q 2 to 3 days until temperature normal for 48 h. Not for treatment of syphilis. [Trade only: For IM use 300/300 and 450/150 (Peds) thousand units/mL procaine/benzathine penicillin (600,000 units/mL); 2 mL syringe.] ▸K ♀B ▸? $$$$ ■

PENICILLIN G Pneumococcal pneumonia and severe infections: 250,000 to 400,000 units/kg/day (8 to 12 million units/day in adult) IV divided q 4 to 6 h. Pneumococcal meningitis: 250,000

(cont.)

to 400,000 units/kg/day (24 million units/day in adult) in 4 to 6 divided doses. Anthrax: see table. ▶K ♀B ▶? $$$$

PENICILLIN V Adults: 250 to 500 mg PO four times per day. Peds: 25 to 50 mg/kg/day divided two to four times per day. AHA doses for pharyngitis: 250 mg (peds 27 kg or less) or 500 mg (adults and peds greater than 27 kg) PO two to three times per day for 10 days. Anthrax: See table. [Generic only: Tabs 250, 500 mg. Oral soln 125, 250 mg/5 mL.] ▶K ♀B ▶? $

PROCAINE PENICILLIN 0.6 to 1 million units IM daily (peak 4 h, lasts 24 h). [Generic: For IM use, 600,000 units/mL; 1, 2 mL syringes.] ▶K ♀B ▶? $$$$$ ■

Penicillins—2nd Generation—Penicillinase-Resistant

DICLOXACILLIN Adult: 250 to 500 mg PO four times per day. Peds: 12.5 to 25 mg/kg/day PO divided four times per day. [Generic only: Caps 250, 500 mg.] ▶KL ♀B ▶? $$

NAFCILLIN Adult: 1 to 2 g IM/IV q 4 h. Peds: 50 to 200 mg/kg/day IM/IV divided q 4 to 6 h. ▶L ♀B ▶? $$$$$

OXACILLIN Adult: 1 to 2 g IM/IV q 4 to 6 h. Peds: 150 to 200 mg/kg/day IM/IV divided q 4 to 6 h. ▶KL ♀B ▶? $$$$$

Penicillins—3rd Generation—Aminopenicillins

AMOXICILLIN (*Amoxil, Moxatag*) Adult, usual dose: 250 to 500 mg PO three times per day or 500 to 875 mg PO two times per day. High-dose for community-acquired pneumonia, acute sinusitis, adults: 1 g PO three times per day. See acute sinusitis table. Chlamydia in pregnancy (CDC alternative regimen): 500 mg PO three times per day for 7 days. See STD table. Lyme disease: 50 mg/kg/day up to 500 mg PO three times per day for 14 days for early disease, 28 days for Lyme arthritis. Group A streptococcal pharyngitis: Treat for 10 days with 50 mg/kg up to 1 g PO once daily; alternate is 25 mg/kg up to 500 mg PO two times per day. Group A streptococcal pharyngitis/tonsillitis, age 12 yo or older: 775 mg ER tab (Moxatag) PO once

(cont.)

daily for 10 days. Usual peds dose: 40 mg/kg/day PO divided three times per day or 45 mg/kg/day divided two times per day. Peds high-dose for otitis media, sinusitis, community-acquired pneumonia: 80 to 90 mg/kg/day (max of 4 g/day) PO divided two times per day. Treat otitis media for 5 to 7 days if age 6 yo and older with mild to moderate symptoms, 7 days for age 2 to 5 yo with mild to moderate symptoms, and 10 days for age younger than 2 yo or children with severe symptoms. See tables for acute otitis media and sinusitis in children. [Generic only: Caps 250, 500 mg. Tabs 500, 875 mg. Chewable tabs 125, 200, 250, 400 mg. Susp 125, 250 mg/5 mL. Susp 200, 400 mg/5 mL. Trade only: Extended-release tabs (Moxatag) 775 mg.] ►K ♀B ▶+ $

AMOXICILLIN-CLAVULANATE (*Augmentin, Augmentin ES-600 Augmentin XR, ✦Clavulin*) Adult, usual dose: 500 to 875 mg PO two times per day or 250 to 500 mg three times per day. Augmentin XR: 2 tabs PO q 12 h with meals. Peds, usual dose: 45 mg/kg/day PO divided two times per day or 40 mg/kg/day divided three times per day. High-dose for community-acquired pneumonia, otitis media, sinusitis: 90 mg/kg/day (max 4 g/day) PO divided two times per day. Treat pneumonia for up to 10 days; sinusitis for 10 to 14 days. Treat otitis media for 5 to 7 days for children 6 yo and older with mild to moderate symptoms, 7 days for children 2 to 5 yo with mild to moderate symptoms, and 10 days for children younger than 2 yo and those with severe symptoms. See tables for acute sinusitis in adults and children and otitis media in children. [Generic/Trade (amoxicillin-clavulanate): Tabs 250/125, 500/125, 875/125 mg. Chewables, Susp 200/28.5, 400/57 mg per tab or 5 mL, 250/62.5 mg per 5 mL. (ES) Susp 600/42.9 mg per 5 mL. Extended-release tabs 1000/62.5 mg. Trade only: Susp 125/31.25 per 5 mL, 250/62.5 mg per 5 mL.] ►K ♀B ▶? $$$

AMPICILLIN Usual dose: 1 to 2 g IV q 4 to 6 h. Sepsis, meningitis: 150 to 200 mg/kg/day IV divided q 3 to 4 h. Peds: 100 to 400 mg/kg/day IM/IV divided q 4 to 6 h. [Generic only: Caps 250, 500 mg. Susp 125, 250 mg/5 mL.] ►K ♀B ▶? $$$$$

UNASYN (ampicillin-sulbactam) Adult: 1.5 to 3 g IM/IV q 6 h. Peds: 100 to 400 mg/kg/day of ampicillin divided q 6 h. ▶K ♀B ▶? $$$

Penicillins—4th Generation—Extended Spectrum

PIPERACILLIN-TAZOBACTAM (Zosyn, ✦Tazocin) Adult: 3.375 to 4.5 g IV q 6 h. Peds appendicitis or peritonitis: 80 mg/kg IV q 8 h for age 2 to 9 mo, 100 mg/kg piperacillin IV q 8 h for age older than 9 mo, use adult dose for wt greater than 40 kg. ▶K ♀B ▶? $$$$$

Quinolones

NOTE: As of 2016, FDA recommends limiting fluoroquinolone treatment of bronchitis, acute sinusitis, and uncomplicated UTI to patients who lack other treatment options. For these indications, the benefit is generally less than the risk of serious adverse events. These include tendonitis/tendon rupture (risk increased by corticosteroids, age over 60 yo, and organ transplant), exacerbation of myasthenia gravis, QT interval prolongation/ torsades, CNS toxicity (eg, seizures, increased intracranial pressure), peripheral neuropathy, hypersensitivity, C. difficile-associated diarrhea, and fluoroquinolone-associated disability (FQAD). FQAD is a rare disabling multi-organ reaction with musculoskeletal symptoms (eg, joint/muscle pain, tendonitis), CNS effects (eg, fatigue, insomnia, anxiety) and/or peripheral neuropathy. It has an onset of hours to weeks and may be irreversible.

CIPROFLOXACIN (Cipro, Cipro XR) Usual adult dose: 200 to 400 mg IV q 8 to 12 h; 250 to 750 mg PO two times per day. Cipro XR for pyelonephritis or complicated UTI: 1000 mg PO daily for 7 to 14 days. Plague: 400 mg IV q 8 to 12 h or 500 to 750 mg PO q 12 h for 14 days. Simple UTI in patients with no other treatment options: 250 mg PO two times per day for 3 days or

(cont.)

Cipro XR 500 mg PO daily for 3 days. Peds. Complicated UTI, pyelonephritis, 1 to 17 yo: 6 to 10 mg/kg (max 400 mg/dose) IV q 8 h, then 10 to 20 mg/kg (max 750 mg/dose) PO q 12 h. Plague, birth to 17 yo: 10 mg/kg IV q8 to 12h or 15 mg/kg (max 500 mg) PO q 8 to 12 h for 10 to 21 days. Anthrax: See table. [Generic/Trade: Tabs 100, 250, 500, 750 mg. Extended-release tabs 500, 1000 mg. Oral susp 250, 500 mg/5 mL.] ▶LK ♀C but teratogenicity unlikely ▶?+ $ ■

GEMIFLOXACIN (*Factive*) Acute exacerbation of chronic bronchitis if no other treatment options, community-acquired pneumonia:320 mg PO daily for 5 days (bronchitis), or 5 to 7 days (pneumonia). [Trade only: Tabs 320 mg.] ▶Feces, K ♀C ▶– $$$$$ ■

LEVOFLOXACIN (*Levaquin*) IV and PO doses are the same. Usual adult dose: 250 to 750 mg daily. Complicated UTI or pyelonephritis: 250 mg once daily for 10 days or 750 mg once daily for 5 days. Community-acquired pneumonia: 750 mg once daily for 5 days or 500 mg once daily for 7 to 14 days. Plague: 500 mg once daily for 10 to 14 days. See table for management of acute sinusitis in adults and children. Simple UTI in patients with no other treatment options: 250 mg once daily for 3 days. Acute exacerbation of chronic bronchitis in patients with no other treatment options: 500 mg once daily for 7 days. Peds. Community-acquired pneumonia: 8 to 10 mg/kg two times per day for age 6 mo to 5 yo; 8 to 10 mg/kg once daily (max 750 mg/ day) for age 5 to 16 yo. Plague, age 6 mo and older: Treat for 10 to 14 days with 8 mg/kg (max 250 mg/dose) two times per day if wt less than 50 kg; 500 mg once daily if wt greater than 50 kg. Anthrax: See table. [Trade/Generic: Tabs 250, 500, 750 mg.] ▶KL ♀C ▶? $$$ ■

MOXIFLOXACIN (*Avelox*) Adults: 400 mg PO/IV daily for 5 days (acute exacerbation of chronic bronchitis if no other treatment options), 5 to 14 days (complicated intra-abdominal infection), 7 days (uncomplicated skin infections), 10 days (acute sinusitis with no other treatment options), 7 to 14 days

(cont.)

(community-acquired pneumonia), 7 to 21 days (complicated skin infections). See tables for management of acute sinusitis and anthrax. [Generic/Trade: Tabs 400 mg.] ▶LK ♀C ▶– $$$$ ■

OFLOXACIN Adult: 200 to 400 mg PO two times per day. [Generic only: Tabs 200, 300, 400 mg.] ▶LK ♀C ▶?+ $$$ ■

Sulfonamides

TRIMETHOPRIM-SULFAMETHOXAZOLE (*Bactrim, cotrimoxazole, Septra, Sulfatrim Pediatric, TMP-SMX*) Adult usual dose: 1 tab PO two times per day, double-strength (DS, 160 mg/800 mg) or single-strength (SS, 80 mg/400 mg). Peds usual dose: 1 mL/kg/day susp PO divided two times per day (up to 20 mL PO two times per day). Use adult dose for wt greater than 40 kg. TMP-SMX is a poor option for otitis media and sinusitis due to high pneumococcus and *H. influenzae* resistance rates; see otitis media and sinusitis treatment tables for alternatives. Community-acquired MRSA skin infections. Adults: 1 to 2 DS tabs PO two times per day for 7 to 10 days; 2 DS tabs PO two times per day for wt 100 kg or greater or BMI of 40 or greater. Peds: 1 to 1.5 mL/kg/day PO divided two times per day. Pneumocystis pneumonia treatment: 15 to 20 mg/kg/day (based on TMP) IV divided q 6 to 8 h or PO divided three times per day for 21 days total. Pneumocystis pneumonia prophylaxis, adults: 1 DS tab PO daily. Risk of hyperkalemia increased by high doses, renal impairment, and drug interactions. [Generic/Trade: Tabs 80 mg TMP/400 mg SMX (SS), 160 mg TMP/800 mg SMX (DS). Susp 40 mg TMP/200 mg SMX per 5 mL. 20 mL susp = 2 SS tabs = 1 DS tab.] ▶K ♀C ▶+ $

Tetracyclines

NOTE: *Tetracyclines can cause photosensitivity, pseudotumor cerebri (avoid with isotretinoin), and may increase INR with warfarin. Use caution in renal dysfunction; doxycycline preferred. Generally avoid in children younger than 8 yo due to risk*

(cont.)

of teeth staining, but benefit of doxycycline for severe infections (e.g., anthrax, Rocky Mountain spotted fever) exceeds potential risk of teeth staining.

DEMECLOCYCLINE Usual dose: 150 mg PO four times per day or 300 mg PO two times per day on empty stomach. SIADH: 600 to 1200 mg/day PO given in 3 to 4 divided doses. [Generic: Tabs 150, 300 mg.] ▸K, feces ♀D ▸?+ $$$$

DOXYCYCLINE (*Acticlate, Adoxa, Avidoxy, Doryx, Doryx MPC, Doxy, Monodox, Oracea, Vibramycin, ✸Doxycin*) See tables for management of acute sinusitis, STDs, and anthrax. 100 mg PO two times per day for 5 to 7 days for community-acquired pneumonia, 7 days for Chlamydia or nongonococcal urethritis, 5 to 10 days for community-acquired skin infection, 14 days for early Lyme disease, 28 days for Lyme arthritis. Acne: Up to 100 mg PO two times per day. Oracea ($$$$$) for inflammatory rosacea: 40 mg PO once q am on empty stomach. Periodontitis: 20 mg PO two times per day. Doryx MPC: 120 mg PO two times per day on day 1, the 120 mg PO once daily. Consider 120 mg PO two times per day for severe infections. Do not crush or chew; not interchangeable with other formulations. Injection: 200 mg IV on 1st day in 1 to 2 infusions, then 100 to 200 mg/day IV in 1 to 2 infusions. Malaria prophylaxis, age 8 yo and older: 2 mg/kg/day up to 100 mg PO daily starting 1 to 2 days before exposure until 4 weeks after. Peds. Severe infections including tickborne rickettsial diseases: 2.2 mg/kg up to 100 mg IV/PO two times per day for any age and wt less than 45 kg; use adult dose for 45 kg or greater. [Monohydrate salt. Generic/Trade: Caps ($$) 50, 75, 100, 150 mg. Tabs ($$$) 50, 75, 100, 150 mg. Susp (Vibramycin) 25 mg/5 mL. Trade only: Delayed-release caps 40 mg (Oracea $$$$$). Generic: Delayed-release caps 40 mg ($$$$$). Hyclate salt. Tabs: Trade only: 75, 150 mg (Acticlate-$$$$$). Generic only: 20, 100mg. Caps: Generic only: 50 mg. Generic/Trade (Vibramycin): 100 mg. Trade only (Acticlate Cap): 75 mg. Delayed-release tabs: Generic only: 75, 100, 150 mg.

(cont.)

Generic/Trade (Doryx $$$$$): 50, 200 mg. Trade only (Doryx MPC $$$$$): 120 mg. Delayed-release caps: Generic only: 75, 100 mg. Calcium salt. Trade only: Syrup (Vibramycin Calcium) 50 mg/5 mL.] ▶LK ♀D ▶?+ varies by therapy

MINOCYCLINE (*Minocin, Solodyn*) Usual dose: 200 mg IV/PO initially, then 100 mg q 12 h. Community-acquired MRSA skin infections: 200 mg PO 1st dose, then 100 mg PO two times per day for 5 to 10 days. Acne (traditional dosing): 50 mg PO two times per day. Solodyn ($$$$$) for inflammatory acne in adults and children 12 yo and older: 1 mg/kg PO once daily. [Generic/Trade: Caps, Tabs ($) 50, 75, 100 mg. Extended-release tabs ($$$$$) 45, 90, 135 mg. Trade only: Extended-release tabs (Solodyn-$$$$$) 55 , 65, 80, 105, 115 mg.] ▶LK ♀D ▶?+ $$

TETRACYCLINE 250 to 500 mg PO four times per day. [Generic only: Caps 250, 500 mg.] ▶LK ♀D ▶?+ $

Other Antimicrobials

AZTREONAM (*Azactam, Cayston*) Gram-negative infections: Adults: 0.5 to 2 g IM/IV q 6 to 12 h. Peds: 30 mg/kg IV q 6 to 8 h. Cystic fibrosis respiratory symptoms, age 7 yo and older: 1 vial Cayston nebulized three times per day for 28 days, followed by cycle of 28 days off treatment. [Trade only (Cayston): 75 mg/vial with diluent for inhalation.] ▶K ♀B ▶+ $$$$$

CHLORAMPHENICOL Usual dose, adult and peds: 50 to 100 mg/kg/day IV divided q 6 h. Aplastic anemia. ▶LK ♀C ▶– $$$$$ ■

CLINDAMYCIN (*Cleocin, ✦Dalacin C*) Usual adult dose: 150 to 450 mg PO four times per day. 600 to 900 mg IV q 8 h. Community-acquired MRSA skin infections: 300 to 450 mg PO three times per day for 5 to 10 days for adults; 10 to 13 mg/kg/dose PO q 6 to 8 h (max 40 mg/kg/day) for peds. Peds usual dose: 20 to 40 mg/kg/day IV divided q 6 to 8 h or give 8 to 25 mg/kg/day susp PO divided q 6 to 8 h. See tables for management of anthrax, and acute sinusitis and otitis media in children. [Generic/Trade: Caps 75, 150, 300 mg. Oral soln 75 mg/5 mL (100 mL).] ▶L ♀B ▶?+ $ ■

DAPTOMYCIN (*Cubicin*) Complicated skin infections (including MRSA): 4 mg/kg IV daily for 7 to 14 days. *S. aureus* bacteremia (including MRSA): 6 mg/kg IV daily for at least 2 to 6 weeks. Infuse over 30 min. Not for pneumonia (inactivated by surfactant). Not approved in children. ▶K ♀B ▷? $$$$$

FOSFOMYCIN (*Monurol*) Simple UTI: One 3 g packet PO single dose. [Trade only: 3 g packet of granules.] ▶K ♀B ▷? $$$

LINEZOLID (*Zyvox*, ✦*Zyvoxam*) Pneumonia, complicated skin infections (including MRSA), vancomycin-resistant *E. faecium* infections: 10 mg/kg up to 600 mg IV/PO q 8 h for age younger than 12 yo; 600 mg IV/PO q 12 h for adults and age 12 yo or older. Anthrax: See table. Myelosuppression, drug interactions due to MAO inhibition. Limit tyramine foods to less than 100 mg/meal. [Generic/Trade: Tabs 600 mg. Susp 100 mg/5 mL.] ▶Oxidation/K ♀C ▷? $$$$$

METRONIDAZOLE (*Flagyl, Flagyl ER*, ✦*Nidazol*) Bacterial vaginosis: 500 mg PO two times per day or Flagyl ER 750 mg PO daily for 7 days. Trichomoniasis: 2 g PO single dose for patient and sex partners (may be used in pregnancy per CDC). See STD table. *H. pylori*: See table in GI section. Anaerobic bacterial infections: Load 1 g or 15 mg/kg IV, then 500 mg or 7.5 mg/kg (up to 4 g/day) IV/PO q 6 to 8 h, each IV dose over 1 h. Peds: 7.5 mg/kg IV q 6 h. *C. difficile*–associated diarrhea: Adults: 500 mg PO three times per day for 10 to 14 days. Peds: 30 mg/kg/day PO divided four times per day for 10 to 14 days. See table for management of *C. difficile* infection in adults. Giardia: 250 mg (5 mg/kg/dose for peds) PO three times per day for 5 to 7 days. [Generic/Trade: Tabs 250, 500 mg. Caps 375 mg. Extended-release tabs: 750 mg.] ▶KL ♀B ▷?– $

NITROFURANTOIN (*Furadantin, Macrodantin, Macrobid*) Uncomplicated UTI: 50 to 100 mg PO four times per day for 7 days. Peds: 5 to 7 mg/kg/day divided four times per day. Macrobid for uncomplicated UTI: 100 mg PO two times per day for 7 days. Take nitrofurantoin with food. [Generic/Trade: Caps

(cont.)

(Macrodantin) 25, 50, 100 mg. Caps (Macrobid) 100 mg. Susp (Furadantin) 25 mg/5 mL.] ▶KL ♀B ▶+? $$

RIFAXIMIN (*Xifaxan*) Traveler's diarrhea: 200 mg PO three times per day for 3 days. Prevention of recurrent hepatic encephalopathy ($$$$$): 550 mg PO two times per day. Irritable bowel syndrome with diarrhea: 550 mg PO three times per day for 14 days. Can retreat up to 2 times if recurrence. [Trade only: Tabs 200, 550 mg.] ▶feces ♀ X/?/? ▶? $$$$

SYNERCID (quinupristin + dalfopristin) Complicated staphylococcal/streptococcal skin infection: 7.5 mg/kg IV q 12 h, each dose over 1 h for at least 7 days. MRSA bacteremia (2nd line): 7.5 mg/kg IV q 8 h. Not active against *E. faecalis*. ▶Bile ♀B ▶? $$$$$

TEDIZOLID (*Sivextro*) Skin infections, including MRSA: 200 mg IV/PO once daily for 6 days. Infuse IV over 1 hour. [Trade only: Tabs 200 mg.] ▶L ♀C ▶? $$$$$

TELITHROMYCIN (*Ketek*) Community-acquired pneumonia: 800 mg PO daily for 7 to 10 days. Not for acute sinusitis or acute exacerbation of chronic bronchitis (risks exceed potential benefit). Contraindicated in myasthenia gravis. [Trade only: Tabs 300, 400 mg.] ▶LK ♀C ▶? $$$$ ■

TIGECYCLINE (*Tygacil*) Complicated skin infections, complicated intra-abdominal infections, community-acquired pneumonia: 100 mg IV 1st dose, then 50 mg IV q 12 h. Infuse over 30 to 60 min. Mortality higher with tigecycline than comparators; do not use unless there are no alternatives. Not indicated for hospital-acquired or ventilator-associated pneumonia or diabetic foot infection. ▶Bile, K ♀D ▶?+ $$$$$ ■

TRIMETHOPRIM (*Primsol*, *✦Proloprim*) 100 mg PO two times per day or 200 mg PO daily. Risk of hyperkalemia increased by high doses, renal impairment, and drug interactions. [Generic only: Tabs 100 mg. Trade only (Primsol-$$$$): Oral soln 50 mg/5 mL.] ▶K ♀C ▶– $

CARDIOVASCULAR

ACE INHIBITOR DOSING

ACE INHIBITOR	HTN		Heart Failure	
	Initial	Max/day	Initial	Max/day
benazepril (*Lotensin*)	10 mg daily*	80 mg	—	—
captopril (*Capoten*)	25 mg bid/tid	450 mg	6.25 mg tid	450 mg
enalapril (*Vasotec*)	5 mg daily*	40 mg	2.5 mg bid	40 mg
fosinopril (*Monopril*)	10 mg daily*	80 mg	5–10 mg daily	40 mg
lisinopril (*Zestril/Prinivil*)	10 mg daily	80 mg	2.5–5 mg daily	40 mg
moexipril (*Univasc*)	7.5 mg daily*	30 mg	—	—
perindopril (*Aceon*)	4 mg daily*	16 mg	2 mg daily	16 mg
quinapril (*Accupril*)	10–20 mg daily*	80 mg	5 mg bid	40 mg
ramipril (*Altace*)	2.5 mg daily*	20 mg	1.25–2.5 mg bid	10 mg
trandolapril (*Mavik*)	1–2 mg daily*	8 mg	1 mg daily	4 mg

bid = two times per day; tid = three times per day.
Data taken from prescribing information and *Circulation* 2013;128:e240–e327.
* May require bid dosing for 24-h BP control.

CARDIOVASCULAR

BETA-BLOCKER DOSING FOR HEART FAILURE REDUCED EJECTION FRACTION (HFrEF; EF 40% or less)

Beta-blocker	Inital	Max/day
bisoprolol	1.25 mg once daily	10 mg once daily
carvedilol	3.125 mg bid	50 mg bid
carvedilol extended-release	10 mg once daily	80 mg once daily
metoprolol succinate extended-release	12.5 to 25 mg once daily	200 mg once daily

bid=two times per day

Data taken from prescribing information and *Circulation* 2013; 128:e240–e327.

CARDIAC PARAMETERS AND FORMULAS

Cardiac output (CO) = heart rate × CVA volume [normal 4 to 8 L/min]

Cardiac index (CI) = CO/BSA [normal 2.8 to 4.2 L/min/m^2]

MAP (mean arterial pressure) = [(SBP − DBP)/3] + DBP [normal 80 to 100 mmHg]

SVR (systemic vascular resistance) = (MAP − CVP) × (80)/CO [normal 800 to 1200 dyne x sec/cm^5]

PVR (pulmonary vasc resisistance) = (PAM − PCWP) × (80)/CO [normal 45 to 120 dyne × sec/cm^5]

QTc = QT/square root of RR [normal 0.38 to 0.42]

Right atrial pressure (central venous pressure) [normal 0 to 8 mmHg]

Pulmonary artery systolic pressure (PAS) [normal 20 to 30 mmHg]

Pulmonary artery diastolic pressure (PAD) [normal 10 to 15 mmHg]

Pulmonary capillary wedge pressure (PCWP) [normal 8 to 12 mmHg (post-MI ~16 mmHg)]

LIPID CHANGE BY CLASS/AGENT[1]

Drug class/agent	LDL-C	HDL-C	TG
Bile acid sequestrants[2]	↓ 15–30%	↑ 3–5%	↑ 0–10%
Cholesterol absorption inhibitor[3]	↓ 18%	↑ 1%	↓ 8%
Fibrates[4]	↓ 5–↑ 20%	↑ 10–20%	↓ 20–50%
Niacin[5]	↓ 5–25%	↑ 15–35%	↓ 20–50%
Omega 3 fatty acids[6]	↓ 6% or ↑ 144%	↓ 5% or ↑ 7%	↓ 19–44%
PCSK9 inhibitors[7]	↓ 40–72%	↑ 0–10%	↓ 0–17%
Statins[8]	↓ 18–55%	↑ 5–15%	↓ 7–30%

(cont.)

LDL-C = low density lipoprotein cholesterol. HDL-C = high density lipoprotein cholesterol. TG = triglycerides.

[1] Adapted from prescribing information.

[2] Cholestyramine (4–16 g), colestipol (5–20 g), colesevelam (2.6–3.8 g).

[3] Ezetimibe (10 mg). When added to statin therapy, will ↓ LDL-C 25%, ↑ HDL-C 3%, ↓ TG 14% in addition to statin effects.

[4] Fenofibrate (145–200 mg), gemfibrozil (600 mg two times per day).

[5] Extended release nicotinic acid (Niaspan® 1–2 g), immediate release (crystalline) nicotinic acid (1.5–3g), sustained release nicotinic acid (Slo-Niacin® 1–2 g).

[6] Epanova® (4 g), Lovaza® (4 g), Vascepa® (4 g).

[7] Alirocumab (75, 150 mg/mL), evolocumab (140 mg/mL).

[8] Atorvastatin (10–80 mg), fluvastatin (20–80 mg), lovastatin (20–80 mg), pravastatin (20–80 mg), rosuvastatin (5–40 mg), simvastatin (20–40 mg).

CHOLESTEROL TREATMENT RECOMMENDATIONS (AGES ≥ 21 YEARS)

Lifestyle changes should be initiated in all patients; reinforce lifestyle changes at each patient encounter.

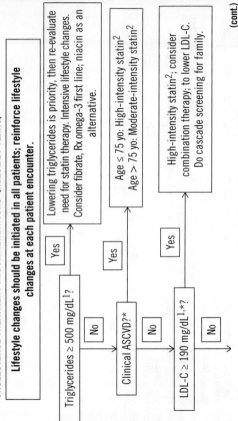

Triglycerides ≥ 500 mg/dL[1]?

Yes → Lowering triglycerides is priority, then re-evaluate need for statin therapy. Intensive lifestyle changes. Consider fibrate, Rx omega-3 first line; niacin as an alternative.*

No →

Clinical ASCVD?*

Yes → Age ≤ 75 yo: High-intensity statin[2]
Age > 75 yo: Moderate-intensity statin[2]

No →

LDL-C ≥ 190 mg/dL[1],*?

Yes → High-intensity statin[2]; consider combination therapy; to lower LDL-C. Do cascade screening for family.

No →

(cont.)

(cont.)

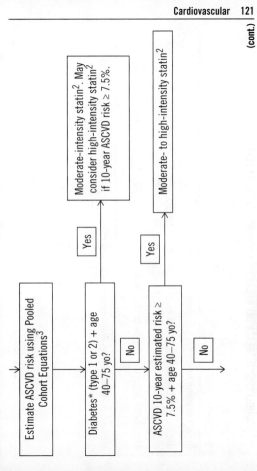

Estimate ASCVD risk using Pooled Cohort Equations[3]

Diabetes* (type 1 or 2) + age 40–75 yo?

No → ASCVD 10-year estimated risk ≥ 7.5% + age 40–75 yo?

Yes → Moderate-intensity statin[2]. May consider high-intensity statin[2] if 10-year ASCVD risk ≥ 7.5%.

ASCVD 10-year estimated risk ≥ 7.5% + age 40–75 yo?

Yes → Moderate- to high-intensity statin[2]

No →

CHOLESTEROL TREATMENT RECOMMENDATIONS (AGES ≥21 YEARS) (*continued*)

No

Benefit of statin therapy is less clear.

Recalculate 10-year ASCVD risk every 4–6 years for patients aged 40–75 yo without clinical ASCVD or diabetes + LDL-C 70–189 mg/dL + not receiving statin therapy.

Assess risk factors + 30-year or lifetime ASCVD risk in those 20–59 yo with low 10-year ASCVD risk.

Consider benefits, risks, drug–drug interactions, adverse effects, and patient preferences before initiating statin therapy.

(cont.)

[1]Rule out secondary causes. If non-fasting triglycerides $\geq$ 500 mg/dL, then a fasting lipid panel is needed.

[2]High-intensity statin = atorvastatin 40, 80 mg; rosuvastatin 20, 40 mg. Moderate-intensity statin is acceptable if patient is not a candidate for high-intensity statin therapy. Moderate-intensity statin = atorvastatin 10, 20 mg; fluvastatin 40 mg twice daily, fluvastatin XL 80 mg; lovastatin 40 mg; pitavastatin 2, 4 mg; pravastatin 40, 80 mg; rosuvastatin 5, 10 mg; simvastatin 20, 40 mg.

[3]Calculator available: http://tools.cardiosource.org/ASCVD-Risk-Estimator/

ASCVD = atherosclerotic cardiovascular disease (includes coronary heart disease, stroke, and peripheral artery disease). DM = Diabetes mellitus. LCL–C = low-density lipoprotein cholesterol. Rx = prescription strength.

Adapted from: *J Am Coll Cardiol.* 2014; 63(25_PA), *Circulation.* 2011; 123: 2292–2333.

*Combination of statin and non-statin therapy to lower LDL–C may be appropriate for patients at high-risk for ASCVD. *J Am Coll Cardiol.* 2016; 68: 92–125.

HTN THERAPY FOR ADULTS ≥ 18 YEARS OLD[1]

Patient Information	BP Target[1] (mm Hg)	Preferred Therapy	Comments
All patients with CKD (with or without diabetes)	< 140/90	Start ACEI or ARB; alone or in combination with a CCB or thiazide[2]	Implement lifestyle interventions; reinforce adherence during patient encounters. Drug treatment strategy based on response and tolerance: Either, titrate first drug to max dose
Any age + diabetes	< 140/90	Start ACEI, ARB, CCB, or thiazide; alone or combination[2]	
Nonblack (no CKD)	Age < 60 yo (no diabetes or CKD)	< 140/90	

(cont.)

	Age ≥ 60 yo (no diabetes or CKD)	< 150/90	before adding second; add second drug before reaching max dose of first drug; or start with 2 drug classes separately or as fixed dose combinations.[3,4]
	Any age + diabetes	<140/90	
Black (no CKD)	Age < 60 yo (no diabetes or CKD)	<140/90	Start CCB or thiazide; alone or combination[2]
	Age ≥ 60 yo (no diabetes or CKD)	< 150/90	

CARDIOVASCULAR

(cont.)

HTN THERAPY FOR ADULTS ≥ 18 YEARS OLD[1]   *(continued)*

[1]These guidelines will be updated in late 2016 or early 2017. The BP targets and treatment recommendations may change based on the results of the SPRINT trial (*N Engl J Med.* 2015;373:2103-16.DOI:10.1056/NEJMoa1511939), which demonstrated fewer fatal and nonfatal major cardiovascular events and death from any cause in patients who were 50 yo or older, at high risk for cardiovascular events, and without diabetes who achieved SBP < 120 mm Hg as compared to SBP < 140 mm Hg. Patients treated to SBP < 120 mm Hg had higher rates of some adverse events (eg, hypotension, syncope, electrolyte abnormalities, acute renal failure).

[2]Do not combine ACEI and ARB therapy.

[3]Consider starting with 2 drugs when SBP is > 160 mmHg and/or DBP is > 100 mm Hg, or if SBP is > 20 mm Hg above goal and/or DBP is > 10 mm Hg above goal. If goal BP is not achieved with 2 drugs, select a third drug from the list. Titrate prn.

[4]If needed, may add another drug (eg, beta-blocker, aldosterone antagonist, others) and/or refer to physician with HTN management expertise.

ACEI = angiotensin converting enzyme inhibitor; ARB = angiotensin-receptor blocker.
CCB = calcium-channel blocker; CKD = chronic kidney disease.

SELECTED DRUGS THAT MAY PROLONG THE QT INTERVAL

alfuzosin	droperidol*	leuprolide	promethazine
amiodarone*	eribulin	levofloxacin*	propofol*
anagrelide*	erythromycin*	lithium	quetiapine
apomorphine	escitalopram*	loperamide*	quinidine*
aripiprazole	ezogabine	(excessive doses)	ranolazine*
arsenic trioxide*	famotidine	methadone*	rilpivirine
asenapine	felbamate	mirabegron	risperidone
atazanavir	fingolimod	mirtazapine	saquinavir
atomoxetine	flecainide*	moexipril/HCTZ	sevoflurane*
azithromycin*	fluconazole*	moxifloxacin*	sotalol*
bedaquiline	foscarnet	nicardipine	tacrolimus
buprenorphine	gemifloxacin	nilotinib	tamoxifen
capecitabine	granisetron	ofloxacin	telithromycin
chloroquine*	halofantrine*	olanzapine	thioridazine*

(cont.)

SELECTED DRUGS THAT MAY PROLONG THE QT INTERVAL (continued)

chlorpromazine*	haloperidol*	ondansetron*	tizanidine
cilostazol*	hydrocodone ER	oxytocin	tolterodine
ciprofloxacin*	ibutilide*	oxaliplatin*	toremifene
citalopram*	iloperidone	paliperidone	tricyclic
clarithromycin*	isradipine	pentamidine*	antidepressants
clozapine	kinase inhibitors	perflutren lipid	vandetanib*
cocaine*		microspheres	vardenafil
dexmedetomidine		pimozide*	venlafaxine
disopyramide*		procainamide*	ziprasidone
dofetilide*			
dolasetron			
donepezil*			
dronedarone*			

(cont.)

NOTE: This table may not include all drugs that prolong the QT interval or cause torsades. Risk of drug-induced QT prolongation may be increased in women, elderly, hypokalemia, hypomagnesemia, bradycardia, starvation, CHF, and CNS injuries. Hepatorenal dysfunction and drug interactions can increase the concentration of QT interval-prolonging drugs. Coadministration of QT interval prolonging drugs can have additive effects. Avoid these (and other) drugs in congenital prolonged QT syndrome (References: prescribing information for individual drugs, www.crediblemeds.org).

*Torsades reported in product labeling/case reports.

HIGH- AND MODERATE-INTENSITY STATIN DOSES

Statin	High-intensity dose (lowers LDL-C at least 50%)	Moderate-intensity dose (lowers LDL-C 30% to 49%)
atorvastatin	40, 80 mg	10, 20 mg
fluvastatin XL	n/a	80 mg
fluvastatin	n/a	40 mg twice daily
lovastatin	n/a	40 mg
pitavastatin	n/a	2, 4 mg
pravastatin	n/a	40, 80 mg
rosuvastatin	20, 40 mg	5, 10 mg
simvastatin	n/a	20, 40 mg

LDL-C = low density lipoprotein cholesterol. Will get ~6% decrease in LDL-C with every doubling of dose.

Adapted from *J Am Coll Cardiol.* 2014; 63(25_PA).

THROMBOLYTIC THERAPY FOR ST-SEGMENT ELEVATION MI (STEMI)

Indications (if high-volume cath lab unavailable)	Clinical history and presentation strongly suggestive of MI within 12 h plus at least 1 of the following: 1 mm ST elevation in at least 2 contiguous leads; new left BBB; or 2 mm ST depression in V1-4 suggestive of true posterior MI.
Absolute contraindications	Previous intracranial hemorrhage; known cerebral vascular lesion arteriovenous malformation); known malignant intracranial neoplasm; recent (<3 months) ischemic CVA (except acute ischemic CVA <4.5 h); aortic dissection; active bleeding or bleeding diathesis (excluding menses); significant closed head or facial trauma (<3 months); intracranial or intraspinal surgery (<2 months); severe uncontrolled HTN (unresponsive to emergency therapy); for streptokinase: prior exposure (<6 months).
Relative contraindications	Severe uncontrolled HTN (>180/110 mm Hg) on presentation or chronic severe HTN; prior ischemic CVA (>3 months), dementia, other intracranial pathology; traumatic/prolonged (>10 min) cardiopulmonary resuscitation; major surgery (<3 weeks); recent (within 2–4 weeks) internal bleeding; puncture of noncompressible vessel; pregnancy; active peptic ulcer disease; current use of anticoagulants.

Reference: *Circulation* 2013;127:e362-425

ACE Inhibitors

NOTE: *See also Antihypertensive Combinations. Contraindicated in pregnancy; with history of angioedema; or with aliskiren in patients with DM. In general, avoid combined use with renin-angiotensin system inhibitors (ie, angiotensin receptor blockers, aliskiren); increases risk of renal impairment, hypotension, and hyperkalemia. Hyperkalemia possible, especially if used concomitantly with other drugs that increase K (including K-containing salt substitutes) and in patients with DM or renal impairment. Concomitant NSAID, including celecoxib, may further deteriorate renal function and decrease antihypertensive effects.*

BENAZEPRIL (*Lotensin*) HTN: Start 10 mg PO daily, usual maintenance dose 20 to 40 mg PO daily or divided two times per day, max 80 mg/day. [Generic/Trade: Tabs, unscored 5, 10, 20, 40 mg.] ▶LK ♀X/X/X, Neonatal harm: Potential anuria, hypotension, renal failure, skull hypoplasia, death. ▶ Do not breastfeed while taking an ACE inhibitor. $$ ■

CAPTOPRIL (*Capoten*) HTN: Start 25 mg PO two to three times per day, usual maintenance dose 25 to 150 mg two to three times per day, max 450 mg/day. Heart failure: Start 6.25 to 12.5 mg PO three times per day, usual dose 50 to 100 mg PO three times per day, max 450 mg/day. Diabetic nephropathy: 25 mg PO three times per day. [Generic only: Tabs, scored 12.5, 25, 50, 100 mg.] ▶LK ♀X/X/X, Neonatal harm: Potential anuria, hypotension, renal failure, skull hypoplasia, death. ▶ Do not breastfeed while taking an ACE inhibitor. $$$ ■

CILAZAPRIL (✦*Inhibace*) Canada only. HTN: 1.25 to 10 mg PO daily. [Generic/Trade: Not available in US. Tabs, scored 1, 2.5, 5 mg.] ▶LK ♀X/X/X, Neonatal harm: Potential anuria, hypotension, renal failure, skull hypoplasia, death. ▶ Do not breastfeed while taking an ACE inhibitor. $ ■

ENALAPRIL (*enalaprilat, Vasotec, Epaned*) HTN: Start 5 mg PO daily, usual maintenance dose 10 to 40 mg PO daily or

(cont.)

divided two times per day, max 40 mg/day. If oral therapy not possible, can use enalaprilat 1.25 mg IV q 6 h over 5 min, and increase up to 5 mg IV q 6 h if needed. Renal impairment or concomitant diuretic therapy: Start 2.5 mg PO daily. Heart failure: Start 2.5 mg PO two times per day, usual dose 10 to 20 mg PO two times per day, max 40 mg/day. [Generic/Trade: Tabs, scored 2.5, 5 mg, unscored 10, 20 mg. Trade only: Oral Soln 1 mg/mL (Epaned-$$$$$).] ▶LK ♀X/X/X, Neonatal harm: Potential anuria, hypotension, renal failure, skull hypoplasia, death. ▶ Do not breastfeed while taking an ACE inhibitor. $$ ■

FOSINOPRIL HTN: Start 10 mg PO daily, usual maintenance dose 20 to 40 mg PO daily or divided two times per day, max 80 mg/day. Heart failure: Start 5 to 10 mg PO daily, usual dose 20 to 40 mg PO daily, max 40 mg/day. [Generic only: Tabs, scored 10 mg, unscored 20, 40 mg.] ▶LK ♀X/X/X, Neonatal harm: Potential anuria, hypotension, renal failure, skull hypoplasia, death. ▶ Do not breastfeed while taking an ACE inhibitor. $$ ■

LISINOPRIL (*Prinivil, Zestril*) HTN: Start 10 mg PO daily, usual maintenance dose 20 to 40 mg PO daily, max 80 mg/day. Heart failure, acute MI: Start 2.5 to 5 mg PO daily, usual dose 5 to 20 mg PO daily, max dose 40 mg. [Generic/Trade: Tabs, unscored (Zestril) 2.5, 5, 10, 20, 30, 40 mg. Tabs, scored (Prinivil) 10, 20, 40 mg.] ▶K ♀X/X/X, Neonatal harm: Potential anuria, hypotension, renal failure, skull hypoplasia, death. ▶ Do not breastfeed while taking an ACE inhibitor. $ ■

MOEXIPRIL (*Univasc*) HTN: Start 7.5 mg PO daily, usual maintenance dose 7.5 to 30 mg PO daily or divided two times per day, max 30 mg/day. [Generic: Tabs, scored 7.5, 15 mg.] ▶LK ♀X/X/X, Neonatal harm: Potential anuria, hypotension, renal failure, skull hypoplasia, death. ▶ Do not breastfeed while taking an ACE inhibitor. $$ ■

PERINDOPRIL (*Aceon, ✦Coversyl*) HTN: Start 4 mg PO daily, usual maintenance dose 4 to 8 mg PO daily or divided two

(cont.)

times per day, max 16 mg/day. Reduction of cardiovascular events in stable CAD: Start 4 mg PO daily for 2 weeks, max 8 mg/day. Elderly (age older than 65 yo): 4 mg PO daily, max 8 mg/day. [Generic/Trade: Tabs, scored 2, 4, 8 mg.] ▶K ♀X/X/X, Neonatal harm: Potential anuria, hypotension, renal failure, skull hypoplasia, death. ▶ Do not breastfeed while taking an ACE inhibitor. $$$ ■

QUINAPRIL (*Accupril*) HTN: Start 10 to 20 mg PO daily (start 10 mg/day if elderly), usual maintenance dose 20 to 80 mg PO daily or divided two times per day, max 80 mg/day. Heart failure: Start 5 mg PO two times per day, usual maintenance dose 10 to 20 mg two times per day. [Generic/Trade: Tabs, scored 5 mg, unscored 10, 20, 40 mg.] ▶LK ♀X/X/X, Neonatal harm: Potential anuria, hypotension, renal failure, skull hypoplasia, death. ▶ Do not breastfeed while taking an ACE inhibitor. $$ ■

RAMIPRIL (*Altace*) HTN: 2.5 mg PO daily, usual maintenance dose 2.5 to 20 mg PO daily or divided two times per day, max 20 mg/day. Heart failure post-MI: Start 2.5 mg PO two times per day, usual maintenance dose 5 mg PO two times per day. Reduce risk of MI, CVA, death from cardiovascular causes: 2.5 mg PO daily for 1 week, then 5 mg daily for 3 weeks, increase as tolerated to max 10 mg/day. [Generic/Trade: Caps 1.25, 2.5, 5, 10 mg.] ▶LK ♀X/X/X, Neonatal harm: Potential anuria, hypotension, renal failure, skull hypoplasia, death. ▶ Do not breastfeed while taking an ACE inhibitor. $ ■

TRANDOLAPRIL (*Mavik*) HTN: Start 1 mg PO daily, usual maintenance dose 2 to 4 mg PO daily or divided two times per day, max 8 mg/day. Heart failure/post-MI: Start 1 mg PO daily, usual maintenance dose 4 mg PO daily. Renal impairment or concomitant diuretic therapy: Start 0.5 mg PO daily. [Generic/Trade: Tabs, scored 1 mg, unscored 2, 4 mg.] ▶LK ♀X/X/X, Neonatal harm: Potential anuria, hypotension, renal failure, skull hypoplasia, death. ▶ Do not breastfeed while taking an ACE inhibitor. $ ■

Aldosterone Antagonists

NOTE: *Hyperkalemia possible, especially if used concomitantly with other drugs that increase K (including K-containing salt substitutes) and in patients with heart failure, DM, or renal impairment.*

EPLERENONE (*Inspra***)** HTN: Start 50 mg PO daily; max 50 mg two times per day. HTN and taking concomitant moderate CYP3A4 inhibitor (eg erythromycin, fluconazole, saquinavir, verapamil): Start 25 mg PO daily ; max 25 mg PO two times daily. Heart failure (with LVEF 40% or less) post MI: Start 25 mg PO daily; titrate to target dose 50 mg daily within 4 weeks, if tolerated. Heart failure (with LVEF 40% or less) post MI and taking concomitant moderate CYP3A4 inhibitor: Do not exceed 25 mg PO daily. Contraindicated in all patients with K+ greater than 5.5 mEq/L; CrCl 30 mL/min or less; strong CYP3A4 inhibitors (eg, clarithromycin, itraconazole, ketoconazole nefazodone, nelfinavir, ritonavir, troleandomycin). Contraindicated in patients treated for HTN with Type 2 DM with microalbuminuria; serum creatinine greater than 2 mg/dL in males or greater than 1.8 mg/dL in females; CrCl < 50 mL/min; or concomitant therapy with K+supplements, K+-sparing diuretics. Measure K+ before initiating, within 1st week, at 1 month after starting treatment or dose adjustment, then prn. Hyperkalemia more common with renal impairment, diabetes, proteinuria, or concomitant ACE inhibitor, ARB, NSAID, or moderate CYP3A inhibitor. Measure serum K+and CrCl 3-7 days of initiation of ACE inhibitor, ARB, NSAID, or moderate CYP3A inhibitor. [Generic/trade: Tabs, unscored 25, 50 mg.] ▶L ♀B ▶? $$$$

SPIRONOLACTONE (*Aldactone***)** HTN: 50 to 100 mg PO daily or divided two times per day (usual dose 25 to 50 mg daily according to ASH-ISH guidelines). Edema: 25 to 200 mg/day. Hypokalemia: 25 to 100 mg PO daily. Primary hyperaldosteronism, maintenance: 100 to 400 mg/day PO.

(cont.)

Heart failure, NYHA III or IV: 25 to 50 mg PO daily. [Generic/Trade: Tabs, unscored 25 mg, scored 50, 100 mg.] ▶LK ♀D ▶+ $ ■

Angiotensin Receptor Blockers (ARBs)

NOTE: *See also Antihypertensive Combinations. Contraindicated in pregnancy; or with aliskiren in patients with DM. In general, avoid combined use with renin-angiotensin system inhibitors (i.e. ACE inhibitors, aliskiren); increases risk of renal impairment, hypotension, and hyperkalemia. Hyperkalemia possible, especially if used concomitantly with other drugs that increase K+ (including K+ containing salt substitutes) and in patients with heart failure, DM, or renal impairment. Concomitant NSAID, including celecoxib, may further deteriorate renal function and decrease antihypertensive effects. May increase lithium levels.*

AZILSARTAN (*Edarbi*) HTN: 80 mg daily. [Trade only: Tabs, unscored 40, 80 mg.] ▶L – ♀D ▶? $$$$ ■

CANDESARTAN (*Atacand*) HTN: Start 16 mg PO daily, max 32 mg/day. Heart failure (NYHA II–IV and LVEF 40% or less): Start 4 mg PO daily, max 32 mg/day. [Generic/Trade: Tabs 4, 8, 16, 32 mg.] ▶K ♀D ▶? $$$ ■

EPROSARTAN (*Teveten*) HTN: Start 600 mg PO daily, max 900 mg/day given daily or divided two times per day. [Generic/Trade: Tabs, unscored 600 mg.] ▶Fecal excretion ♀D ▶? $$$$ ■

IRBESARTAN (*Avapro*) HTN: Start 150 mg PO daily, max 300 mg/day. Type 2 diabetic nephropathy: Start 150 mg PO daily, target dose 300 mg daily. [Generic/Trade: Tabs, unscored 75, 150, 300 mg.] ▶L ♀D ▶? $ ■

LOSARTAN (*Cozaar*) HTN: Start 50 mg PO daily, max 100 mg/day given daily or divided two times per day. Volume-depleted patients or history of hepatic impairment: Start 25 mg PO daily. CVA risk reduction in patients with HTN and LV hypertrophy (may not be effective in black patients): Start 50 mg PO

(cont.)

daily. If need more BP reduction, add HCTZ 12.5 mg PO daily, then increase losartan to 100 mg/day, then increase HCTZ to 25 mg/day. Type 2 diabetic nephropathy: Start 50 mg PO daily, target dose 100 mg daily. [Generic/Trade: Tabs, unscored 25, 50, 100 mg.] ▶L ♀D ▶? $ ■

OLMESARTAN (*Benicar*, *✦Olmetec*) HTN: Start 20 mg PO daily, max 40 mg/day. [Trade only: Tabs, unscored 5, 20, 40 mg.] ▶K ♀D ▶? $$$$ ■

TELMISARTAN (*Micardis*) HTN: Start 40 mg PO daily, max 80 mg/day. Cardiovascular risk reduction: Start 80 mg PO daily, max 80 mg/day. [Generic/Trade: Tabs, unscored 20, 40, 80 mg.] ▶L ♀D ▶? $$$$ ■

VALSARTAN (*Diovan*) HTN: Start 80 to 160 mg PO daily, max 320 mg/day. Heart failure: Start 40 mg PO two times per day, target dose 160 mg two times per day. Reduce mortality/morbidity post-MI with LV systolic dysfunction/failure: Start 20 mg PO two times per day, target dose 160 mg two times per day. [Generic/Trade: Tabs, scored 40 mg, unscored 80, 160, 320 mg.] ▶L ♀D ▶? $$$$ ■

Antiadrenergic Agents

CLONIDINE — CARDIOVASCULAR (*Catapres, Catapres-TTS, ✦Dixarit*) HTN, immediate-release: Start 0.1 mg PO two times per day, usual maintenance dose 0.2 to 0.6 mg/day in 2 to 3 divided doses, max 2.4 mg daily. Rebound HTN with abrupt discontinuation, taper dose slowly. HTN, transdermal (Catapres-TTS): Start 0.1 mg/24 h patch once a week, titrate to desired effect, max effective dose 0.6 mg/24 h (two 0.3 mg/24 h patches). Transdermal Therapeutic System (TTS) is designed for 7-day use so that a TTS-1 delivers 0.1 mg/day for 7 days. May supplement 1st dose of TTS with oral for 2 to 3 days while therapeutic level is achieved. Menopausal flushing: 0.1 to 0.4 mg/day PO divided two to three times per day. Transdermal system applied weekly: 0.1 mg/day. May cause dizziness, drowsiness, or lightheadedness.

(cont.)

Monitor for bradycardia when taking concomitant digitalis, nondihydropyridine calcium channel blockers, or beta-blockers. [Generic/Trade: Tabs, immediate-release, unscored (Catapres) 0.1, 0.2, 0.3 mg. Transdermal weekly patch ($$$$$) 0.1 mg/day (TTS-1), 0.2 mg/day (TTS-2), 0.3 mg/day (TTS-3).] ▶LK ♀C ▶? $

DOXAZOSIN (*Cardura, Cardura XL*) BPH, immediate-release: Start 1 mg PO at bedtime, max 8 mg/day. BPH, extended-release (not approved for HTN): 4 mg PO q am with breakfast, max 8 mg/day. HTN, immediate-release: Start 1 mg PO at bedtime, max 16 mg/day. Take 1st dose at bedtime to minimize orthostatic hypotension. [Generic/Trade: Tabs, scored 1, 2, 4, 8 mg. Trade only (Cardura XL): Tabs, extended-release, 4, 8 mg.] ▶L ♀ 0/0/0; Data in pregnant women are limited and not sufficient to inform a drug-associated risk for major birth defects and miscarriage. ▶ No information available. $$ ■

GUANFACINE—CARDIOVASCULAR (*Tenex*) HTN: Start 1 mg PO at bedtime, may increase by 1 mg at bedtime every 3 to 4 weeks, max 3 mg/day. [Generic/Trade: Tabs, unscored 1, 2 mg.] ▶K ♀B ▶? $

METHYLDOPA HTN: Start 250 mg PO 2 to 3 times daily, max 3000 mg/day. May be used to manage BP during pregnancy. [Generic only: Tabs, unscored 250, 500 mg.] ▶LK ♀B ▶+ $

PRAZOSIN (*Minipress*) HTN: Start 1 mg PO two to three times per day, max 40 mg/day. Take 1st dose at bedtime to minimize orthostatic hypotension. [Generic/Trade: Caps 1, 2, 5 mg.] ▶L ♀C ▶? $$ ■

RESERPINE HTN: Start 0.05 to 0.1 mg PO daily or 0.1 mg PO every other day, max dose 0.25 mg/day. [Generic only: Tabs, scored 0.1, 0.25 mg.] ▶LK ♀C ▶- $$

TERAZOSIN HTN: Start 1 mg PO at bedtime, usual effective dose 1 to 5 mg PO daily or divided two times per day, max 20 mg/day. Take 1st dose at bedtime to minimize orthostatic hypotension. BPH: Start 1 mg PO at bedtime, usual effective dose 10 mg/day, max 20 mg/day. [Generic only: Caps 1, 2, 5, 10 mg.] ▶LK ♀C ▶? $$ ■

Antidysrhythmics/Cardiac Arrest

ADENOSINE (*Adenocard*) PSVT conversion (not A-fib): Adult and peds wt 50 kg or greater: 6 mg rapid IV and flush, preferably through a central line. If no response after 1 to 2 min, then 12 mg. A 3rd dose of 12 mg may be given prn. Peds wt less than 50 kg: Initial dose 50 to 100 mcg/kg, subsequent doses 100 to 200 mcg/kg q 1 to 2 min prn up to a max single dose of 300 mcg/kg or 12 mg, whichever is less. Half-life is less than 10 sec. Give doses by rapid IV push followed by NS flush. Need higher dose if on theophylline or caffeine, lower dose if on dipyridamole or carbamazepine ▶Plasma ♀C ▶? $

AMIODARONE (*Pacerone, Cordarone*) Proarrhythmic. Life-threatening ventricular arrhythmia without cardiac arrest: Load 150 mg IV over 10 min, then 1 mg/min for 6 h, then 0.5 mg/min for 18 h. Mix in D5W. Oral loading dose 800 to 1600 mg PO daily for 1 to 3 weeks, reduce to 400 to 800 mg PO daily for 1 month when arrhythmia is controlled, reduce to lowest effective dose thereafter, usually 200 to 400 mg PO daily. Photosensitivity with oral therapy. Pulmonary and hepatic toxicity. Hypo- or hyperthyroidism possible. Coadministration of fluoroquinolones, macrolides, loratadine, trazodone, azoles, or Class IA and III antiarrhythmic drugs may prolong QTc. Initiating ledipasvir/sofosbuvir or sofosbuvir with simeprevir may cause serious symptomatic bradycardia, some requiring pacemaker insertion; monitor heart rate in patients taking or recently discontinuing amiodarone when starting antiviral treatment. May increase digoxin levels; discontinue digoxin or decrease dose by 50%. May increase INR with warfarin; decrease warfarin dose by 33 to 50%. Do not use with grapefruit juice. Do not use with simvastatin dose greater than 20 mg/day, lovastatin dose greater than 40 mg/day; may increase atorvastatin level; increases risk of myopathy and rhabdomyolysis. Caution with beta-blockers and calcium channel blockers. IV therapy may cause hypotension. Contraindicated in cardiogenic shock and

CARDIOVASCULAR

(cont.)

in profound/symptomatic bradycardia (whether from AV block or sinus-node dysfunction) in the absence of a functioning pacemaker. [Trade only (Pacerone): Tabs, unscored 100 mg. Generic/Trade: Tabs, scored 200, 400 mg.] ▶L ♀X/X/X; Neonatal harm: Potential cardiac, growth, neurodevelopmental, neurological, thyroid effects. ▶ Do not breastfeed while taking amiodarone. $$$$ ■

ATROPINE (*AtroPen*) Bradyarrhythmia/CPR: 0.5 to 1 mg IV q 3 to 5 min to max 0.04 mg/kg (3 mg). Peds: 0.02 mg/kg/ dose, minimum single dose 0.1 mg, max cumulative dose 1 mg. Treatment of muscarinic symptoms of insecticide or nerve agent poisonings: Mild symptoms: 1 injection of 2 mg auto-injector pen, 2 additional injections after 10 min may be given in rapid succession if severe symptoms develop. Severe symptoms: 3 injections of 2 mg pen in rapid succession. Administer in mid-lateral thigh. Max 3 injections. [Trade only: Prefilled auto-injector pen: 0.25 mg (yellow), 0.5 mg (blue), 1 mg (dark red), 2 mg (green).] ▶K ♀C ▶– $

DIGOXIN (*Lanoxin, Digitek, ✦Toxolin*) Proarrhythmic. Systolic heart failure/rate control of chronic A-fib: Younger than 70 yo: 0.25 mg PO daily; age 70 yo or older: 0.125 mg PO daily; impaired renal function: 0.0625 to 0.125 mg PO daily. Rapid A-fib: Total loading dose (TLD), 10 to 15 mcg/kg IV/PO, give in 3 divided doses q 6 to 8 h; give ~50% TLD for 1 dose, then ~25% TLD for 2 doses (eg, 70 kg with normal renal function: 0.5 mg, then 0.25 mg q 6 to 8 h for 2 doses). Impaired renal function, 6 to 10 mcg/kg IV/PO TLD, given in 3 divided doses of 0.125 to 0.375 mg IV/PO daily. Consider patient-specific characteristics (lean/ ideal wt, CrCl, age, concomitant disease states, concomitant medications, and factors likely to alter pharmacokinetic/ dynamic profile of digoxin) when dosing; see prescribing information for alterations based on wt, renal function, or drug interactions. Assess electrolytes, renal function, levels periodically. Adjust dose based on response and therapeutic serum levels; the risk of adverse events increases when the

(cont.)

serum level is more than 1.2 ng/mL. Nausea, vomiting, visual disturbances, and cardiac arrhythmias may indicate toxicity. [Generic/Trade: Tabs, scored (Lanoxin, Digitek) 0.125, 0.25 mg. Generic only: Elixir 0.05 mg/mL.] ▶KL ♀C ▶+ $

DIGOXIN IMMUNE FAB (*Digibind, DigiFab*) Digoxin toxicity: Acute ingestion of known amount: 1 vial binds approximately 0.5 mg digoxin. Acute ingestion of unknown amount: 10 vials IV, may repeat once. Toxicity during chronic therapy: 6 vials usually adequate; one formula is: Number vials = (serum dig level in ng/mL) × (kg)/100. ▶K ♀C ▶? $$$$$

DISOPYRAMIDE (*Norpace, Norpace CR*) Proarrhythmic. Rarely indicated, consult cardiologist. Ventricular arrhythmia: 400 to 800 mg PO daily in divided doses (immediate-release is divided q 6 h: extended-release is divided q 12 h). [Generic/Trade: Caps, immediate-release 100, 150 mg. Trade only: Caps, extended-release 100, 150 mg.] ▶KL ♀C ▶+ $$$ ■

DOFETILIDE (*Tikosyn*) Proarrhythmic. Conversion of A-fib/flutter: Specialized dosing based on CrCl and QTc interval. [Generic/Trade: Caps, 0.125, 0.25, 0.5 mg.] ▶KL ♀C ▶– $$$$$ ■

DRONEDARONE (*Multaq*) Proarrhythmic. Reduce hospitalization risk for patients with A-fib who are in sinus rhythm and have a history of paroxysmal or persistent A-fib: 400 mg PO two times per day with morning and evening meals. Do not use with permanent atrial fibrillation, NYHA Class IV heart failure or NYHA Class II to III heart failure with recent decompensation requiring hospitalization or referral to heart failure clinic, 2nd or 3rd degree AV block or sick sinus syndrome without functioning pacemaker, bradycardia less than 50 bpm, QTc Bazett interval greater than 500 msec, liver or lung toxicity related to previous amiodarone use, severe hepatic impairment, pregnancy, lactation, grapefruit juice, drugs or herbals that increase QT interval, Class I or III antiarrhythmic agents, potent inhibitors of CYP3A4 enzyme system (clarithromycin, itraconazole, ketoconazole, nefazodone, ritonavir, voriconazole), or inducers of CYP3A4 enzyme system (carbamazepine, phenytoin,

(cont.)

CARDIOVASCULAR

phenobarbital, rifampin, St. John's wort). Correct hypo/hyperkalemia and hypomagnesemia before giving. Monitor ECG q 3 months; if in A-fib, then either discontinue dronedarone or cardiovert. May initiate or worsen heart failure symptoms. May be associated with hepatic injury; discontinue if hepatic injury is suspected. Serum creatinine may increase during 1st weeks, but does not reflect change in renal function; reversible when discontinued. Monitor renal function periodically. Give with appropriate antithrombotic therapy. May increase INR when used with warfarin. May increase dabigatran level. May increase digoxin level; discontinue digoxin or decrease dose by 50%. Use cautiously with beta-blockers (BB) and calcium channel blockers (CCB); initiate lower doses of BB or CCB; initiate at low dose and monitor ECG. Do not use with more than 10 mg of simvastatin. May increase level of sirolimus, tacrolimus, or CYP3A4 substrates with narrow therapeutic index. [Trade only: Tabs, unscored 400 mg.] ▶L ♀X ▶– $$$$$ ■

FLECAINIDE Proarrhythmic. Prevention of paroxysmal atrial fib/flutter or PSVT, with symptoms and no structural heart disease: Start 50 mg PO q 12 h, may increase by 50 mg two times per day q 4 days, max 300 mg/day. Use with AV nodal slowing agent (beta-blocker, verapamil, diltiazem) to minimize risk of 1:1 atrial flutter. Life-threatening ventricular arrhythmias without structural heart disease: Start 100 mg PO q 12 h, may increase by 50 mg two times per day q 4 days, max 400 mg/day. With CrCl <35 mL/min: Start 50 mg PO two times per day. [Generic: Tabs, unscored 50 mg, scored 100, 150 mg.] ▶K ♀C ▶– $$$$ ■

IBUTILIDE (*Corvert*) Proarrhythmic. Recent onset A-fib/flutter: 0.01 mg/kg up to 1 mg IV over 10 min, may repeat once if no response after 10 min. Keep on cardiac monitor at least 4 h. ▶K ♀C ▶? $$$$$ ■

ISOPROTERENOL (*Isuprel*) Refractory bradycardia or 3rd degree AV block: bolus method: 0.02 to 0.06 mg IV: infusion method, dilute 2 mg in 250 mL D5W (8 mcg/mL); a rate of 37.5 mL/h

(cont.)

delivers 5 mcg/min. Peds infusion method: 0.05 to 2 mcg/kg/min. Using the same concentration as adult for a 10 kg child, a rate of 8 mL/h delivers 0.1 mcg/kg/min. ▶LK ♀C ▶? $$$$$

LIDOCAINE (*Xylocaine, Xylocard*) Ventricular arrhythmia: Load 1 mg/kg IV, then 0.5 mg/kg q 8 to 10 min prn to max 3 mg/kg. IV infusion: 4 g in 500 mL D5W (8 mg/mL) run at rate of 7.5 to 30 mL/h to deliver 1 to 4 mg/min. Peds: 20 to 50 mcg/kg/min. ▶LK ♀B ▶? $

MEXILETINE (*Mexitil*) Proarrhythmic. Rarely indicated, consult cardiologist. Ventricular arrhythmia: Start 200 mg PO q 8 h with food or antacid, max dose 1200 mg/day. [Generic only: Caps 150, 200, 250 mg.] ▶L ♀C ▶– $$$$ ■

PROCAINAMIDE Proarrhythmic. Ventricular arrhythmia: Loading dose: 100 mg IV q 10 min or 20 mg/min (150 mL/h) until QRS widens more than 50%, dysrhythmia suppressed, hypotension, or total of 17 mg/kg or 1000 mg delivered. Infusion: dilute 2 g in 250 mL D5W (8 mg/mL) rate of 15 to 45 mL/h to deliver 2 to 6 mg/min. ▶LK ♀C ▶? $$ ■

PROPAFENONE (*Rythmol, Rythmol SR*) Proarrhythmic. Prevention of paroxysmal A-fib/flutter or PSVT, with symptoms and no structural heart disease; or life-threatening ventricular arrhythmias: Start (immediate-release) 150 mg PO q 8 h, may increase after 3 to 4 days to 225 mg PO q 8 h, max 900 mg/day. Prolong time to recurrence of symptomatic A-fib without structural heart disease: 225 mg SR PO q 12 h, may increase after 5 days to 325 mg SR PO q 12 h, max 425 mg SR PO q 12 h. Consider using with AV nodal blocking agent (beta-blocker, verapamil, diltiazem) to minimize risk of 1:1 atrial flutter. Do not use with amiodarone, quinidine, or the combination of CYP3A4 and CYP2D6 inhibitors (or CYP2D6 deficiency). May increase digoxin, warfarin, beta-blocker levels. CYP1A2, 2D6, or 3A4 inhibitors; cimetidine; fluoxetine may increase level. Rifampin reduces level. Orlistat reduces level; taper orlistat withdrawal in patients stabilized on propafenone. Concomitant lidocaine increases risk of CNS side effects.

(cont.)

[Generic/Trade: Tabs, immediate-release scored 150, 225 mg. Caps, sustained-release, (SR-$$$$$) 225, 325, 425 mg. Generic only: Tabs, immediate-release, scored 300 mg.] ▶L ♀C ▶? $$ ■

QUINIDINE Proarrhythmic. Arrhythmia: Gluconate, extended-release: 324 to 648 mg PO q 8 to 12 h; sulfate, immediate-release: 200 to 400 mg PO q 6 to 8 h; sulfate, extended-release: 300 to 600 mg PO q 8 to 12 h. [Generic only: Gluconate, Tabs ($$$$), extended-release, unscored 324 mg. Sulfate, Tabs ($), scored immediate-release 200, 300 mg, Tabs, extended-release, ($$$$) 300 mg.] ▶LK ♀C ▶+ $ ■

SODIUM BICARBONATE Severe acidosis: 1 mEq/kg IV up to 50 to 100 mEq/dose. ▶K ♀C ▶? $

SOTALOL (*Betapace, Betapace AF, Sotylize, ✦Rylosol*) Proarrhythmic. Ventricular arrhythmia (Sotylize, Betapace): Start 80 mg PO two times per day, Sotylize max 320 mg/day, Betapace max 640 mg/day. A-fib/A-flutter (Sotylize, Betapace AF): Start 80 mg PO two times per day, Sotylize max 160 mg/day, Betapace AF max 640 mg/day. Initiate or re-initiate this product in a facility with cardiac resuscitation capacity, continuous EKG and CrCl monitoring. Do not substitute Betapace for Betapace AF. Adjust dose if CrCl <60 mL/min. [Generic/Trade: Tabs, scored 80, 120, 160, 240 mg. Tabs, scored (Betapace AF) 80, 120, 160 mg. Trade only: 5 mg/mL (Sotylize).] ▶K ♀B ▶– $$$$ ■

Antihyperlipidemic Agents—Bile Acid Sequestrants

CHOLESTYRAMINE (*Questran, Questran Light, Prevalite, ✦Olestyr*) Elevated LDL-C: Powder: Start 4 g PO daily to two times per day before meals, increase up to max 24 g/day. [Generic/Trade: Powder for oral susp, 4 g cholestyramine resin/9 g powder (Questran), 4 g cholestyramine resin/5 g powder (Questran Light), 4 g cholestyramine resin/5.5 g powder (Prevalite). Each available in bulk powder and single-dose packets.] ▶Not absorbed ♀C ▶+ $$$$

COLESEVELAM (*Welchol, ★Lodalis*) LDL-C reduction or glycemic control of type 2 diabetes: 3.75 g once daily or 1.875 g PO two times per day, max 3.75 g/day. Give with meal and 4 to 8 ounces of water, fruit juice, or diet soft drink. 3.75 g is equivalent to 6 tabs; 1.875 g is equivalent to 3 tabs. Powder packets contain phenylalanine. [Trade only: Tabs, unscored 625 mg. Powder single-dose packets 3.75 g.] ▶Not absorbed ♀B ▶+ $$$$$

COLESTIPOL (*Colestid, Colestid Flavored*)   Elevated LDL-C: Tabs: Start 2 g PO daily to two times per day with full glass of liquid, max 16 g/day. Granules: Start 5 g PO daily to two times per day, max 30 g/day. Mix granules in at least 90 mL of non-carbonated liquid. Administer other drugs at least 1 h before or 4 to 6 h after colestipol. [Generic/Trade: Tabs 1 g. Granules for oral susp, 5 g/7.5 g powder. Available in bulk powder and individual packets.] ▶Not absorbed ♀B ▶+ $$$

Antihyperlipidemic Agents—Fibrates

NOTE: *Contraindicated with active liver disease, gall bladder disease, and/or severe renal impairment (see prescribing information and guidelines for product specific information). Evaluate renal function (SrCr and estimated glomerular filtration rate [eGFR] based on creatinine) at baseline, within 3 months after initiation, q 6 months thereafter. Monitor LFTs (baseline, periodically). Use in combination with statin therapy is generally discouraged and not proven to reduce risk of CV events beyond stain monotherapy. Increased risk of myopathy and rhabdomyolysis when used with a statin or colchicine. May cause paradoxical decrease in HDL. May increase cholesterol excretion into bile, leading to cholelithiasis. May increase the effect of warfarin; monitor INR. Take either at least 2 h before or 4 h after bile acid sequestrants.*

BEZAFIBRATE (*★Bezalip SR*)   Canada only. Hyperlipidemia/hypertriglyceridemia: 400 mg of sustained-release PO daily. [Canada Trade only: Sustained-release tabs 400 mg.] ▶K ♀D ▶- $$$

FENOFIBRATE (*TriCor, Antara, Fenoglide, Lipofen, Triglide, ✦Lipidil Micro, Lipidil Supra, Lipidil EZ*) Hypertriglyceridemia: TriCor tabs: 48 to 145 mg PO daily, max 145 mg daily. Antara: 30 to 90 mg PO daily; max 130 mg daily. Fenoglide: 40 to 120 mg PO daily; max 120 mg daily. Lipofen: 50 to 150 mg PO daily, max 150 mg daily. Triglide: 50 to 160 mg PO daily, max 160 mg daily. Generic tabs: 54 to 160 mg, max 160 mg daily. Generic caps: 67 to 200 mg PO daily; max 200 mg daily. Hypercholesterolemia/mixed dyslipidemia: TriCor tabs: 145 mg PO daily. Antara: 130 mg PO daily. Fenoglide: 120 mg daily. Lipofen: 150 mg daily. Triglide: 160 mg daily. Generic tabs: 160 mg daily. Generic caps 200 mg PO daily. Reduce dose for mild to moderate renal insufficiency. All formulations, except Antara, TriCor, and Triglide, should be taken with food. May consider concomitant therapy with a low- or moderate-intensity statin if the benefits from triglyceride lowering (when 500 mg/dL or more) outweigh the risk of adverse effects. May increase serum creatinine level without changing eGFR.   [Generic only: Tabs, unscored 54, 160 mg. Generic caps 67, 134, 200 mg. Generic/ Trade: Tabs (TriCor), unscored 48, 145 mg. Caps (Antara) 30, 90 mg. Tabs (Fenoglide), unscored 40, 120 mg. Trade only: Tabs (Lipofen), unscored 50, 150 mg. Tabs (Triglide), unscored 50, 160 mg.] ▶LK ♀C ▶– $$$

FENOFIBRIC ACID (*Fibricor, Trilipix*) Hypertriglyceridemia: Fibricor: 35 to 105 mg PO daily, max 105 mg daily. Trilipix: 45 to 135 mg PO daily, max 135 mg daily. Hypercholesterolemia/ mixed dyslipidemia: Fibricor: 105 mg PO daily. Trilipix: 135 mg PO daily. Renal impairment: Fibricor: 35 mg PO daily. TriLipix 45 mg PO daily. May increase serum creatinine level without changing eGFR. [Generic/Trade: Caps (Trilipix), delayed-release 45, 135 mg. Trade only: Tabs (Fibricor) 35, 105 mg. Generic only: Tabs 35, 105 mg.] ▶LK ♀C ▶– $$$

GEMFIBROZIL (*Lopid*) Hypertriglyceridemia/primary prevention of CAD: 600 mg PO two times per day 30 min before meals. Do not use with statin; increases risk of myopathy and rhabdomyolysis. [Generic/Trade: Tabs, scored 600 mg.] ▶LK ♀C ▶? $

Antihyperlipidemic Agents—HMG-CoA Reductase Inhibitors ("Statins") and combinations

NOTE: *Each statin has restricted maximum doses that are lower than typical maximum doses when used with certain interacting medications; see prescribing information for complete information. Consider patient characteristics that may modify the decision to use higher-intensity statin therapy, including history of hemorrhagic stroke or Asian descent. Muscle issues: Evaluate muscle symptoms before initiating statin therapy and at each follow-up visit. Measure creatinine kinase before starting statin, if patient at risk for adverse muscle events. Risk of muscle issues increases with advanced age (65 yo or older), female gender, uncontrolled hypothyroidism, low vitamin D level, renal impairment, higher statin doses, history of muscle disorders, and concomitant use of certain medicines (eg, fibrates, niacin 1 gram or more, colchicine, or ranolazine). Teach patients to report promptly unexplained muscle pain, tenderness, or weakness; rule out common causes; discontinue if myopathy diagnosed or suspected. Obtain creatine kinase, TSH, vitamin D level when patient complains of muscle soreness, tenderness, weakness, or pain. Hepatotoxicity: Rare. Monitor ALT before initiating statin therapy and as clinically indicated thereafter. Discontinue statin with persistent ALT elevations more than 3 times the upper limit of normal or objective evidence of liver injury. Diabetes: Measure A1c before starting statin, if diabetes status unknown. Statins may increase the risk of hyperglycemia and type 2 diabetes in patients with risk factors for diabetes; benefit usually outweighs risk. Cognition: The 2013 ACC/AHA cholesterol guidelines expert panel did not find evidence that statins adversely affect cognition. If patient complains of confusion or memory impairment while on statin therapy, consider all possible causes, including other drugs (eg, sleep aids, analgesics, OTC antihistamines) and medical conditions (eg, depression, anxiety, sleep apnea) that affect memory.*

ATORVASTATIN (*Lipitor*)   Hyperlipidemia/prevention of cardiovascular events: Start 10 to 40 mg PO daily, max 80 mg/day. Do not give with cyclosporine or tipranavir + ritonavir. Use with caution and lowest dose necessary with lopinavir + ritonavir. Do not exceed 20 mg/day when given with clarithromycin, itraconazole, other protease inhibitors (saquinavir + ritonavir, darunavir + ritonavir, fosamprenavir, or fosamprenavir + ritonavir). Do not exceed 40 mg/day when given with boceprevir or nelfinavir.   [Generic/Trade: Tabs, unscored 10, 20, 40, 80 mg.] ▶L ♀X ▶– $

CADUET (amlodipine + atorvastatin)   Simultaneous treatment of HTN and hypercholesterolemia: Establish dose using component drugs first. See component drugs for other dose restrictions. Dosing interval: Daily.   [Generic/Trade: Tabs, 2.5/10, 2.5/20, 2.5/40, 5/10, 5/20, 5/40, 5/80, 10/10, 10/20, 10/40, 10/80 mg.] ▶L ♀X ▶– $$$$$

FLUVASTATIN (*Lescol, Lescol XL*)   Hyperlipidemia: Start 20 to 80 mg PO at bedtime, max 80 mg daily (XL) or divided two times per day. Post-percutaneous coronary intervention: 80 mg of extended-release PO daily, max 80 mg daily. Do not exceed 20 mg/day when given with cyclosporine or fluconazole. [Generic/Trade: Caps 20, 40 mg. Trade only: Tabs, extended-release, unscored 80 mg.] ▶L ♀X ▶– $$$$

LIPTRUZET (ezetimibe + atorvastatin)   Hyperlipidemia: Start 10/10 or 10/20 mg PO daily, max 10/80 mg/day. See component drug for other dose restrictions.   [Trade only: Tabs, unscored ezetimibe/atorvastatin 10/10, 10/20, 10/40, 10/80 mg.] ▶L – ♀X ▶– $$$$

LOVASTATIN (*Altoprev*)   Hyperlipidemia/prevention of cardiovascular events: Start 20 mg PO q pm, max 80 mg/day daily or divided two times per day. Do not use with clarithromycin, cobicistat-containing products, cyclosporine, erythromycin, gemfibrozil, grapefruit juice, HIV protease inhibitors, itraconazole, ketoconazole, nefazodone, posaconazole, telithromycin or voriconazole; increases risk of

(cont.)

myopathy. Do not exceed 20 mg/day when used with danazol, diltiazem, dronedarone, verapamil, or CrCl <30 mL/min. Do not exceed 40 mg/day when used with amiodarone. [Generic: Tabs, unscored 10, 20, 40 mg. Trade only: Tabs, extended-release (Altoprev) 20, 40, 60 mg.] ▶L ♀X ▶– $$$

PITAVASTATIN (*Livalo*) Hyperlipidemia: Start 2 mg PO at bedtime, max 4 mg daily. CrCl 15 to 59 mL/min or on dialysis: Max start 1 mg PO daily, max 2 mg daily. Do not use with ciclosporine. Do not exceed 1 mg/day when given with erythromycin. Do not exceed 2 mg/day when given with rifampin. [Trade only: Tabs 1, 2, 4 mg.] ▶L – ♀X ▶– $$$$$

PRAVASTATIN (*Pravachol*) Hyperlipidemia/prevention of cardiovascular events: Start 40 mg PO daily, max 80 mg/day. Do not exceed 20 mg/day when given with cyclosporine. Do not exceed 40 mg/day when given with clarithromycin. [Generic/Trade: Tabs, unscored 20, 40, 80 mg. Generic: Tabs, unscored 10 mg.] ▶L ♀X/X/X; Contraindicated during pregnancy. ▶ Do not breastfeed while taking this medication. $$$

ROSUVASTATIN (*Crestor*) Hyperlipidemia/slow progression of atherosclerosis/primary prevention of cardiovascular disease: Start 10 to 20 mg PO daily, max 40 mg/day. Renal impairment (CrCl <30 mL/min and not on hemodialysis): Start 5 mg PO daily, max 10 mg/day. Asians: Start 5 mg PO daily. When given with atazanavir with or without ritonavir, lopinavir with ritonavir, or simeprevir, do not exceed 10 mg/day. When given with cyclosporine, do not exceed 5 mg/day. Avoid using with gemfibrozil; if used concomitantly, do not exceed 10 mg/day. When given with colchicine, do not exceed 5 mg/day. [Generic/Trade only: Tabs, unscored 5, 10, 20, 40 mg.] ▶L ♀X ▶– $$$$$

SIMVASTATIN (*Zocor*) Do not initiate therapy with or titrate to 80 mg/day; only use 80 mg/day in patients who have taken this dose for more than 12 months without evidence of muscle toxicity. Hyperlipidemia: Start 10 to 20 mg PO q pm, max 40 mg/day. Reduce cardiovascular mortality/events in high risk for coronary heart disease event: Start 40 mg PO q pm, max

(cont.)

40 mg/day. Severe renal impairment: Start 5 mg/day, closely monitor. Chinese patients: Do not exceed 20 mg/day with niacin 1 g or more daily. Do not use with clarithromycin, cobicistat-containing products, cyclosporine, danazol, erythromycin, gemfibrozil, grapefruit juice, HIV protease inhibitors, itraconazole, ketoconazole, nefazodone, posaconazole, strong CYP3A4 inhibitors, telithromycin, voriconazole; increases risk of myopathy. Do not exceed 10 mg/day when used with diltiazem, dronedarone, or verapamil. Do not exceed 20 mg/day when used with amiodarone, amlodipine or ranolazine. Do not exceed 20 mg/day when used with lomitapide; if patient has been on simvastatin 80 mg/day for at least 1 year without muscle toxicity, do not exceed 40 mg/day when used with lomitapide. [Generic/Trade: Tabs, unscored 5, 10, 20, 40, 80 mg.] ▶L ♀X ▶— $

VYTORIN (ezetimibe + simvastatin) Hyperlipidemia: Start 10/10 or 10/20 mg PO q pm, max 10/40 mg/day. Restrict the use of the 10/80 mg dose to patients who have taken it at least 12 months without muscle toxicity. See simvastatin monograph for other dose restrictions. [Trade only: Tabs, unscored ezetimibe/simvastatin 10/10, 10/20, 10/40, 10/80 mg.] ▶L ♀X ▶— $$$$

Antihyperlipidemic Agents—Omega Fatty Acids

NOTE: *FDA-approved fish oil. Swallow whole. May prolong bleeding time, may potentiate warfarin. Monitor AST/ALT if hepatic impairment. Use caution in patients with known hypersensitivity to fish and/or shellfish.*

ICOSAPENT ETHYL (*Vascepa*) Hypertriglyceridemia (500 mg/dL or above): 2 caps PO twice daily. Contains EPA. [Trade only: Caps 1 g.] ▶L ♀C ▶? $$$$$

OMEGA-3-ACID ETHYL ESTERS (*Omtryg, Lovaza*) Hypertriglyceridemia (500 mg/dL or above): 4 caps PO daily or divided two times per day. Contains EPA + DHA. [Generic/Trade (Lovaza): Caps 1 g. Trade only (Omtryg): Caps 1.2 g.] ▶L ♀C ▶? $$$$$

OMEGA-3-CARBOXYLIC ACIDS (*Epanova*) Hypertriglyceridemia (500 mg/dL or above): 2 to 4 capsules PO daily. Contains EPA + DHA. [Trade only: Caps 1 g.] ▶L ♀C ▶? $$$$$

Antihyperlipidemic Agents—Other

ALIROCUMAB (*Praluent*) Reduce LDL-C as adjunct to diet and maximally tolerated statin with heterozygous familial hypercholesterolemia or clinical atherosclerotic cardiovascular disease: Start 75 mg SC q 2 weeks; max 150 mg q 2 weeks. Human monoclonal antibody. Give in abdomen, upper arm, or thigh. Store in a refrigerator at 36-46° F; can be out of refrigeration for no more than 24 hours. The prefilled syringe or pen should warm to room temperature for 30-40 minutes before use. Tell patient that it may take up to 20 seconds to inject full dose. ▶N/A ♀?/?/?; Consider possible risks to fetus before prescribing to pregnant women. ▶ No information available. $$$$$

EVOLOCUMAB (*Repatha*) Reduce LDL-C as adjunct to diet and maximally tolerated statin with heterozygous familial hypercholesterolemia or clinical atherosclerotic cardiovascular disease: 140 mg SC every 2 weeks or 420 mg SQ once monthly. Reduce LDL-C as adjunct to diet and other lipid lowering therapies with homozygous familial hypercholesterolemia: 420 mg SQ once monthly. Human monoclonal antibody. Give in abdomen, upper arm, or thigh. Ideally store in a refrigerator at 36-46° F;can be kept at room temperature (77° F) for up to 30 days. Tell patient that it may take up to 15 seconds to inject full dose. [Trade only: Single prefilled syringe 140 mg/mL. Multi Dose (x2 Sureclick) prefilled syringe 140 mg/mL. Monthly injection (Pushtronex with on body infusion device) 420 mg/3.5 mL.] ▶N/A ♀?/?/?; Consider possible risks to fetus before prescribing to pregnant women. ▶ No information available. $$$$$ ∎

EZETIMIBE (*Zetia*, ✦*Ezetrol*) Hyperlipidemia: 10 mg PO daily. [Trade only: Tabs, unscored 10 mg.] ▶L ♀C ▶? $$$$

Antihypertensive Combinations

NOTE: *In general, establish dose using component drugs first. See component drugs for metabolism, pregnancy, and lactation.*

ANTIHYPERTENSIVE COMBINATIONS

BY TYPE:	
ACEI + Diuretic	*Accuretic, Capozide, ✽Inhibace Plus, Lotensin HCT, Monopril HCT, Prinzide, Uniretic, Vaseretic, Zestoretic*
ACEI + CCB	*Lotrel, Prestalia, Tarka*
ARB + Beta-blocker	*Byvalson*
ARB + CCB	*Azor, Exforge, Twynsta*
ARB + Diuretic	*Atacand HCT, ✽Atacand Plus, Avalide, Benicar HCT, Diovan HCT, Edarbyclor, Hyzaar, Micardis HCT, ✽Micardis Plus, Teveten HCT*
ARB + CCB + Diuretic	*Exforge HCT, Tribenzor*
Beta-blocker + Diuretic	*Corzide, Dutoprol, Inderide, Lopressor HCT, Tenoretic, Ziac*
CCB + Statin	*Caduet*
Direct renin inhibitor + Diuretic	*✽Rasilez HCT, Tekturna HCT*
Diuretic combinations	*Aldactazide, Dyazide, Maxzide, ✽Moduret, Moduretic, ✽Triazide*

(cont.)

ANTIHYPERTENSIVE COMBINATIONS (*continued*)

BY TYPE:	
Diuretic + miscellaneous antihypertensive	*Aldoril, Clorpres, Minizide*

ACEI = ACE Inhibitor. ARB = angiotensin receptor blocker.
CCB = calcium channel blocker.

BY NAME: *Accuretic* (quinapril + HCTZ): Generic/Trade: Tabs, scored 10/12.5, 20/12.5, unscored 20/25 mg. *Aldactazide* (spironolactone + HCTZ): Generic/Trade: Tabs, unscored 25/25, scored 50/50 mg. *Aldoril* (methyldopa + HCTZ): Generic: Tabs, unscored 250/15, 250/ 25 mg. *Atacand* HCT (candesartan + HCTZ, ✸ *Atacand Plus*): Generic/Trade: Tab, unscored 16/12.5, 32/12.5, 32/25 mg. *Avalide* (irbesartan + HCTZ): Generic/Trade: Tabs, unscored 150/12.5, 300/ 12.5 mg. *Azor* (amlodipine + olmesartan): Trade only: Tabs, unscored 5/20, 5/40, 10/20, 10/40 mg. *Benicar HCT* (olmesartan + HCTZ): Trade only: Tabs, unscored 20/12.5, 40/12.5, 40/25 mg. *Byvalson (valsartan + nebivolol)*: Trade only: Tabs, unscored 80/5 mg. *Caduet* (amlodipine + atorvastatin): Generic/Trade: 2.5/10, 2.5/20, 2.5/40, 5/10, 5/20, 5/40, 5/80, 10/10, 10/20, 10/40, 10/80 mg. *Capozide* (captopril + HCTZ): Generic only: Tabs, scored 25/15, 25/25, 50/15, 50/25 mg. *Clorpres* (clonidine—cardiovascular + chlorthalidone): Trade only: Tabs, scored 0.1/15, 0.2/15, 0.3/15 mg. *Corzide* (nadolol + bendroflumethiazide): Generic/Trade: Tabs 40/5, 80/5 mg. *Diovan* HCT (valsartan + HCTZ): Generic/Trade: Tabs, unscored 80/12.5, 160/12.5, 160/25, 320/12.5, 320/25 mg. *Dutoprol* (metoprolol succinate + HCTZ): Trade only: Tabs, unscored 25/12.5, 50/12.5, 100/12.5 mg. *Dyazide* (triamterene + HCTZ): Generic/Trade: Caps, (Dyazide)

(cont.)

ANTIHYPERTENSIVE COMBINATIONS (*continued*)

37.5/25, (generic only) 50/25 mg. *Edarbyclor* (azilsartan + chlorthalidone): Trade only: Tabs, unscored 40/12.5, 40/25 mg. *Exforge* (amlodipine + valsartan): Generic/Trade only: Tabs, unscored 5/160, 5/320, 10/160, 10/320 mg. *Exforge HCT* (amlodipine + valsartan + HCTZ): Generic/Trade only: Tabs, unscored 5/160/12.5, 5/160/25, 10/160/12.5, 10/160/25, 10/320/25 mg. *Hyzaar* (losartan + HCTZ): Generic/Trade: Tabs, unscored 50/12.5, 100/12.5, 100/25 mg. *Inderide* (propranolol + HCTZ): Generic only: Tabs, scored 40/25, 80/25 mg. ✳*Inhibace Plus* (cilazapril + HCTZ): Trade only: Tabs, scored 5/12.5 mg. *Lopressor HCT* (metoprolol tartrate + HCTZ): Generic/Trade: Tabs, scored 50/25, 100/25 mg. Generic: Tabs, scored 100/50 mg. *Lotensin HCT* (benazepril + HCTZ): Generic/ Trade: Tabs, scored 5/6.25, 10/12.5, 20/12.5, 20/25 mg. *Lotrel* (amlodipine + benazepril): Generic/Trade: Cap, 2.5/10, 5/10, 5/20, 10/20 mg, 5/40, 10/40 mg. *Maxzide* (triamterene + HCTZ, ✳*Triazide*): Generic/Trade: Tabs, scored (Maxzide-25) 37.5/25, (Maxzide) 75/50 mg. *Micardis HCT* (telmisartan + HCTZ, ✳*Micardis Plus*): Generic/Trade: Tabs, unscored 40/12.5, 80/12.5, 80/25 mg. *Minizide* (prazosin + polythiazide): Trade only: Caps, 1/0.5, 2/0.5, 5/0.5 mg. *Moduretic* (amiloride + HCTZ, ✳*Moduret*): Generic only: Tabs, scored 5/50 mg. *Monopril HCT* (fosinopril + HCTZ): Generic only: Tabs, unscored 10/12.5, scored 20/12.5 mg. *Prestalia* (perindopril + amlodipine): Trade: Tabs, unscored 3.5/2.5, 7.5/5 14/10 mg. *Prinzide* (lisinopril + HCTZ): Generic/Trade: Tabs, unscored 10/12.5, 20/12.5, 20/25 mg. *Tarka* (trandolapril + verapamil): Trade only: Tabs, unscored 2/180, 1/240, 2/240, 4/240 mg. *Tekturna HCT* (aliskiren + HCTZ, ✳*Rasilez HCT*): Trade only: Tabs, unscored 150/12.5, 150/25, 300/12.5, 300/25 mg.

(cont.)

ANTIHYPERTENSIVE COMBINATIONS (*continued*)

Tenoretic (atenolol + chlorthalidone): Generic/Trade: Tabs, scored 50/25, unscored 100/25 mg. *Teveten HCT* (eprosartan + HCTZ): Trade only: Tabs, unscored 600/12.5, 600/25 mg. *Tribenzor* (amlodipine + olmesartan + HCTZ): Trade only: Tabs, unscored 5/20/12.5, 5/40/12.5, 5/40/25 10/40/12.5, 10/40/25 mg. *Twynsta* (amlodipine + telmisartan): Generic/Trade: Tabs,unscored 5/40, 5/80, 10/40, 10/80 mg. *Uniretic* (moexipril + HCTZ): Generic/ Trade: Tabs, scored15/12.5, 15/25 mg. Generic: Tabs, scored 7.5/12.5. *Vaseretic* (enalapril + HCTZ): Generic/Trade:Tabs, unscored 5/12.5, 10/25 mg. *Zestoretic* (lisinopril HCTZ): Generic/Trade: Tabs, unscored10/12.5, 20/12.5, 20/25 mg. *Ziac* (bisoprolol + HCTZ): Generic/Trade: Tabs, unscored 2.5/6.25, 5/6.25, 10/6.25 mg.

Antihypertensives—Other

ALISKIREN (*Tekturna*, ✦*Rasilez*) HTN: 150 mg PO daily, max 300 mg/day. Contraindicated in pregnancy; or with ACE inhibitors or angiotensin receptor blocks in patients with DM. Avoid use with ACE inhibitors or angiotensin receptor blockers, particularly in patients with <60 mL/min; increases risk of renal impairment, hypotension, and hyperkalemia. Do not use with cyclosporine or itraconazole. Concomitant NSAID, including celecoxib, may further deteriorate renal function and decrease antihypertensive effects. Hyperkalemia possible, especially if used concomitantly with other drugs that increase K+ (including K+-containing salt substitutes) and in patients with heart failure, DM, or renal impairment. Monitor potassium and renal function periodically. [Trade only: Tabs, unscored 150, 300 mg.] ▶LK ♀D ▶–? $$$$ ■

FENOLDOPAM (*Corlopam*) Severe HTN: 10 mg in 250 mL D5W (40 mcg/mL), start at 0.1 mcg/kg/min titrate q 15 min, usual effective dose 0.1 to 1.6 mcg/kg/min. ▶LK ♀B ▶? $$$$

HYDRALAZINE (*Apresoline*) Hypertensive emergency: 10 to 20 mg IV or 10 to 50 mg IM, repeat prn. HTN: Start 10 mg PO two to four times per day, max 300 mg/day. Headaches, peripheral edema, systemic lupus erythematosus–like syndrome. [Generic only: Tabs, unscored 10, 25, 50, 100 mg.] ▶LK ♀C ▶+ $$$

NITROPRUSSIDE (*Nitropress*) Hypertensive emergency: Dilute 50 mg in 250 mL D5W (200 mcg/mL), rate of 6 mL/h for 70 kg adult delivers starting dose of 0.3 mcg/kg/min. Max 10 mcg/kg/min. Protect from light. Cyanide toxicity with high doses (10 mcg/kg/min), hepatic/renal impairment, and prolonged infusions (longer than 3 to 7 days); check thiocyanate levels. ▶RBCs ♀C ▶– $$$$$ ∎

PHENTOLAMINE (*Regitine*, *✦Rogitine*) Extravasation: 5 to 10 mg in 10 mL NS, inject 1 to 5 mL SC (in divided doses) around extravasation site. ▶Plasma ♀C ▶? $$$$

Antiplatelet Drugs

ABCIXIMAB (*ReoPro*) Platelet aggregation inhibition, percutaneous coronary intervention: 0.25 mg/kg IV bolus via separate infusion line before procedure, then 0.125 mcg/kg/min (max 10 mcg/min) IV infusion for 12 h. ▶Plasma ♀C ▶? $$$$$

AGGRENOX (**acetylsalicylic acid + dipyridamole**) Prevention of CVA after TIA/CVA: 1 cap PO two times per day. Headache is a common adverse effect. [Generic/Trade: Caps 25 mg aspirin/200 mg extended-release dipyridamole.] ▶LK ♀D ▶? $$$$$

CANGRELOR (*Kengreal*) Adjunct to percutaneous coronary intervention (PCI) to reduce thrombotic events, including periprocedural MI, repeat coronary revascularization, and stent thrombosis, in patients who have not been treated with P2Y12 platelet inhibitor and glycoprotein IIb/IIIa inhibitor: Load 30 mcg/kg IV prior to PCI, then IV infusion 4 mcg/kg/min for at least 2 hours or duration of procedure, whichever

(cont.)

is longer. Use dedicated IV line. Maintain platelet inhibition with oral P2Y12 inhibitor: Give clopidogrel or prasugrel loading dose immediately after discontinuing cangrelor infusion, or give ticagrelor loading dose during cangrelor infusion or immediately after discontinuing infusion.   ▶degraded chemically ♀C ▶? $$$$$

CLOPIDOGREL (*Plavix*)   Reduction of thrombotic events, recent acute MI/CVA, established peripheral arterial disease: 75 mg PO daily. Non-ST segment elevation acute coronary syndrome: 300 to 600 mg loading dose, then 75 mg PO daily in combination with aspirin. ST segment elevation MI: Start with/without 300 mg loading dose, then 75 mg PO daily in combination with aspirin, with/without thrombolytic. Allergic cross-reactivity may occur among thienopyridines (clopidogrel, prasugrel, ticlopidine). Avoid drugs that are strong or moderate CYP2C19 inhibitors (eg, omeprazole, esomeprazole, cimetidine, etravirine, felbamate, fluconazole, fluoxetine, fluvoxamine, ketoconazole, voriconazole). Concomitant aspirin, SSRI, or SNRI increases bleeding risk.   [Generic/Trade: Tabs, unscored 75, 300 mg.] ▶LK ♀B ▶? $ ■

DIPYRIDAMOLE (*Persantine*)   Antithrombotic: 75 to 100 mg PO four times per day. [Generic/Trade: Tabs, unscored 25, 50, 75 mg.] ▶L ♀B ▶? $$$

EPTIFIBATIDE (*Integrilin*)   Acute coronary syndrome: Load 180 mcg/kg IV bolus, then infuse 2 mcg/kg/min for up to 72 h. Discontinue infusion prior to CABG. Percutaneous coronary intervention: Load 180 mcg/kg IV bolus just before procedure, followed by infusion of 2 mcg/kg/min and a 2nd 180 mcg/kg IV bolus 10 min after the first bolus. Continue infusion for up to 18 to 24 h (minimum 12 h) after procedure. CrCl <50 mL/min not on dialysis: Reduce infusion rate to 1 mcg/kg/min. Dialysis: contraindicated. Thrombocytopenia possible; monitor platelets. ▶K ♀B ▶? $$$$$

PRASUGREL (*Effient*)   Reduction of thrombotic events after acute coronary syndrome managed with percutaneous coronary

CARDIOVASCULAR

(cont.)

intervention (PCI): 60 mg loading dose, then 10 mg PO daily in combination with aspirin. Wt less than 60 kg: Consider lower maintenance dose of 5 mg PO daily. May cause significant, fatal bleeding. Do not use with active bleeding or history of TIA or CVA. Generally not recommended for patients 75 yo and older. Risk factors for bleeding: Body wt less than 60 kg, propensity to bleed, concomitant medications that increase bleeding risk. Allergic cross-reactivity may occur among thienopyridines (clopidogrel, prasugrel, ticlopidine).   [Trade only: Tabs, unscored 5, 10 mg.] ▶LK ♀?/?/?; Consider possible risks to fetus before prescribing to pregnant women. ▶ Consider possible risks to breastfed child before prescribing to the nursing woman. $$$$$ ■

TICAGRELOR (*Brilinta*)   Reduction of thrombotic events in patients with acute coronary syndrome (MI or unstable angina) or history of MI: 180 mg loading dose, then 90 mg PO two times daily for first year post-acute coronary syndrome event, then 60 mg PO two times daily. Give with aspirin; after any initial dose, use with aspirin 75 to 100 mg max per day. Do not use with history of intracranial hemorrhage, active bleeding, severe hepatic impairment, strong CYP3A inhibitors, or CYP3A inducers. Monitor digoxin levels when initiating or changing ticagrelor therapy. Do not use with strong CYP3A inhibitors (eg, clarithromycin, HIV protease inhibitors, itraconazole, ketoconazole, nefazodone, telithromycin, voriconazole), CYP3A inducers (eg, carbamazepine, dexamethasone, phenobarbital, phenytoin, rifampin), or severe hepatic impairment. P-glycoprotein inhibitors (eg, cyclosporine) increase ticagrelor levels.   [Trade only: Tabs, unscored 60, 90 mg.] ▶L – ♀?/?/?; Consider possible risks to fetus before prescribing to pregnant women. ▶ Do not breastfeed while taking this medication. $$$$$ ■

TICLOPIDINE Due to high incidence of neutropenia and thrombotic thrombocytopenia purpura, other antiplatelet agents preferred. Platelet aggregation inhibition/reduction

(cont.)

of thrombotic CVA: 250 mg PO twice daily with food. Allergic cross-reactivity may occur among thienopyridines (clopidogrel, prasugrel, ticlopidine). [Generic: Tabs, unscored 250 mg.] ▶L ♀B ▶? $$$$ ■

TIROFIBAN (*Aggrastat*) Non-ST segment elevation acute coronary syndromes: Give 25 mcg/kg within 5 min, then 0.15 mcg/kg/min for up to 18 h. Renal impairment (CrCl 60 mL/min or less): Give 25 mcg/kg within 5 min, then 0.075 mcg/kg/min. ▶K ♀B ▶? $$$$$

VORAPAXAR (*Zontivity*) Reduction of thrombotic events in patients with history of MI or with peripheral artery disease: 2.08 mg PO daily. Do not use with active bleeding or history of CVA or stroke. Avoid use with strong CYP3A4 inhibitors or inducers. Store in original container with desiccant. [Trade only: Tabs, unscored 2.08 mg.] ▶L ♀B ▶– $$$$$ ■

Beta-Blockers

NOTE: *See also Antihypertensive Combinations. Not first line for HTN (unless concurrent angina, post MI, or heart failure with reduced ejection fraction). Atenolol may be less effective for HTN than other beta-blockers. Non-selective beta-blockers, including carvedilol and labetalol, are contraindicated with asthma; use agents with beta-1 selectivity and monitor cautiously; beta-1 selectivity diminishes at high doses. Contraindicated with acute decompensated heart failure, sick sinus syndrome without pacer, cardiogenic shock, heart block greater than first degree, or severe bradycardia. Agents with intrinsic sympathomimetic activity (eg, pindolol) are contraindicated post acute MI. Abrupt cessation may precipitate angina, MI, arrhythmias, tachycardia, rebound HTN; or with thyrotoxicosis, thyroid storm; discontinue by tapering over 1 to 2 weeks. Do not routinely stop chronic beta-blocker therapy prior to surgery. Discontinue beta-blocker several days before discontinuing concomitant clonidine to minimize the risk of rebound HTN. Patients actively*

CARDIOVASCULAR

(cont.)

using cocaine should avoid beta-blockers with unopposed alpha-adrenergic vasoconstriction, because this will promote coronary artery vasoconstriction/spasm (carvedilol or labetalol have additional alpha-1-blocking effects and are safer). Concomitant amiodarone, disopyramide, clonidine, digoxin, or nondihydropyridine calcium channel blockers may increase risk of bradycardia. Monitor for heart failure exacerbation and hypotension (particularly orthostatic) when titrating dose. All beta-blockers, except carvedilol, may increase blood glucose or mask tachycardia occurring with hypoglycemia. May aggravate psoriasis or symptoms of arterial insufficiency. Intraoperative floppy iris syndrome may occur during cataract surgery, if patient is on or has previously taken agents with alpha-1-blocking activity.

ACEBUTOLOL (*Sectral, ✦Rhotral*) HTN: Start 400 mg PO daily or 200 mg PO two times per day, max 1200 mg/day. Beta-1 receptor selective; has mild intrinsic sympathomimetic activity. [Generic/Trade: Caps 200, 400 mg.] ▶LK ♀B ▶– $$ ■

ATENOLOL (*Tenormin*) Acute MI: 50 to 100 mg PO daily or in divided doses. HTN: Start 25 to 50 mg PO daily or divided two times per day, max 100 mg/day. Beta-1 receptor selective. May be less effective for HTN and lowering CV event risk than other beta-blockers. [Generic/Trade: Tabs, unscored 25, 100 mg; scored 50 mg.] ▶K ♀D ▶– $ ■

BETAXOLOL (*Kerlone*) HTN: Start 5 to 10 mg PO daily, max 20 mg/day. Beta-1 receptor selective. [Generic/Trade: Tabs, scored 10 mg; unscored 20 mg.] ▶LK ♀C ▶? $ ■

BISOPROLOL (*Zebeta, ✦Monocor*) HTN: Start 2.5 to 5 mg PO daily, max 20 mg/day. Highly beta-1 receptor selective. [Generic/Trade: Tabs, scored 5 mg; unscored 10 mg.] ▶LK ♀C ▶? $$ ■

CARVEDILOL (*Coreg, Coreg CR*) Heart failure, immediate-release: Start 3.125 mg PO two times per day, double dose q 2 weeks as tolerated up to max of 25 mg two times per day (for

(cont.)

wt 85 kg or less) or 50 mg two times per day (for wt greater than 85 kg). Heart failure, sustained-release: Start 10 mg PO daily, double dose q 2 weeks as tolerated up to max of 80 mg/day. LV dysfunction following acute MI, immediate-release: Start 3.125 to 6.25 mg PO two times per day, double dose q 3 to 10 days as tolerated to max of 25 mg two times per day. LV dysfunction following acute MI, sustained-release: Start 10 to 20 mg PO daily, double dose q 3 to 10 days as tolerated to max of 80 mg/day. HTN, immediate-release: Start 6.25 mg PO two times per day, double dose q 7 to 14 days as tolerated to max 50 mg/day. HTN, sustained-release: Start 20 mg PO daily, double dose q 7 to 14 days as tolerated to max 80 mg/day. Take with food to decrease orthostatic hypotension. Give Coreg CR in the morning. Alpha-1, beta-1, and beta-2 receptor blocker. [Generic/Trade: Tabs, immediate-release, unscored 3.125, 6.25, 12.5, 25 mg. Trade only: Caps, extended-release 10, 20, 40, 80 mg.] ▶L ♀C ▶? $$$ ■

ESMOLOL (*Brevibloc*) SVT/HTN emergency: Load 500 mcg/kg over 1 min (dilute 5 g in 500 mL to make a soln of 10 mg/mL and give 3.5 mL to deliver 35 mg bolus for 70 kg patient), then start infusion 50 to 200 mcg/kg/min (42 mL/h delivers 100 mcg/kg/min for 70 kg patient). Half-life is 9 min. Beta-1 receptor selective. ▶K ♀C ▶? $$$$$ ■

LABETALOL (*Trandate*) HTN: Start 100 mg PO two times per day, max 2400 mg/day. HTN emergency: Start 20 mg IV slow injection, then 40 to 80 mg IV q 10 min prn up to 300 mg or IV infusion 0.5 to 2 mg/min. Peds: Start 0.3 to 1 mg/kg/dose (max 20 mg). May be used to manage BP during pregnancy. Alpha-1, beta-1, and beta-2 receptor blocker. [Generic/Trade: Tabs, scored 100, 200, 300 mg.] ▶LK ♀C ▶+ $$$ ■

METOPROLOL (*Lopressor, Toprol-XL, ✦Betaloc*) Acute MI: 50 to 100 mg PO q 12 h; or 5-mg increments IV q 5 to 15 min up to 15 mg followed by oral therapy. HTN (immediate-release): Start 100 mg PO daily or in divided doses, increase prn up to 450 mg/day; may require multiple daily doses to maintain

(cont.)

24 h BP control. HTN (extended-release): Start 25 to 100 mg PO daily, increase prn up to 400 mg/day. Heart failure: Start 12.5 to 25 mg (extended-release) PO daily, double dose q 2 weeks as tolerated up to max 200 mg/day. Angina: Start 50 mg PO two times per day (immediate-release) or 100 mg PO daily (extended-release), increase prn up to 400 mg/day. IV to PO conversion: 1 mg IV is equivalent to 2.5 mg PO (divided four times per day). Immediate-release form is metoprolol tartrate; extended-release form is metoprolol succinate. The immediate-release and extended-release products may not give same clinical response on mg:mg basis; monitor response and side effects when interchanging between metoprolol products. Extended-release tabs may be broken in half, but do not chew or crush. Beta-1 receptor selective. Take with food. [Generic/Trade: Tabs, immediate release, tartrate, scored 50, 100 mg, extended-release, succinate, 25, 50, 100, 200 mg. Generic only: Tabs, extended-release, tartrate, scored 25 mg.] ▶L ♀C ▶? $$ ■

NADOLOL (*Corgard*) HTN: Start 20 to 40 mg PO daily, max 320 mg/day. Prevent rebleeding esophageal varices: 40 to 160 mg PO daily; titrate dose to reduce heart rate to 25% below baseline. Beta-1 and beta-2 receptor blocker. [Generic/Trade: Tabs, scored 20, 40, 80 mg.] ▶K ♀C ▶– $$$$

NEBIVOLOL (*Bystolic*) HTN: Start 5 mg PO daily, max 40 mg/day. At doses of 10 mg or less or for extensive metabolizers: beta-1 receptor selective. At doses greater than 10 mg or poor metabolizers: beta-1 and beta-2 receptor blocker. [Trade only: Tabs, unscored 2.5, 5, 10, 20 mg.] ▶L ♀C ▶– $$$ ■

PINDOLOL HTN: Start 5 mg PO two times per day, max 60 mg/day. Has intrinsic sympathomimetic activity (partial beta-agonist activity); beta-1 and beta-2 receptor blocker. [Generic only: Tabs, scored 5, 10 mg.] ▶K ♀B ▶? $$$

PROPRANOLOL (*Inderal, Inderal LA, InnoPran XL*) HTN: Start 20 to 40 mg PO two times per day or 60 to 80 mg PO daily, max 640 mg/day; extended-release (Inderal LA) max 640 mg/day; extended-release (InnoPran XL) 80 mg at bedtime (10 pm),

(cont.)

max 120 mg at bedtime (chronotherapy). Supraventricular tachycardia or rapid atrial fibrillation/flutter: 1 mg IV q 2 min. Max of 2 doses in 4 h. Migraine prophylaxis: Start 40 mg PO two times per day or 80 mg PO daily (extended-release), max 240 mg/day. Prevent rebleeding esophageal varices: 20 to 180 mg PO two times per day; titrate dose to reduce heart rate to 25% below baseline. Beta-1 and beta-2 receptor blocker. [Generic/Trade: Caps, extended-release 60, 80, 120, 160 mg. Generic only: Soln 20, 40 mg/5 mL. Tabs, scored 10, 20, 40, 60, 80 mg. Trade only: (InnoPran XL at bedtime) 80, 120 mg.] ▶L ♀C ▶+ $$ ■

TIMOLOL (*Blocadren*) HTN: Start 10 mg PO two times per day, max 60 mg/day. Beta-1 and beta-2 receptor blocker. [Generic only: Tabs, 5, 10, 20 mg.] ▶LK ♀C ▶+ $$$ ■

Calcium Channel Blockers (CCBs)—Dihydropyridines

NOTE: *See also Antihypertensive Combinations. Avoid in decompensated heart failure. May increase edema. Extended/controlled/sustained-release forms: swallow whole; do not chew or crush. Avoid grapefruit juice.*

AMLODIPINE (*Norvasc*) HTN: Start 5 mg PO daily, max 10 mg/day. Elderly, small, frail, or with hepatic insufficiency: Start 2.5 PO daily. [Generic/Trade: Tabs, unscored 2.5, 5, 10 mg.] ▶L ♀C ▶− $

CLEVIDIPINE (*Cleviprex*) HTN: Start 1 to 2 mg/h IV, titrate q 1.5 to 10 min to BP response, usual maintenance dose 4 to 6 mg/h, max 32 mg/h IV. An increase of 1 to 2 mg/h will decrease SBP approximately 2 to 4 mmHg. ▶KL ♀C ▶? $$$$$

FELODIPINE (*Plendil*, ✦*Renedil*) HTN: Start 2.5 to 5 mg PO daily, max 10 mg/day. [Generic/Trade: Tabs, extended-release, unscored 2.5, 5, 10 mg.] ▶L ♀C ▶? $$

ISRADIPINE HTN: Start 2.5 mg PO two times per day, max 20 mg/day (max 10 mg/day in elderly). [Generic only: Immediate-release caps 2.5, 5 mg.] ▶L ♀C ▶? $$$$

NICARDIPINE (*Cardene, Cardene SR*) HTN emergency: Begin IV infusion at 5 mg/h, titrate to effect, max 15 mg/h. HTN: Start 20

CARDIOVASCULAR

mg PO three times per day, max 120 mg/day. Sustained-release: Start 30 mg PO two times per day, max 120 mg/day. Short-term management of HTN, patient receiving PO nicardipine: If using 20 mg PO q 8 h, give 0.5 mg/h IV; if using 30 mg PO q 8 h, give 1.2 mg/h IV; if using 40 mg PO q 8 h, give 2.2 mg/h. [Generic/Trade: Caps, immediate-release 20, 30 mg. Trade only: Caps, sustained-release 30, 45, 60 mg.] ▶L ♀C ▶? $$$

NIFEDIPINE (*Procardia, Adalat, Procardia XL, Adalat CC, Afeditab CR, ✦Adalat XL*) HTN/angina: Extended-release: 30 to 60 mg PO daily, max 120 mg/day. Angina: Immediate-release: Start 10 mg PO three times per day, max 120 mg/day. Avoid sublingual administration, may cause excessive hypotension, acute MI, CVA. Do not use immediate-release caps for treating HTN, hypertensive emergencies, or ST-elevation MI. Preterm labor: Loading dose: 10 mg PO q 20 to 30 min if contractions persist, up to 40 mg within the 1st h. Maintenance dose: 10 to 20 mg PO q 4 to 6 h or 60 to 160 mg extended-release PO daily. [Generic/Trade: Caps 10, 20 mg. Tabs, extended-release (Adalat CC, Afeditab CR, Procardia XL) 30, 60 mg; (Adalat CC, Procardia XL) 90 mg.] ▶L ♀C ▶– $$

NISOLDIPINE (*Sular*) HTN: Start 17 mg PO daily, max 34 mg/day. Take on an empty stomach. [Generic/Trade: Tabs, extended-release 8.5, 17, 25.5, 34 mg. These replace the former 10, 20, 30, 40 mg tabs. Generic only: Tabs, extended-release 20, 30, 40 mg.] ▶L ♀C ▶? $$$$$

Calcium Channel Blockers (CCBs)—Non-Dihydropyridines

NOTE: *See also Antihypertensive Combinations. Avoid in decompensated heart failure, 2nd/3rd degree heart block without pacemaker, acute MI and pulmonary congestion, or systolic blood pressure <90 mm Hg systolic.*

DILTIAZEM (*Cardizem, Cardizem LA, Cardizem CD, Cartia XT, Dilacor XR, Diltiazem CD, Diltzac, Diltia XT, Matzim LA, Tiazac, Taztia XT*) Atrial fibrillation/flutter, PSVT: Bolus 20 mg

(cont.)

(0.25 mg/kg) IV over 2 min. Rebolus 15 min later (if needed) 25 mg (0.35 mg/kg). Infusion 5 to 15 mg/h. HTN, once daily, extended-release: Start 120 to 240 mg PO daily, max 540 mg/day. HTN, once daily, graded extended-release (Cardizem LA): Start 180 to 240 mg PO daily, max 540 mg/day. HTN, twice daily, sustained-release: Start 60 to 120 mg PO two times per day, max 360 mg/day. Angina, immediate-release: Start 30 mg PO four times per day, max 360 mg/day divided three to four times per day. Angina, extended-release: Start 120 to 240 mg PO daily, max 540 mg/day. Angina, once daily, graded extended-release (Cardizem LA): Start 180 mg PO daily, doses more than 360 mg may provide no additional benefit. [Generic/Trade: Tabs, immediate-release, unscored (Cardizem) 30 mg, scored 60, 90, 120 mg. Caps, extended-release (Cardizem CD, Cartia XT daily) 120, 180, 240, 300, 360 mg, (Diltzac, Taztia XT, Tiazac daily) 120, 180, 240, 300, 360, 420 mg, (Dilacor XR, Diltia XT) 120, 180, 240 mg. Tabs, extended-release (Cardizem LA daily, Matzim LA) 180, 240, 300, 360, 420 mg. Generic only: Caps, extended release (twice daily) 60, 90, 120 mg. Trade only: Tabs, extended-release (Cardizem LA daily) 120 mg.] ▶L ♀C ▶+ $$

VERAPAMIL (*Isoptin SR, Calan, Calan SR, Verelan, Verelan PM*) SVT adults: 5 to 10 mg IV over 2 min. SVT peds (age 1 to 15 yo): 2 to 5 mg (0.1 to 0.3 mg/kg) IV, max dose 5 mg. Angina, immediate-release: start 40 to 80 mg PO three to four times per day, max 480 mg/day. Angina, sustained-release: Start 120 to 240 mg PO daily, max 480 mg/day (use twice daily dosing for doses greater than 240 mg/day with Isoptin SR and Calan SR). HTN: Same as angina, except (Verelan PM) 100 to 200 mg PO at bedtime, max 400 mg/day; immediate-release tabs should be avoided in treating HTN. Use cautiously with impaired renal/hepatic function. [Generic/Trade: Tabs, immediate-release, scored (Calan) 40, 80, 120 mg. Tabs, sustained-release, unscored (Isoptin SR, Calan SR) 120 mg, scored 180, 240 mg. Caps, sustained-release (Verelan) 120, 180, 240, 360 mg. Caps, extended-release (Verelan PM) 100, 200, 300 mg.] ▶L ♀C ▶– $$

Diuretics—Loop

NOTE: Thiazides are preferred diuretics for HTN. With decreased renal function (CrCl <30 mL/min), loop diuretics may be more effective than thiazides for HTN. Rare hypersensitivity in patients allergic to sulfa-containing drugs, except ethacrynic acid. For diuretics given twice daily, give second dose in mid-afternoon to avoid nocturia.

BUMETANIDE (*Bumex, ✦Burinex*) Edema: 0.5 to 1 mg IV/IM; 0.5 to 2 mg PO daily. 1 mg bumetanide is roughly equivalent to 40 mg furosemide. [Generic only: Tabs, scored 0.5, 1, 2 mg.] ▸K ♀C ▶? $

ETHACRYNIC ACID (*Edecrin*) Can be safely used in patients with true sulfa allergy. Edema: 0.5 to 1 mg/kg IV, max 100 mg/dose; 25 to 100 mg PO daily to two times per day. [Trade only: Tabs, scored 25 mg.] ▸K ♀B ▶? $$$$$

FUROSEMIDE (*Lasix*) HTN: Start 10 to 40 mg PO two times per day, max 600 mg daily. Edema: Start 20 to 80 mg IV/IM/PO, increase dose by 20 to 40 mg in 6 to 8 h until desired response is achieved, max 600 mg/day. Ascites: 40 mg PO daily in combination with spironolactone; may increase dose after 2 to 3 days if no response. [Generic/Trade: Tabs, unscored 20, scored 40, 80 mg. Generic only: Oral soln 10 mg/mL, 40 mg/5 mL.] ▸K ♀C ▶? $

TORSEMIDE (*Demadex*) HTN: Start 5 mg PO daily, increase prn q 4 to 6 weeks, max 10 mg daily. Edema: 10 to 20 mg IV/PO daily, max 200 mg IV/PO daily. [Generic/Trade: Tabs, scored 5, 10, 20, 100 mg.] ▸LK ♀B ▶? $

Diuretics—Potassium-Sparing

NOTE: See also antihypertensive combinations and aldosterone antagonists. May cause hyperkalemia. Use cautiously with other agents that may cause hyperkalemia (ie, ACE inhibitors, ARBs, aliskiren, potassium containing salt substitutes).

AMILORIDE (*Midamor*) Edema/HTN: Start 5 mg PO daily in combination with another diuretic, usually a thiazide for HTN, max 20 mg/day. [Generic only: Tabs, unscored 5 mg.] ▶LK ♀B ▶? $$$

TRIAMTERENE (*Dyrenium*) Edema (cirrhosis, nephrotic syndrome, heart failure): Start 100 mg PO two times per day, max 300 mg/day. [Trade only: Caps 50, 100 mg.] ▶LK ♀B ▶– $$$

Diuretics—Thiazide Type

NOTE: *See also Antihypertensive Combinations. Possible hypersensitivity in sulfa allergy. Should be used for most patients with HTN, alone or combined with other antihypertensive agents. Thiazides are not recommended for gestational HTN. Coadministration with NSAIDs, including selective COX-2 inhibitors, may reduce the antihypertensive, diuretic, and natriuretic effects of thiazides. Thiazide-induced hypokalemia is associated with increased fasting blood glucose and new-onset DM; keep potassium ≥4.0 mg/dL to minimize risk; may use thiazide in combination with oral potassium supplementation, ACE inhibitor, ARB, or potassium-sparing diuretic to maintain K level. Lithium level may increase with concomitant use; monitor lithium level.*

CHLOROTHIAZIDE (*Diuril*) HTN: Start 125 to 250 mg PO daily or divided two times per day, max 1000 mg/day divided two times per day. [Trade only: Susp 250 mg/5 mL. Generic only: Tabs, scored 250, 500 mg.] ▶L ♀C, D if used in pregnancy-induced HTN ▶+ $

CHLORTHALIDONE HTN: 12.5 to 25 mg PO daily, max 50 mg/day. Edema: 50 to 100 mg PO daily, max 200 mg/day. Nephrolithiasis (unapproved use): 25 to 50 mg PO daily. [Generic only: Tabs, unscored 25, 50 mg.] ▶L ♀B, D if used in pregnancy-induced HTN ▶+ $

HYDROCHLOROTHIAZIDE (*HCTZ, Oretic, Microzide*) HTN: 12.5 to 25 mg PO daily, max 50 mg/day. Edema: 25 to 100 mg PO

(cont.)

daily, max 200 mg/day. [Generic/Trade: Tabs, scored 25, 50 mg. Caps 12.5 mg.] ▸L ♀B, D if used in pregnancy-induced HTN▸+ $

INDAPAMIDE (★Lozide) HTN: 1.25 to 5 mg PO daily, max 5 mg/day. Edema: 2.5 to 5 mg PO q am. [Generic only: Tabs, unscored 1.25, 2.5 mg.] ▸L ♀B, D if used in pregnancy-induced HTN▸? $

METHYCLOTHIAZIDE (Enduron) HTN: Start 2.5 mg PO daily, usual maintenance dose 2.5 to 5 mg/day. [Generic only: Tabs, scored, 5 mg.] ▸L ♀B, D if used in pregnancy-induced HTN▸? $$$

METOLAZONE Edema: 5 to 10 mg PO daily, max 10 mg/day in heart failure, 20 mg/day in renal disease. If used with loop diuretic, start with 2.5 mg PO daily. [Generic: Tabs 2.5, 5, 10 mg.] ▸L ♀B, D if used in pregnancy-induced HTN▸? $$$

Nitrates

NOTE: *Avoid if systolic BP below 90 mmHg, severe bradycardia, tachycardia, or right ventricular infarction. Avoid if patient takes PDE-5 inhibitor (eg, avanafil, sildenafil, tadalafil, vardenafil) or guanylate cyclase stimulators (eg, riociguat).*

ISOSORBIDE DINITRATE (Isordil, Dilatrate-SR) Angina prophylaxis: 5 to 40 mg PO three times per day (7 am, noon, 5 pm), sustained-release: 40 to 80 mg PO two times per day (8 am, 2 pm). [Generic/Trade: Tabs, scored 5 mg. Trade only: Tabs, scored (Isordil) 40 mg. Caps, extended-release (Dilatrate-SR) 40 mg. Generic only: Tabs, scored 10, 20, 30 mg. Tabs, scored, sustained-release 40 mg.] ▸L ♀C ▸? $$$

ISOSORBIDE MONONITRATE Angina: 20 mg PO two times per day (8 am and 3 pm). Extended-release: Start 30 to 60 mg PO daily, max 240 mg/day. Do not use for acute angina. [Generic only: Tabs, 10, 20 mg. Tabs, extended-release, scored 30, 60; unscored 120 mg.] ▸L ♀C ▸? $

NITROGLYCERIN INTRAVENOUS INFUSION Perioperative HTN, acute MI/heart failure, acute angina: Mix 50 mg in 250 mL D5W (200 mcg/mL), start at 10 to 20 mcg/min (3 to 6 mL/h), then titrate upward by 10 to 20 mcg/min prn. ▸L ♀C ▸? $

NITROGLYCERIN OINTMENT (*Nitro-BID*) Angina prophylaxis: Start 0.5 inch q 8 h, maintenance 1 to 2 inch q 8 h, max 4 inch q 4 to 6 h; 15 mg/inch. Allow for a nitrate-free period of 10 to 14 h to avoid nitrate tolerance. 1 inch ointment contains about 15 mg. Do not use for acute angina attack. [Trade only: Oint, 2%, tubes 1, 30, 60 g (Nitro-BID).] ▶L ♀C ▶? $$$

NITROGLYCERIN SPRAY (*Nitrolingual, NitroMist*) Acute angina: 1 to 2 sprays under the tongue prn, max 3 sprays in 15 min. [Generic/Trade: Nitrolingual soln, 4.9, 12 g. 0.4 mg/spray (60 or 200 sprays/canister). NitroMist aerosol, 4.1, 8.5 g; 0.4 mg/spray (90 or 200 sprays/canister).] ▶L ♀C ▶? $$$$$

NITROGLYCERIN SUBLINGUAL (*Nitrostat, GONITRO*) Acute angina, sublingual tabs: 0.4 mg SL, repeat dose q 5 min prn up to 3 doses in 15 min. Acute angina, sublingual powder: 0.4 to 0.8 mg SL, repeat dose q 5 min prn up to 1.2 mg total in 15 min. [Trade only: SL tabs, unscored (Nitrostat) 0.3, 0.4, 0.6 mg; in bottles of 100 or package of 4 bottles with 25 tabs each. SL powder packets (GONITRO) 0.4 mg; in boxes of 12, 36, 96 packets each.] ▶L ♀B ▶? $

NITROGLYCERIN SUSTAINED RELEASE Angina prophylaxis: Start 2.5 mg PO two to three times per day, then titrate upward prn. [Generic only: Caps, extended-release 2.5, 6.5, 9 mg.] ▶L ♀C ▶? $$

NITROGLYCERIN TRANSDERMAL (*Minitran, Nitro-Dur, ✦Trinipatch, Transderm-Nitro*) Angina prophylaxis: 1 patch 12 to 14 h each day. Allow for a nitrate-free period of 10 to 14 h each day to avoid nitrate tolerance. Do not use for acute angina attack. [Generic/Trade: Transdermal system 0.1, 0.2, 0.4, 0.6 mg/h. Trade only: (Nitro-Dur) 0.3, 0.8 mg/h.] ▶L ♀C ▶? $$

Pressors/Inotropes

DOBUTAMINE Inotropic support: Start 0.5 to 1 mcg/kg/min; titrate based on response; usual dose 2 to 20 mcg/kg/min. For short-term use, up to 48 h. Continuously monitor BP and EKG. Dilute 250 mg in 250 mL D5W (1 mg/mL); a rate of 21 mL/h delivers 5 mcg/kg/min for a 70 kg patient. ▶Plasma ♀D ▶– $

DOPAMINE Pressor: Start at 5 mcg/kg/min, increase prn by 5 to 10 mcg/kg/min increments at 10-min intervals, max 50 mcg/kg/min. Mix 400 mg in 250 mL D5W (1600 mcg/mL); a rate of 13 mL/h delivers 5 mcg/kg/min in a 70 kg patient. Doses in mcg/kg/min: 2 to 4 (traditional renal dose, apparently ineffective) dopaminergic receptors; 5 to 10 (cardiac dose) dopaminergic and beta-1 receptors; more than 10 dopaminergic, beta-1, and alpha-1 receptors. ▶Plasma ♀C ▶– $ ■

EPHEDRINE Pressor: 10 to 25 mg IV slow injection, with repeat doses q 5 to 10 min prn, max 150 mg/day. Orthostatic hypotension: 25 mg PO daily to four times per day. Bronchospasm: 25 to 50 mg PO q 3 to 4 h prn. [Generic only: Caps, 50 mg.] ▶K ♀C ▶? $

EPINEPHRINE (*EpiPen, EpiPen Jr, Adrenalin*) Cardiac arrest: 1 mg IV q 3 to 5 min. Anaphylaxis: 0.3 to 0.5 mg SC/IM, may repeat q 5 to 10 min. Acute asthma and hypersensitivity reactions: Adults: 0.1 to 0.3 mg of 1:1000 soln SC or IM. Peds: 0.01 mg/kg (up to 0.3 mg) of 1:1000 soln SC or IM. [Soln for injection: 1:1000 (1 mg/mL in 1 mL amps or 10 mL vial-$). Trade only: EpiPen autoinjector delivers one 0.3 mg (1:1000, 0.3 mL) IM/SC dose. EpiPen Jr. autoinjector delivers one 0.15 mg (1:2000, 0.3 mL) IM/SC dose. 3 mL) EpiPen available in a 2-pack ($$$$$).] ▶Plasma ♀C ▶– varies by therapy

MIDODRINE (✹*Amatine*) Orthostatic hypotension: 10 mg PO three times per day. The last daily dose should be no later than 6 pm to avoid supine HTN during sleep. [Generic: Tabs, scored 2.5, 5, 10 mg.] ▶LK ♀C ▶? $$$$$ ■

MILRINONE Systolic heart failure (NYHA class III, IV): Load 50 mcg/kg IV over 10 min, then begin IV infusion of 0.375 to 0.75 mcg/kg/min. ▶K ♀C ▶? $$

NOREPINEPHRINE (*Levophed*) Acute hypotension: Start 8 to 12 mcg/min, adjust to maintain BP, average maintenance rate 2 to 4 mcg/min. Mix 4 mg in 500 mL D5W (8 mcg/mL); a rate of 22.5 mL/h delivers 3 mcg/min. Ideally through central line. ▶Plasma ♀C ▶? $ ■

PHENYLEPHRINE—INTRAVENOUS Severe hypotension: Infusion: 20 mg in 250 mL D5W (80 mcg/mL), start 100 to 180 mcg/min (75 to 135 mL/h), usual dose once BP is stabilized 40 to 60 mcg/min. ▶Plasma ♀C ▶– $ ■

VASOPRESSIN (*Vasostrict, ADH, ✹Pressyn AR*) Diabetes insipidus: 5 to 10 units IM/SC two to four times per day prn. Cardiac arrest: 40 units IV; may repeat if no response after 3 min. Septic shock: 0.01 to 0.04 units/min. Variceal bleeding: 0.2 to 0.4 units/min initially (max 0.8 units/min). ▶LK ♀C ▶? $$$$$

Pulmonary Arterial Hypertension

AMBRISENTAN (*Letairis, ✹Volibris*) Pulmonary arterial hypertension: Start 5 mg PO daily; max 10 mg/day. Titrate at 4 week intervals as needed and tolerated. May give with tadalafil to improve exercise ability and decrease disease progression and hospitalizations. Contraindicated with idiopathic pulmonary fibrosis or pregnancy. Monitor hemoglobin. If pulmonary edema occurs, consider veno-occlusive disease; if confirmed, discontinue therapy. Not recommended with moderate or severe hepatic impairment. Do not exceed 5 mg when given with cyclosporine. May reduce sperm count. Do not split, crush, or chew tablets. Only available through restricted program; prescribers, pharmacies, female patients must enroll. [Trade only: Tabs, unscored 5, 10 mg.] ▶L ♀X ▶– $$$$$ ■

BOSENTAN (*Tracleer*) Pulmonary arterial hypertension: Start 62.5 mg PO two times per day for 4 weeks, increase to 125 mg two times per day maintenance dose. Only available through restricted program; prescribers, pharmacies, patients must enroll. Hepatotoxicity; monitor LFTs. Contraindicated in pregnancy. If pulmonary edema occurs, consider veno-occlusive disease; if confirmed, discontinue therapy. Monitor hemoglobin. May reduce sperm count. Many drug interactions; see prescribing information. [Trade only: Tabs, unscored 62.5, 125 mg.] ▶L ♀X ▶–? $$$$$ ■

EPOPROSTENOL (*Flolan, Veletri*) Pulmonary arterial hypertension: Start 2 ng/kg/min IV infusion via central venous catheter. Adjust dose based on response. Avoid abrupt dose decreases or cessation. If pulmonary edema occurs, consider veno-occlusive disease; if confirmed, discontinue therapy. ▶Plasma ♀B ▶? $$$$$

ILOPROST (*Ventavis*) Pulmonary arterial hypertension: Start 2.5 mcg/dose by inhalation (as delivered at mouthpiece); if well tolerated, increase to 5 mcg/dose by inhalation (as delivered at mouthpiece). Use 6 to 9 times a day (minimum of 2 h between doses) while awake. Only administer with I-neb AAD Systems. Avoid contact with skin/eyes or oral ingestion. Monitor vital signs when initiating therapy. Do not initiate therapy if SBP less than 85 mmHg. Discontinue therapy if pulmonary edema occurs; this may be sign of pulmonary venous hypertension. May induce bronchospasm. ▶L ♀C ▶? $$$$$

MACITENTAN (*Opsumit*) Pulmonary arterial hypertension: 10 mg PO daily. Contraindicated with pregnancy. Only available through restricted program; prescribers, pharmacies, female patients must enroll. [Trade: Tabs 10 mg.] ▶L ♀X ▶– $$$$$ ■

RIOCIGUAT (*Adempas*) Pulmonary arterial hypotension: Start 1 mg PO three times daily; max 2.5 mg three times daily. Contraindicated with pregnancy, nitrates, nitric oxide donors, PDE-5 inhibitors (eg, sildenafil, tadalafil, vardenafil), nonspecific PDE inhibitors (eg, dipyridamole, theophylline). Only available through restricted program; prescribers, pharmacies, female patients must enroll. [Trade: Tabs 0.5, 1, 1.5, 2, 2.5 mg.] ▶LK ♀X ▶– $$$$$ ■

SELEXIPAG (*Uptravi*) Pulmonary arterial hypertension: Start 200 mcg PO two times daily, increase by 200 mcg PO two times daily each week to highest tolerated dose, max 1600 mcg PO two times daily. With moderate hepatic impairment (Childs-Pugh class B): Start 200 mcg PO daily, increase by 200 mcg PO daily each week to highest tolerated dose, max 1600 mcg PO daily. Avoid concomitant strong CYP2C8 inhibitors (eg,

(cont.)

gemfibrozil). Avoid with severe hepatic impairment (Childs-Pugh class C). If pulmonary edema occurs, consider veno-occlusive disease. [Trade only: Tabs, unscored 200, 400, 600, 800, 1000, 1200, 1400, 1600 mcg.] ▶L ♀?/?/?; Animal reproduction studies showed no clinically relevant effects on embryo fetal development and survival. ▶ Do not breastfeed while taking this medication. $$$$$

SILDENAFIL—CARDIOVASCULAR (*Revatio*) Pulmonary arterial hypertension: 5 mg or 20 mg PO three times per day, with doses 4 to 6 h apart; or 2.5 mg or 10 mg IV three times per day. Contraindicated with nitrates or guanylate cyclase stimulators (eg, riociguat). Coadministration is not recommended with ritonavir, potent CYP3A4 inhibitors, or other phosphodiesterase-5 inhibitors. Teach patients to seek medical attention for vision loss, hearing loss, or in men if erections last longer than 4 h. [Generic/Trade: Tabs 20 mg. Trade only: Susp 10 mg/mL.] ▶LK ♀B▶– $$$$

TADALAFIL (*Adcirca*) Pulmonary arterial hypertension: 40 mg PO daily. Contraindicated with nitrates or guanylate cyclase stimulators (eg, riociguat). Coadministration is not recommended with potent CYP3A inhibitors (itraconazole, ketoconazole), potent CYP3A inducers (rifampin), other phosphodiesterase-5 inhibitors. Caution with ritonavir, see prescribing info for specific dose adjustments. Teach patients to seek medical attention for vision loss, hearing loss, or in men if erections last longer than 4 h. [Trade only (Adcirca): Tabs 20 mg.] ▶L ♀B▶– $$$$

TREPROSTINIL SODIUM—INJECTABLE (*Remodulin*) Pulmonary arterial hypertension: Continuous SC (preferred) or central IV infusion. Start 1.25 ng/kg/min based on ideal body wt. Dose based on clinical response and tolerance. Avoid abruptly lowering the dose or cessation. Use cautiously in the elderly and those with liver or renal dysfunction. Initiate in setting with personnel and equipment for physiological monitoring and emergency care. Administer by continuous infusion using

CARDIOVASCULAR

(cont.)

infusion pump. May potentiate bleeding risk for patients on anticoagulants. May potentiate hypotensive effects of other medications. ▸KL ♀B ▸? $$$$$

TREPROSTINIL—INHALED SOLUTION (*Tyvaso*) Pulmonary arterial hypertension: Start 3 breaths (18 mcg) per treatment session four times per day while awake; treatments should be at least 4 h apart; max 9 breaths (54 mcg) per treatment four times per day. Administer undiluted with the Tyvaso Inhalation System. Avoid contact with skin/eyes or oral ingestion. May need to adjust doses if CYP2C8 inducers or CYP2C8 inhibitors are added or withdrawn. Use cautiously in the elderly and those with liver or renal dysfunction. Inhibits platelet aggregation and increases risk of bleeding; may potentiate bleeding risk of anticoagulants. May potentiate hypotensive effects of other medications. Efficacy not established with existing lung disease (asthma, COPD). Monitor patients with acute pulmonary infections for worsening of lung disease and loss of drug effect. [1.74 mg in 2.9 mL inhalation soln.] ▸KL – ♀B ▸? $$$$$

TREPROSTINIL—ORAL (*Orenitram*) Pulmonary artery hypertension: Start 0.25 mg PO two times daily; increase by 0.25 to 0.5 mg two times daily or 0.125 mg three times daily q 3 to 4 days as tolerated. Use lower starting dose with mild hepatic impairment or with strong CYP2C8 inhibitor. To transition from intravenous (IV) or subcutaneous (SC) treprostinil, simultaneously decrease IV/SC infusion rate up to 30 ng/kg/min per day and increase the oral treprostinil dose up to 6 mg per day (2 mg TID). Take with food. Swallow whole. Do not abruptly discontinue. Avoid use with moderate or severe hepatic impairment. [Trade: Extended-release tabs 0.125, 0.25, 1, 2.5 mg.] ▸L ♀C ▸? $$$$$

Thrombolytics

ALTEPLASE (*TPA, t-PA, Activase, Cathflo, ✦Activase rt-PA*) Acute MI: wt 67 kg or less, give 15 mg IV bolus, then

(cont.)

0.75 mg/kg (max 50 mg) over 30 min, then 0.5 mg/kg (max 35 mg) over the next 60 min; wt greater than 67 kg, give 15 mg IV bolus, then 50 mg over 30 min, then 35 mg over the next 60 min. Acute ischemic stroke with symptoms 3 h or less: 0.9 mg/kg (max 90 mg); give 10% of total dose as an IV bolus, and the remainder IV over 60 min. Multiple exclusion criteria. Acute pulmonary embolism: 100 mg IV over 2 h, then restart heparin when PTT twice normal or less. Occluded central venous access device: 2 mg/mL in catheter for 2 h. May use 2nd dose if needed. ▶L ♀C ▶? $$$$$

RETEPLASE (*Retavase*) Acute MI: 10 units IV over 2 min; repeat once in 30 min. ▶L ♀C ▶? $$$$$

STREPTOKINASE (*Streptase, Kabikinase*) Acute MI: 1.5 million units IV over 60 min. ▶L ♀C ▶? $$$$$

TENECTEPLASE (*TNKase*) Acute MI: Single IV bolus dose over 5 sec based on body wt: Wt less than 60 kg: 30 mg; wt 60 kg to 69 kg: 35 mg; wt 70 to 79 kg: 40 mg; wt 80 to 89 kg: 45 mg; wt 90 kg or more: 50 mg. ▶L ♀C ▶? $$$$$

Volume Expanders

ALBUMIN (*Albuminar, Buminate, Albumarc, ✦Plasbumin*) Shock, burns: 500 mL of 5% soln IV infusion as rapidly as tolerated, repeat in 30 min if needed. ▶L ♀C ▶? $$$$

DEXTRAN (*Rheomacrodex, Gentran, Macrodex*) Shock/hypovolemia: up to 20 mL/kg in 1st 24 h, then up to 10 mL/kg for 4 days. ▶K ♀C ▶? $$

HETASTARCH (*Hespan, Hextend, Voluven*) Shock/hypovolemia: 500 to 1000 mL IV infusion. Hespan, Hextend: usually should not exceed 20 mL/kg/day. Voluven: Do not exceed 50 mL/kg/day. ▶K ♀C ▶? $$ ■

PLASMA PROTEIN FRACTION (*Plasmanate, Protenate, Plasmatein*) Shock/hypovolemia: 5% soln 250 to 500 mL IV prn. ▶L ♀C ▶? $$$$

CARDIOVASCULAR

Other

BIDIL (hydralazine + isosorbide dinitrate) Heart failure (adjunct to standard therapy in black patients): Start 1 tab PO three times per day, increase as tolerated to max 2 tabs three times per day. May decrease to ½ tab three times per day with intolerable side effects. [Trade only: Tabs, scored 37.5/20 mg.] ▶LK ♀C ▶? $$$$$

CILOSTAZOL (Pletal) Intermittent claudication: 100 mg PO two times per day on empty stomach. 50 mg PO two times per day with CYP3A4 inhibitors (eg, ketoconazole, itraconazole, erythromycin, diltiazem) or CYP2C19 inhibitors (eg, omeprazole). Contraindicated in heart failure of any severity due to decreased survival. [Generic/Trade: Tabs 50, 100 mg.] ▶L ♀C ▶? $$$$ ■

ENTRESTO (sacubitril + valsartan) Reduce cardiovascular death and hospitalization for heart failure with chronic heart failure (NYHA Class II–IV) and reduced ejection fraction: Start 49/51 mg PO two times per day, double dose after 2 to 4 weeks as tolerated, target maintenance dose 97/103 mg PO two times daily. Patients not currently taking ACE inhibitor or angiotensin receptor blocker or previously taking low dose of these agents, severe renal impairment (eGFR less than 30 mL/min/1.73 m^2), moderate hepatic impairment (Child-Pugh B): Start 24/26 mg PO two times per day, double dose after 2 to 4 weeks as tolerated; target maintenance dose 97/103 mg PO two times daily. Usually given with other heart failure therapies, in place of ACE inhibitor or other angiotensin receptor blocker. If switching from ACE inhibitor, allow 36 hours washout period between administration of the drugs. Do not use with severe hepatic impairment. Contraindicated with pregnancy, concomitant ACE inhibitor, concomitant aliskiren in patients with DM, or previous angioedema with ACE inhibitor or angiotensin receptor blocker. Combined use with renin-angiotensin system inhibitors (ie, ACE inhibitors, aliskiren, other angiotensin receptor

(cont.)

blocker) increases risk of renal impairment, hypotension, and hyperkalemia. Hyperkalemia possible, especially if used concomitantly with other drugs that increase K+ (including K+-containing salt substitutes) and in patients with heart failure, DM, or renal impairment. Concomitant NSAID, including celecoxib, may further deteriorate renal function and decrease antihypertensive effects. May increase lithium levels. [Trade: Tabs, unscored 24/26, 49/51, 97/103 mg.] ▶esterases ♀D ▶– $$$$$ ■

IVABRADINE (*Corlanor*) Stable, symptomatic heart failure with ejection fraction less than or equal to 35%, sinus rhythm with heart rate of at least 70 beats per minute, and either maximally tolerated beta-blocker dose or intolerant to beta-blocker: Start 5 mg PO two times per day, max 15 mg/day. With conduction defect or if bradycardia could lead to hemodynamic compromise, start 2.5 mg PO two times daily. Fetal toxicity; females should use effective contraception. Contraindicated with strong CYP3A4 inhibitors (eg, azole antifungals, macrolide antibiotics, HIV protease inhibitors, nefazodone); acute decompensated heart failure; BP less than 90/50 mmHg; sick sinus syndrome, sinoatrial block, or 3rd degree AV block without functioning pacemaker; resting heart rate less than 60 bpm prior to treatment; severe hepatic impairment; or pacemaker dependent. Monitor for atrial fibrillation, bradycardia. Not recommended with 2nd degree heart block or with demand pacemakers set to at least 60 beats per minute. Avoid concomitant CYP3A4 inhibitors or CYP3A4 inducers. Negative chronotropes increase risk of bradycardia; monitor heart rate. [Trade only: Tabs, unscored 5, 7.5 mg.] ▶L ♀? ▶– $$$$$

NESIRITIDE (*Natrecor*) Hospitalized patients with decompensated heart failure with dyspnea at rest: 2 mcg/kg IV bolus over 1 min, then 0.01 mcg/kg/min IV infusion for up to 48 h. Do not initiate at higher doses. Limited experience with increased doses. Mix 1.5 mg vial in 250 mL D5W (6 mcg/mL);

(cont.)

CARDIOVASCULAR

a bolus of 23.3 mL is 2 mcg/kg for a 70 kg patient; infusion set at rate 7 mL/h delivers a 0.01 mcg/kg/min for a 70 kg patient. Contraindicated with cardiogenic shock or SBP less than 100 mmHg. Symptomatic hypotension. May increase mortality. Not indicated for outpatient infusion, for scheduled repetitive use, to improve renal function, or to enhance diuresis. May worsen renal impairment. ▶K, Plasma ♀C ▶? $$$$$

PENTOXIFYLLINE Intermittent claudication: 400 mg PO three times per day with meals. Contraindicated with recent cerebral/retinal bleed. [Generic: Tabs, extended-release 400 mg.] ▶L ♀C ▶? $$$

RANOLAZINE (*Ranexa*) Chronic angina: 500 mg PO two times per day, max 1000 mg two times per day. Max 500 mg two times per day, if used with diltiazem, verapamil, or moderate CYP3A inhibitors. Baseline and follow-up ECGs; may prolong QT interval. If CrCl <60 mL/min at baseline, monitor renal function; discontinue ranolazine if acute renal failure occurs. Contraindicated with hepatic cirrhosis, potent CYP3A4 inhibitors, CYP3A inducers. Increases level of cyclosporine, digoxin, lovastatin, simvastatin, sirolimus, tacrolimus, antipsychotics, TCA(s). Swallow whole; do not crush, break, or chew. Teach patients to report palpitations or fainting spells. [Trade only: Tabs, extended-release 500, 1000 mg.] ▶LK ♀C ▶? $$$$$

CONTRAST MEDIA

MRI Contrast—Gadolinium-Based

NOTE: *Avoid gadolinium-based contrast agents if severe renal insufficiency (GFR <30 mL/min/1.73 m) due to risk of nephrogenic systemic fibrosis/nephrogenic fibrosing dermopathy. Similarly avoid in acute renal insufficiency of any severity due to hepatorenal syndrome or during the perioperative phase of liver transplant.*

GADOBENATE (*MultiHance*) ▶K ♀C ▶? $$$$ ■
GADOBUTROL (*Gadavist*, ✦*Gadavist*) ▶K –♀C ▶? $$$$ ■
GADODIAMIDE (*Omniscan*) ▶K ♀C ▶? $$$$ ■
GADOPENTETATE (*Magnevist*) ▶K ♀C ▶? $$$ ■
GADOTERIDOL (*ProHance*) ▶K ♀C ▶? $$$$ ■
GADOVERSETAMIDE (*OptiMARK*) ▶K ♀C ▶– $$$$ ■

MRI Contrast—Other

FERUMOXSIL (*GastroMARK*) Non-iodinated, nonionic, iron-based, oral GI contrast for MRI: 600 mL (105 mg Fe) administered orally at a rate of about 300 mL over 15 minutes (max 900 mL or 157.5 mg Fe). Take after fasting at least 4 hours. Shake bottles for vigorously for 1 min before use. [300 mL bottles] ▶L ♀B ▶? $$$$

MANGAFODIPIR (*Teslascan*) Non-iodinated manganese-based IV contrast for MRI. ▶L ♀– ▶– $$$$

Radiography Contrast

NOTE: *Beware of allergic or anaphylactoid reactions. Avoid IV contrast in renal insufficiency or dehydration. Hold metformin (Glucophage) prior to or at the time of iodinated contrast dye use and for 48 h after procedure. Restart after procedure only if renal function is normal.*

(cont.)

BARIUM SULFATE Noniodinated GI (eg, oral, rectal) contrast: Dosage depends on indication and form, see package insert. ▶Not absorbed ♀? ▶+ $

DIATRIZOATE (*Cystografin, Gastrografin, Hypaque, MD-Gastroview, RenoCal, Reno-DIP, Reno-60, Renografin*) Iodinated, ionic, high-osmolality IV or GI contrast: Dosage varies based on study and form, see package insert. Oral contrast for abdominal CT: typical dose is 250 mL of solution made by mixing 25 mL of GI formulation (Gastrografin, MD-Gastroview) in one liter of water. Have patient complete drinking 30 minutes prior to study. Avoid use if there is a risk of aspiration. ▶K ♀C ▶? $

IODIXANOL (*Visipaque*) Iodinated, nonionic, iso-osmolar IV contrast. ▶K ♀B ▶? $$$

IOHEXOL (*Omnipaque*) Iodinated, nonionic, low-osmolality for IV, intrathecal, and oral/body cavity contrast. Dosages vary depending on forms and type of study, see package insert. Oral pass-thru examination of the GI tract: Dosages vary depending on forms, however one example dose would be to mix 50 mL of Omnipaque 350 into one liter of water and have patient drink 500 mL one hour prior to study and remainder 30 min prior to study. [Omnipaque 140, 180, 240, 300, 350] ▶K ♀B ▶? $$$

IOPAMIDOL (*Isovue*) Iodinated, nonionic, low-osmolality IV contrast. ▶K ♀? ▶? $$

IOPROMIDE (*Ultravist*) Iodinated, nonionic, low-osmolality IV contrast. ▶K ♀B ▶? $$$

IOTHALAMATE (*Conray, ✦Vascoray*) Iodinated, ionic, high-osmolality IV contrast. ▶K ♀B ▶– $

IOVERSOL (*Optiray*) Iodinated, nonionic, low-osmolality IV contrast. ▶K ♀B ▶? $$

IOXAGLATE (*Hexabrix*) Iodinated, ionic, low-osmolality IV contrast. ▶K ♀B ▶– $$$

IOXILAN (*Oxilan*) Iodinated, nonionic, low-osmolality IV contrast. ▶K ♀B ▶– $$$

DERMATOLOGY

CORTICOSTEROIDS: TOPICAL

Potency*	Generic	Trade Name**	Forms	Frequency
Low	alclometasone dipropionate	Aclovate	0.05% C/O	bid-tid
Low	clocortolone pivalate	Cloderm	0.1% C	tid
Low	desonide	DesOwen, Desonate, LoKara, Verdeso	0.05% C/L/O/F/G	bid-tid
Low	hydrocortisone	Hytone, others	0.5% C/L/O; 1% C/L/O; 2.5% C/L/O	bid-qid
Low	hydrocortisone acetate	Cortaid, Corticaine	0.5% C/O; 1% C/O/Sp	bid-qid
Medium	betamethasone valerate	Luxiq	0.1% C/L/O; 0.12% F (Luxiq)	qd-bid
Medium	desoximetasone‡	Topicort, LP Topicort	0.25% C	bid

(cont.)

CORTICOSTEROIDS: TOPICAL (*continued*)

Potency*	Generic	Trade Name**	Forms	Frequency
Medium	fluocinolone	Synalar, Dermasmoothe FS Scalp Oil	0.01% C/S; 0.025% C/O	bid-qid
Medium	flurandrenolide	Cordran	0.025% C/O; 0.05% C/L/O/T	bid-qid
Medium	fluticasone propionate	Cutivate	0.005% O; 0.05% C/L	daily-bid
Medium	hydrocortisone butyrate	Locoid	0.1% C/O/S	bid-tid
Medium	hydrocortisone valerate	Westcort	0.2% C/O	bid-tid
Medium	mometasone furoate	Elocon	0.1% C/L/O	qd

(cont.)

Medium	triamcinolone[‡]	Aristocort, Kenalog	0.025% C/L/O; 0.1% C/L/O/S	bid-tid
High	amcinonide	Cyclocort	0.1% C/L/O	bid-tid
High	betamethasone dipropionate[‡]	Maxivate, others	0.05% C/L/O (non-Diprolene)	qd-bid
High	desoximetasone[‡]	Topicort	0.05% G; 0.25% C/O	bid
High	diflorasone diacetate[‡]	Maxiflor	0.05% C/O	bid
High	fluocinonide	Lidex, Vanos	0.1% C	bid-qid
High	halcinonide	Halog	0.1% C/O	bid-tid
High	triamcinolone[‡]	Aristocort, Kenalog	0.5% C/O	bid-tid
Very high	betamethasone dipropionate[‡]	Diprolene, Diprolene AF	0.05% C/G/L/O	qd-bid

(cont.)

CORTICOSTEROIDS: TOPICAL (*continued*)

Potency*	Generic	Trade Name**	Forms	Frequency
Very high	clobetasol	Temovate, Cormax, Olux, Temovate E	0.05% C/G/O/L/S/Sp/F (0lux)	bid
Very high	diflorasone diacetate‡	Psorcon	0.05% C/O	qd-tid
Very high	halobetasol propionate	Ultravate	0.05% C/O	qd-bid

bid = two times per day; tid = three times per day; qid = four times per day.

*Potency based on vasoconstrictive assays, which may not correlate with efficacy. Not all available.

**Not all brand name products are commercially available, but generic versions are marketed. products are listed, including those lacking potency ratings.

‡These drugs have formulations in more than once potency category.

C, cream; O, ointment; L, lotion; T, tape; F, foam; S, solution; G, gel; Sp, spray

Acne Preparations

ACANYA (clindamycin—topical + benzoyl peroxide) Apply daily. [Trade only: Gel (clindamycin 1.2% + benzoyl peroxide 2.5%) 50 g.] ▸K ♀C ▸+ $$$$$

ADAPALENE (*Differin*) Apply at bedtime. [OTC: Gel 0.1%. Rx only, Trade/Generic: Cream 0.1% (45 g). Gel 0.3% (45 g). Trade only: Soln 0.1% (59 mL). Generic only: Soln 0.1% (59 mL)] ▸bile ♀C ▸? $$$$

AZELAIC ACID (*Azelex, Finacea, Finevin*) Apply two times per day. [Trade only: Cream 20%, 30, 50 g (Azelex). Gel 15% 50 g (Finacea). Foam 15% 50g (Finacea).] ▸K ♀B ▸? $$$$$

BENZACLIN (clindamycin—topical + benzoyl peroxide) Apply two times per day. [Generic/Trade: Gel (clindamycin 1% + benzoyl peroxide 5%) 25, 50 g (jar). Trade only: 35 g (pump) and 50 g (pump).] ▸K ♀C ▸+ $$$$$

BENZAMYCIN (erythromycin—topical + benzoyl peroxide) Apply two times per day. [Generic/Trade: Gel (erythromycin 3% + benzoyl peroxide 5%) 23.3, 46.6 g. Trade only: Benzamycin Pak, #60 gel pouches.] ▸LK ♀C ▸? $$$

BENZOYL PEROXIDE (*Benzac, Benzagel 10%, Desquam, Clearasil, ✦Solugel*) Apply once daily; increase to two to three times per day if needed. [OTC and Rx generic: Liquid 2.5, 5, 10%. Bar 5, 10%. Mask 5%. Lotion 4, 5, 8, 10%. Cream 5, 10%. Gel 2.5, 4, 5, 6, 10, 20%. Pad 3, 4, 6, 8, 9%. Other strengths available.] ▸LK ♀C ▸? $

CLINDAMYCIN—TOPICAL (*Cleocin T, Clindagel, Evoclin, ✦Dalacin T*) Apply daily (Evoclin, Clindagel, ClindaMax) or two times per day (Cleocin T). [Generic/Trade: Gel 1% 30, 60 g. Lotion 1% 60 mL. Soln 1% 30, 60 mL. Foam 1% 50, 100 g. Pads 1% 60 ct.] ▸L ♀B ▸− $$$

✦ **DIANE-35** (cyproterone + ethinyl estradiol) Canada only. 1 tab PO daily for 21 consecutive days, stop for 7 days, repeat cycle. [Canada Generic/Trade: Blister pack of 21 tabs 2 mg cyproterone acetate/0.035 mg ethinyl estradiol.] ▸L ♀X ▸− $$

DUAC **(clindamycin—topical + benzoyl peroxide, ✦*Clindoxyl*)** Apply at bedtime. [Generic/Trade: Gel (clindamycin 1% + benzoyl peroxide 5%) 45 g.] ▶K ♀C ▶+ $$$$$

EPIDUO **(adapalene + benzoyl peroxide, *Epiduo Forte, ✦Tactuo*)** Apply daily. [Trade only: Epiduo, Tactuo Gel (0.1% adapalene + benzoyl peroxide 2.5%) 45 g. Epiduo Forte (0.3% adapalene + benzoyl peroxide 2.5%) 15, 30, 45, 60, 70 g.] ▶bile, K ♀C ▶? $$$$$

ERYTHROMYCIN—TOPICAL (*Eryderm, Erycette, Erygel, A/T/S, ✦Sans-Acne, Ery-Sol*) Apply two times per day. [Generic/Trade: Soln 2% 60 mL. Pads 2%. Gel 2% 30, 60 g.] ▶L ♀B ▶? $$

ISOTRETINOIN (*Absorica, Amnesteem, Claravis, Sotret, Myorisan, Zenatane, ✦Accutane Roche, Clarus*) 0.5 to 2 mg/kg/day PO divided two times per day for 15 to 20 weeks. Typical target dose is 1 mg/kg/day. Potent teratogen; use extreme caution. Can only be prescribed by healthcare professionals who are registered with the iPLEDGE program. May cause depression. Not for long-term use. [Generic: Caps 10, 20, 40 mg. Generic only: Caps (Absorica) 25, 35 mg. Caps (Sotret, Absorica, Claravis, and Zenatane) 30 mg.] ▶LK ♀X ▶– $$$$$

ONEXTON **(clindamycin—topical + benzoyl peroxide)** Apply once daily to the face. [Trade only: Gel (clindamycin 1.2% + benzoyl peroxide 3.75%) 50 g.] ▶K ♀C ▶+ $$$$

SALICYLIC ACID (*Akurza, Clearasil Cleanser, Stridex Pads*) Apply/wash area up to three times per day. [OTC Generic/Trade: Pads, Gel, Lotion, Liquid, Mask scrub, 0.5%, 1%, 2%. Rx Trade only (Akurza): Cream 6% 340 g. Lotion 6%, 355 mL.] ▶not absorbed ♀? ▶? $

SULFACET-R **(sulfacetamide—topical + sulfur)** Apply one to three times per day. [Generic/Trade: Lotions, cleansers, washes.] ▶K ♀C ▶? $$$

SULFACETAMIDE—TOPICAL (*Klaron*) Apply two times per day. [Generic/Trade: Lotion 10% 118 mL.] ▶K ♀C ▶? $$$$

TAZAROTENE (*Tazorac, Avage, Fabior*) Acne: Apply 0.1% cream (Tazorac) or foam (Fabior) at bedtime. Psoriasis: Apply 0.05%

(cont.)

cream at bedtime, increase to 0.1% prn. Wrinkles: Apply 0.1% cream (Avage) once daily. [Trade only: Cream (Tazorac) 0.05% and 0.1% 30, 60 g. Foam (Fabior) 0.1% 50, 100 g. Gel 0.05% and 0.1% 30, 100 g. Trade only: Cream (Avage) 0.1% 15, 30 g.] ▶L ♀X ▶? $$$$

TRETINOIN—TOPICAL (*Retin-A, Retin-A Micro, Renova, Retisol-A, Atralin,✦Stieva-A, Rejuva-A, Vitamin A Acid Cream*) Acne, wrinkles: Apply at bedtime. [Generic/Trade: Cream 0.025% 20, 45 g; 0.05% 20, 45 g; 0.1% 20, 45 g. Gel 0.01% 15, 45 g; 0.025% 15, 45 g; 0.05% 45 g. Micro gel 0.04%, 0.1% 20, 45, 50 g pump; 0.08% 50 g pump. Trade only: Renova cream 0.02% 40, 60 g.] ▶LK ♀C ▶? $$$

VELTIN (clindamycin—topical + tretinoin—topical) Apply at bedtime. [Trade: Gel clindamycin 1.2% + tretinoin 0.025%, 30, 60 g.] ▶LK ♀C ▶? $$$$$

ZIANA (clindamycin—topical + tretinoin—topical) Apply at bedtime. [Trade only: Gel clindamycin 1.2% + tretinoin 0.025% 30, 60 g.] ▶LK ♀C ▶? $$$$$

Actinic Keratosis Preparations

DICLOFENAC—TOPICAL (*Solaraze, Voltaren, Pennsaid*) Actinic/solar keratoses: Apply two times per day to lesions for 60 to 90 days (Solaraze). Osteoarthritis of areas amenable to topical therapy: 2 g (upper extremities) to 4 g (lower extremities) four times per day (Voltaren). 40 gtts to knee(s) four times daily (Pennsaid). [Generic/Trade: Gel 3% (Solaraze) 100 g. Soln 1.5% (Pennsaid) 150 mL. Trade only: Gel 1% (Voltaren) 100 g. Soln 2.0% Pump (Pennsaid) 112 g.] ▶L ♀C Category D at 30 weeks gestation and beyond. Avoid use starting at 30 weeks gestation. ▶? $$$ ∎

FLUOROURACIL—TOPICAL (*5-FU, Tolak, Carac, Efudex, Fluoroplex*) Actinic keratoses: Apply two times per day for 2 to 6 weeks or once daily to face, ear or scalp for 4 weeks (Tolak).

(cont.)

DERMATOLOGY

Superficial basal cell carcinomas: Apply 5% cream/soln two times per day. [Trade only: Cream 1% 30 g (Fluoroplex $$$$$). Generic/Trade: Cream 0.5% 30 g (Carac $$$$$). Soln 2%, 5% 10 mL (Efudex $$$$$). Cream 5% 40 g. Cream 4% 40 g (Tolak $$$$$).] ▶L ♀X ▶– $$$$$

INGENOL (*Picato*) Apply 0.015% gel to affected area on face and scalp once daily for 3 days or 0.05% gel on affected areas of trunk and extremities once daily for 2 days. [Trade: Gel 0.015% 0.25 g, 0.05% 0.25 g.] ▶not absorbed ♀C ▶? $$$$$

METHYL AMINOLEVULINATE (*Metvix, Metvixia*) Actinic keratosis: Apply cream to non-hyperkeratotic actinic keratoses lesion and surrounding area on face or scalp; cover with dressing for 3 h; remove dressing and cream and perform illumination therapy. Repeat in 7 days. [Trade only: Cream 16.8%, 2 g tube.] ▶not absorbed ♀C ▶?

Antibacterials (Topical)

BACITRACIN—TOPICAL Apply daily to three times per day. [OTC Generic/Trade: Oint 500 units/g 1, 15, 30 g.] ▶not absorbed ♀C ▶? $

✦FUSIDIC ACID—TOPICAL (*✦Fucidin*) Canada only. Apply three to four times per day. [Canada trade only: Cream 2% fusidic acid 5, 15, 30 g. Oint 2% sodium fusidate 5, 15, 30 g.] ▶L ♀? ▶? $

GENTAMICIN—TOPICAL Apply three to four times per day. [Generic only: Oint 0.1% 15, 30 g. Cream 0.1% 15, 30 g.] ▶K ♀D ▶? $$$

MAFENIDE (*Sulfamylon*) Apply one to two times per day. [Trade only: Topical soln 50 g packets. Cream 5% 57, 114, 454 g.] ▶LK ♀C ▶? $$$

METRONIDAZOLE—TOPICAL (*Noritate, MetroCream, MetroGel, MetroLotion, ✦Rosasol*) Rosacea: Apply daily (1%) or two times per day (0.75%). [Trade only: Cream (Noritate) 1% 60 g. Generic/Trade: Gel (MetroGel) 1% 45, 60 g. Gel 0.75% 45 g. Cream 0.75% 45 g. Lotion (MetroLotion) 0.75% 59 mL.] ▶KL ♀B (– in 1st trimester) ▶– $$$$

MUPIROCIN (*Bactroban, Centany*) Impetigo/infected wounds: Apply three times per day. Nasal MRSA eradication: 0.5 g of nasal formulation only in each nostril two times per day for 5 days. [Generic/Trade: Oint 2% 22 g. Nasal oint 2% 1 g single-use tubes (for MRSA eradication). Trade only: Cream 2% 15, 30 g.] ▶not absorbed ♀B ▷? $$

NEOSPORIN CREAM **(neomycin—topical + polymyxin— topical + bacitracin—topical)** Apply one to three times per day. [OTC Trade only: neomycin 3.5 mg/g + polymyxin 10,000 units/g; 15 g and unit dose 0.94 g.] ▶K ♀C ▷? $

NEOSPORIN OINTMENT **(bacitracin—topical + neomycin— topical + polymyxin—topical)** Apply one to three times per day. [OTC Generic/Trade: bacitracin 400 units/g + neomycin 3.5 mg/g + polymyxin 5000 units/g 15, 30 g and "to go" 0.9 g packets.] ▶K ♀C ▷? $

POLYSPORIN **(bacitracin—topical + polymyxin—topical, ✦*Polytopic*)** Apply one to three times per day. [OTC Trade only: Oint 15, 30 g and unit dose 0.9 g. Powder 10 g.] ▶K ♀C ▷? $

RETAPAMULIN (*Altabax*) Impetigo: Apply thin layer two times per day for 5 days. [Trade only: Oint 1% 15, 30 g.] ▶not absorbed ♀B ▷? $$$$

SILVER SULFADIAZINE (*Silvadene, ✦Flamazine*) Apply one to two times per day. [Generic/Trade: Cream 1% 20, 50, 85, 400, 1000 g.] ▶LK ♀B ▷– $$

Antifungals (Topical)

BUTENAFINE (*Lotrimin Ultra, Mentax*) Treatment of tinea pedis: Apply daily for 4 weeks or two times per day for 7 days. Tinea corporis, tinea versicolor, or tinea cruris: Apply daily for 2 weeks. [Rx Trade only: Cream 1% 15, 30 g (Mentax). OTC Trade only: Cream 1% 12, 24 g (Lotrimin Ultra).] ▶L ♀B ▷? $

CICLOPIROX (*Loprox, Loprox TS, Penlac, ✦Stieprox shampoo*) Tinea pedis, tinea cruris, tinea corporis, tinea versicolor, and candidiasis (cream, lotion): Apply two times per day. Fungal

(cont.)

nail infection (Penlac): Apply daily to affected nails; apply over previous coat; remove with alcohol every 7 days. Seborrheic dermatitis (Loprox shampoo): Shampoo two times per week for 4 weeks. [Generic/Trade: Shampoo (Loprox) 1% 120 mL. Nail soln (Penlac) 8% 6.6 mL. Generic only: Gel 0.77% 30, 45, 100 g. Cream (Loprox) 0.77% 15, 30, 90 g. Lotion (Loprox TS) 0.77% 30, 60 mL.] ▶K ♀B ▶? $$$$

CLOTRIMAZOLE—TOPICAL (*Lotrimin AF, Mycelex, ✤Canesten, Clotrimaderm*) Treatment of tinea pedis, tinea cruris, tinea corporis, tinea versicolor, and cutaneous candidiasis: Apply two times per day. [Note that different Lotrimin brand name products may contain clotrimazole, miconazole, or butenafine. Rx Generic only: Cream 1% 15, 30, 45 g. Soln 1% 10, 30 mL. OTC Generic/Trade (Lotrimin AF): Cream 1% 12, 24 g.] ▶L ♀B ▶? $

ECONAZOLE (*Ecoza*) Tinea pedis, tinea cruris, tinea corporis, tinea versicolor: Apply daily. Cutaneous candidiasis: Apply two times per day. [Generic only: Cream 1% 15, 30, 85 g. Trade only: Foam 1% 70 g (Ecoza-$$$$$).] ▶not absorbed ♀C ▶? $$

EFINACONAZOLE (*Jublia*) Onychomycosis of toenail: Apply once daily to affected toenail for 48 weeks. [Trade: Soln 1% 4, 8 mL brush applicator.] ▶minimal absorption ♀C ▶ $$$$$

KETOCONAZOLE—TOPICAL (*Extina, Nizoral, Nizoral AD, Xolegel, ✤Ketoderm*) Tinea/candidal infections: Apply daily. Seborrheic dermatitis: Apply cream one to two times per day for 4 weeks or gel daily for 2 weeks or foam two times per day for 4 weeks. Dandruff (Nizoral AD): Apply shampoo twice a week. Tinea versicolor: Apply shampoo to affected area, leave on for 5 min, rinse. [Generic/Trade: Shampoo 2% 120 mL. Generic only: Cream 2% 15, 30, 60 g. Trade only: Shampoo 1% 125, 200 mL (OTC Nizoral AD). Gel 2% 45 g (Xolegel). Foam 2% 50, 100 g (Extina).] ▶L ♀C ▶? $$

LULICONAZOLE (*Luzu*) Tinea pedis: Apply once daily for 2 weeks. Tinea cruris, tinea corporis: Apply once daily for 1 week. [Trade: 1% cream, 60 g.] ▶minimal absorption ♀C ▶? $$$$$

MICONAZOLE—TOPICAL (*Micatin, Lotrimin AF, Zeasorb AF*) Tinea, candida: Apply two times per day. [OTC Generic only: Cream 2% 15, 45 g. OTC Trade only: Powder 2% 70, 160 g. Spray powder 2% 90, 100, 140 g. Spray liquid 2% 90, 105 mL. Gel 2% 24 g.] ▶L ♀+ ▶? $

NAFTIFINE (*Naftin*) Tinea: Apply daily (cream) or two times per day (gel). [Generic/Trade: Cream 1% 60, 90 g. Cream 2% 45, 60 g. Trade only: Cream 1% Pump 90 g. Gel 1% 40, 60, 90 g. Gel 2% 45, 60 g.] ▶LK ♀B ▶? $$$$$

NYSTATIN—TOPICAL (*Mycostatin, Nyamyc, ✦Nyaderm*) Candidiasis: Apply two to three times per day. [Generic only: Cream, Oint 100,000 units/g 15, 30 g. Generic/Trade: Powder 100,000 units/g 15, 30, 60 g.] ▶not absorbed ♀C ▶? $$

OXICONAZOLE (*Oxistat, Oxizole*) Tinea pedis, tinea cruris, and tinea corporis: Apply one to two times per day. Tinea versicolor (cream only): Apply daily. [Generic/Trade : Cream 1% 30, 60, 90 g. Trade only: Lotion 1% 30, 60 mL.] ▶minimal absorption ♀B ▶? $$$$$

SERTACONAZOLE (*Ertaczo*) Tinea pedis: Apply two times per day. [Trade only: Cream 2% 60 g.] ▶minimal absorption ♀C ▶? $$$$$

TERBINAFINE—TOPICAL (*Lamisil, Lamisil AT*) Tinea: Apply one to two times per day. [OTC Generic/Trade (Lamisil AT): Cream 1% 12, 24 g. OTC Trade only: Spray pump soln 1% 30 mL. Gel 1% 6, 12 g.] ▶L ♀B ▶? $

TOLNAFTATE (*Tinactin*) Apply two times per day. [OTC Generic/Trade: Cream 1% 15, 30 g. Soln 1% 10 mL. Powder 1% 45 g. OTC Trade only: Gel 1% 15 g. Powder 1% 90 g. Spray powder 1% 100, 133, 150 g. Spray liquid 1% 100, 113 mL.] ▶? ♀? ▶? $

Antiparasitics (Topical)

BENZYL ALCOHOL (*Ulesfia*) Lice: Apply to dry hair to saturate scalp and hair. Rinse after 10 minutes. Reapply in 7 to 10 days. Flammable. [Trade only: Lotion 5% 60 mL and in 2-pack with nit comb.] ▶not absorbed – ♀B ▶? $$$$

CROTAMITON (*Eurax*) Scabies: Apply cream/lotion topically from chin to feet, repeat in 24 h, bathe 48 h later. Pruritus: Massage prn. [Trade only: Cream 10% 60 g. Lotion 10% 60, 480 mL.] ▶? ♀C ▶? $$$$$

LINDANE Other drugs preferred. Scabies: Apply 30 to 60 mL of lotion, wash after 8 to 12 h. Lice: 30 to 60 mL of shampoo, wash off after 4 min. Can cause seizures in epileptics or if overused/misused in children. Not for infants. [Generic only: Lotion 1% 60 mL. Shampoo 1% 60 mL.] ▶L ♀B ▶? $$$$

MALATHION (*Ovide*) Lice: Apply to dry hair, let dry naturally, wash off in 8 to 12 h. Repeat in 7 to 10 days, if lice present. Flammable. [Generic/Trade only: Lotion 0.5% 59 mL.] ▶? ♀B ▶? $$$$

PERMETHRIN (*Elimite, Acticin, Nix, ★Kwellada-P*) Scabies: Apply cream from head (avoid mouth/nose/eyes) to soles of feet and wash after 8 to 14 h. 30 g is typical adult dose. Repeat in 7 days. Lice: Saturate hair and scalp with 1% rinse, wash after 10 min. Do not use in age younger than 2 mo. May repeat therapy in 7 days, as necessary. [Generic/Trade: Cream (Elimite, Acticin) 5% 60 g. OTC Generic/Trade: Liquid creme rinse (Nix) 1% 60 mL.] ▶L ♀B ▶? $$

★R&C (pyrethrins + piperonyl butoxide) Lice: Apply shampoo, wash after 10 min. Reapply in 5 to 10 days. A-200 brand name no longer available. [OTC Generic/Trade: Shampoo (0.33% pyrethrins, 4% piperonyl butoxide) 60, 120 mL.] ▶L ♀C ▶? $

RID (pyrethrins + piperonyl butoxide) Lice: Apply shampoo/mousse, wash after 10 min. Reapply in 5 to 10 days prn. [OTC Generic/Trade: Shampoo 60, 120, 240 mL. OTC Trade only: Mousse 5.5 oz.] ▶L ♀C ▶? $

SPINOSAD (*Natroba*) Lice: Apply to dry hair/scalp to cover. Leave on 10 min then rinse. Retreat if live lice seen after 7 days. [Generic/Trade: Topical susp, 0.9%, 120 mL.] ▶not absorbed – ♀B ▶? $$$$$

Antipsoriatics

ACITRETIN (*Soriatane*) 25 to 50 mg PO daily. Avoid pregnancy during therapy and for 3 years after discontinuation. [Generic/Trade: Caps 10, 17.5, 25 mg.] ▶L ♀X ▶– $$$$$

ANTHRALIN (*Zithranol*) Scalp psoriasis: Apply shampoo to scalp 3 to 4 times a week. Lather and leave on for 3 to 5 min. Rinse. Psoriasis of skin or scalp: Apply cream once a day. Initially use short contact times (5 to 15 min) and gradually increase to 30 min. Wash off. [Trade: Shampoo 1% (Zithranol shampoo) 85 g. Cream 1.2% (Zithranol RR cream) 15, 45 g.] ▶minimal absorption ♀C ▶? $$$$$

ANTHRALIN (*Drithocreme*) Apply daily. Short contact periods (ie, 15 to 20 min) followed by removal may be preferred. [Trade only: Cream 0.5, 1% 50 g.] ▶? ♀C ▶– $$$

CALCIPOTRIENE (*Dovonex, Sorilux*) Apply two times per day. [Trade only: Oint 0.005% 30, 60, 100 g (Dovonex). Cream 0.005% 30, 60, 100 g (Dovonex). Foam for scalp 0.005% 60, 120 g (Sorilux). Generic/Trade: Scalp soln 0.005% 60 mL.] ▶L ♀C ▶? $$$$

✦DOVOBET (calcipotriol + betamethasone—topical) Canada only. Apply once daily for up to 4 weeks (severe scalp psoriasis) or up to 8 weeks (mild to moderate plaque psoriasis of body). [Rx: Trade: Gel (50 mcg/g calcipotriol and 0.5 mg/g betamethasone) 30g, 60g.] ▶L ♀D ▶? $$$$$

ENSTILAR (calcipotriene + betamethasone dipropionate) Apply to affected area once daily for up to 4 weeks. Discontinue when control is achieved. Do not use more than 60 g every 4 days. Flammable. [Foam (0.005% calcipotriene + 0.064% betamethasone dipropionate) 60 g.] ▶L ♀C ▶– $$$$$

IXEKIZUMAB (*Taltz*) Moderate to severe plaque psoriasis: 160 mg SC at week 0, then 80 mg SQ at weeks 2, 4, 6, 8, 10, and 12, then 80 mg SC every 4 weeks. [Trade only: prefilled autoinjector 80 mg, prefilled syringe 80 mg.] ▶proteolysis ♀?/?/? ▶? $$$$$

TACLONEX (calcipotriene + betamethasone—topical) Apply daily for up to 4 weeks. [Calcipotriene 0.005% +

(cont.)

betamethasone dipropionate 0.064%. Generic/Trade: Oint 60, 100 g. Trade only: Topical susp (Taclonex) 60, 120 g.] ▶L ♀C ▶? $$$$$

USTEKINUMAB (*Stelara*) Severe plaque psoriasis, active psoriatic arthritis, wt less than or equal to 100 kg: 45 mg SC initially and again 4 weeks later, followed by 45 mg SC q 12 weeks. For wt greater than 100 kg and psoriatic arthritis with moderate to severe plaque psoriasis: 90 mg SC initially and again 4 weeks later, followed by 90 mg SC q 12 weeks. [Trade only: 45 and 90 mg prefilled syringe and vial.] ▶L ♀B ▶? $$$$$

Antivirals (Topical)

ACYCLOVIR—TOPICAL (*Zovirax*) Herpes genitalis: Apply ointment q 3 h (6 times per day) for 7 days. Recurrent herpes labialis: Apply cream 5 times per day for 4 days. [Generic/Trade: Oint 5% 5, 15, 30 g. Trade only: Cream 5% 5 g.] ▶K ♀C ▶? $$$$$

DOCOSANOL (*Abreva*) Oral-facial herpes (cold sores): Apply 5 times per day until healed. [OTC Trade only: Cream 10% 2 g.] ▶not absorbed ♀B ▶? $

IMIQUIMOD (*Aldara, Zyclara, ✦Vyloma*) Genital/perianal warts: Apply once daily for up to 8 weeks. Wash off after 8 h. Non-hyperkeratotic, non-hypertrophic actinic keratoses on face/scalp in immunocompetent adults: Apply two times per week overnight for 16 weeks (Aldara) or once daily for two 2-week periods separated by a 2-week break (Zyclara). Wash off after 8 h. Primary superficial basal cell carcinoma: Apply 5 times a week for 6 weeks (Aldara). Wash off after 8 h. [Generic/Trade: Cream 5% (Aldara) single-use packets. Trade only: Cream 3.75% (Zyclara-$$$$$) single-use packets, box of 28 and 7.5 g pump. Cream 2.5% 7.5 g pump.] ▶not absorbed ♀C ▶? $$$

PENCICLOVIR (*Denavir*) Herpes labialis (cold sores): Apply cream q 2 h while awake for 4 days. [Trade only: Cream 1% tube 5 g.] ▶not absorbed ♀B ▶? $$$$$

PODOFILOX (*Condylox,* ✦*Condyline, Wartec*) External genital warts (gel and soln) and perianal warts (gel only): Apply two times per day for 3 consecutive days of the week and repeat for up to 4 weeks. [Generic/Trade: Soln 0.5% 3.5 mL. Trade only: Gel 0.5% 3.5 g.] ▶? ♀C ▶? $$$

PODOPHYLLIN (*Podocon-25, Podofin, Podofilm*) Warts: Apply by physician. [Not to be dispensed to patients. For hospital/clinic use; not intended for outpatient prescribing. Trade only: Liquid 25% 15 mL.] ▶? ♀– ▶– $$$

SINECATECHINS (*Veregen*) Apply three times per day to external genital and perianal warts for up to 16 weeks. [Rx Trade only: Oint 15% 30 g.] ▶minimal absorption ♀C ▶? $$$$$

Atopic Dermatitis Preparations

NOTE: *Potential risk of cancer. Should only be used as 2nd-line agent for short-term and intermittent treatment of atopic dermatitis in those unresponsive to or intolerant of other treatments.*

PIMECROLIMUS (*Elidel*) Apply two times per day. [Trade only: Cream 1% 30, 60, 100 g.] ▶L ♀C ▶? $$$$$ ∎

TACROLIMUS—TOPICAL (*Protopic*) Apply two times per day. [Generic/Trade: Oint 0.03%, 0.1% 30, 60, 100 g.] ▶minimal absorption ♀C ▶? $$$$$ ∎

Corticosteroid/Antimicrobial Combinations

CORTISPORIN (neomycin—topical + polymyxin—topical + hydrocortisone—topical) Apply two to four times per day. [Trade only: Cream 7.5 g. Oint (also contains bacitracin) 15 g.] ▶LK ♀C ▶? $$$$

✦**FUCIDIN-H** (fusidic acid—topical + hydrocortisone—topical) Canada only. Apply three times per day. [Canada Trade only: Cream (2% fusidic acid, 1% hydrocortisone acetate) 30 g.] ▶L ♀? ▶? $$

LOTRISONE (clotrimazole—topical + betamethasone—topical, ★Lotriderm) Apply two times per day. Do not use for diaper rash. [Generic/Trade: Cream (clotrimazole 1% + betamethasone 0.05%) 15, 45 g. Lotion (clotrimazole 1% + betamethasone 0.05%) 30 mL.] ▶L ♀C ▶? $$$

MYCOLOG II (nystatin—topical + triamcinolone—topical) Apply two times per day. [Generic only: Cream, Oint 15, 30, 60 g.] ▶L ♀C ▶? $$$$$

Hemorrhoid Care

ANALPRAM-HC (hydrocortisone—topical + pramoxine—topical, Epifoam, Proctofoam HC, Pramosone) [Generic/Trade: Cream (Analpram-HC 1% hydrocortisone + 1% pramoxine, 2.5% hydrocortisone + 1% pramoxine) 4, 30 g. Trade only: Topical aerosol foam (Proctofoam HC, Epifoam 1% hydrocortisone + 1% pramoxine) 10 g. Lotion (Analpram-HC, Pramosone 2.5% hydrocortisone + 1% pramoxine) 60, 120 mL. Lotion (Pramosone 1% hydrocortisone + 1% pramoxine) 60, 120, 240 mL. Oint (Pramosone 1% hydrocortisone + 1% pramoxine, 2.5% hydrocortisone + 1% pramoxine) 28 g.] ▶L ♀C ▶? $$$

DIBUCAINE (Nupercainal) Apply three to four times per day prn. [OTC Generic/Trade: Oint 1% 30, 60 g.] ▶L ♀? ▶? $

PRAMOXINE—TOPICAL (Tucks Hemorrhoidal Ointment, Fleet Pain Relief, ProctoFoam NS) Apply up to 5 times per day prn. [OTC Trade only: Oint (Tucks Hemorrhoidal Ointment) 30 g. Pads (Fleet Pain Relief) 100 each. Aerosol foam (ProctoFoam NS) 15 g.] ▶not absorbed ♀+ ▶+ $

STARCH (Tucks Suppositories) 1 suppository up to 6 times per day prn. [OTC Trade only: Supp (51% topical starch; vegetable oil, tocopheryl acetate) 12, 24 each.] ▶not absorbed ♀+ ▶+ $

WITCH HAZEL (Tucks) Apply to anus/perineum up to 6 times per day prn. [OTC Generic/Trade: Pads 50% 12, 40, 100 ea, generically available in various quantities.] ▶? ♀+ ▶+ $

Other Dermatologic Agents

ALITRETINOIN (*Panretin*, ✦*Toctino*) Apply two to four times per day to cutaneous Kaposi's lesions. [Trade only: Gel 0.1% 60 g.] ▶not absorbed ♀D ▶– $$$$$

ALUMINUM CHLORIDE (*Drysol, Certain Dri*) Apply at bedtime. [Rx Trade only: Soln 20% 37.5 mL bottle, 35, 60 mL bottle with applicator. OTC Trade only (Certain Dri): Soln 12.5% 36 mL bottle.] ▶K ♀? ▶? $

BECAPLERMIN (*Regranex*) Diabetic ulcers: Apply daily. [Trade only: Gel 0.01%, 15 g.] ▶minimal absorption ♀C ▶? $$$$$ ■

BRIMONIDINE—TOPICAL (*Mirvaso*) Persistent erythema associated with rosacea: Apply once daily to chin, forehead, nose, and each cheek. [0.33% gel, 30, 45 g.] ▶L ♀B ▶– $$$$$

CALAMINE Apply three to four times per day prn for poison ivy/oak or insect bite itching. [OTC Generic only: Lotion 120, 240, 480 mL.] ▶? ♀? ▶? $

CAPSAICIN (*Zostrix, Zostrix-HP, Qutenza*) Arthritis, post-herpetic or diabetic neuralgia: Apply three to four times per day. Post-herpetic neuralgia: 1 patch (Qutenza) applied for 1 hour in medical office, may repeat q 3 months. [Rx: Patch 8% (Qutenza). OTC Generic/Trade: Cream 0.025% 60 g, 0.075% (HP) 60 g. OTC Generic only: Lotion 0.025% 59 mL, 0.075% 59 mL.] ▶? ♀? ▶? $

COAL TAR (*Polytar, Tegrin, Cutar, Tarsum*) Seborrheic dermatitis: Apply shampoo at least twice a week. Psoriasis: Apply one to four times per day. [OTC Generic/Trade: Shampoo, cream, ointment, gel, lotion, liquid, oil, soap.] ▶? ♀? ▶? $

DEET (*Off, Cutter, Repel, Ultrathon, n-n-diethyl-m-toluamide*) Mosquito repellant: 10% to 50% every 2 to 6 h. Higher concentration products do not work better, but have a longer duration of action. [OTC Generic/Trade: Spray, lotion, towelette 4.75% to 100%.] ▶L ♀+ ▶+ $

DEOXYCHOLIC ACID (*Kybella*) Reduction of chin (submental) fullness: 0.2 mL injections 1 cm apart until all of planned

(cont.)

treatment areas have been injected. [Injectable solution.] ▶not absorbed ♀? ▶? $$$$$

DOXEPIN—TOPICAL (*Prudoxin, Zonalon*) Pruritus: Apply four times per day for up to 8 days. [Trade only: Cream 5% 30, 45 g.] ▶L ♀B ▶– $$$$$

EFLORNITHINE (*Vaniqa*) Reduction of facial hair: Apply to face two times per day. [Trade only: Cream 13.9% 30, 45 g.] ▶K ♀C ▶? $$$

HYALURONIC ACID (*Bionect, Restylane, Perlane*) Moderate to severe facial wrinkles: Inject into wrinkle/fold (Restylane, Perlane). Protection of dermal ulcers: Apply gel/cream/spray two or three times per day (Bionect). [OTC Trade only: Cream 2% 15, 30 g. Rx Generic/Trade: Soln 3% 30 mL. Gel 4% 30 g. Cream 4% 15, 30, 60 g. Injectable gel 2%.] ▶? ♀? ▶? $$$

HYDROQUINONE (*Eldopaque, Eldoquin, Eldoquin Forte, EpiQuin Micro, Esoterica, Glyquin, Lustra, Melanex, Solaquin, Claripel, ✦Ultraquin*) Hyperpigmentation: Apply two times per day. [OTC Trade only: Cream 2% 15, 30 g. Rx Generic/Trade: Soln 3% 30 mL. Gel 4% 30 g. Cream 4% 15, 30, 60 g.] ▶? ♀C ▶? $

IVERMECTIN—TOPICAL (*Sklice, Soolantra*) Lice (Sklice): Apply lotion to dry hair and scalp. Rinse after 10 min. Single application only. Rosacea (Soolantra): Apply cream to affected area once daily. [Trade: Lotion (Sklice) 0.5%, 120 mL. Cream (Soolantra) 1% 30, 45, 60 g.] ▶minimal absorption – ♀C ▶? $$$$$

LACTIC ACID (*Lac-Hydrin, AmLactin, ✦Dermalac*) Apply two times per day. [Trade only: Lotion 12% 150, 360 mL. OTC: Cream 12% 140, 385 g. AmLactin AP is lactic acid (12%) with pramoxine (1%).] ▶? ♀? ▶? $$

LIDOCAINE—TOPICAL (*Xylocaine, Lidoderm, Numby Stuff, LMX, Zingo, ✦Maxilene*) Apply prn. Dose varies with anesthetic procedure, degree of anesthesia required, and individual patient response. Postherpetic neuralgia: Apply up to 3 patches to affected area at once for up to 12 h within

(cont.)

a 24-h period. Apply 30 min prior to painful procedure (ELA-Max 4%). Discomfort with anorectal disorders: Apply prn (ELA-Max 5%). Intradermal powder injection for venipuncture/IV cannulation, 3 to 18 yo (Zingo): 0.5 mg to site 1 to 10 min prior. [For membranes of mouth and pharynx: Spray 10%, Oint 5%, Liquid 5%, Soln 2%, 4%, Dental patch. For urethral use: Jelly 2%. Patch (Lidoderm $$$$$) 5%. Intradermal powder injection system: 0.5 mg (Zingo). OTC Trade only: Liposomal lidocaine 4% (ELA-Max).] ▶LK ♀B ▶+ $ − varies by therapy

MINOXIDIL—TOPICAL (*Rogaine, Women's Rogaine, Rogaine Extra Strength, Minoxidil for Men***)** Androgenetic alopecia in men or women: 1 mL to dry scalp two times per day (2% soln) or once daily (5% soln). [OTC Generic/Trade: Soln 2% 60 mL (Rogaine, Women's Rogaine). Soln 5% 60 mL (Rogaine Extra Strength, Theroxidil Extra Strength—for men only). Foam 5% 60 g (Rogaine Extra Strength).] ▶K ♀C ▶− $

OATMEAL (*Aveeno***)** Pruritus from poison ivy/oak, varicella: Apply lotion four times per day prn. Also bath packets for tub. [OTC Generic/Trade: Lotion. Bath packets.] ▶not absorbed ♀? ▶? $

PLIAGLIS (tetracaine—topical + lidocaine—topical) Superficial dermatological procedures: Apply 20 to 30 min prior procedure. Tattoo removal: Apply 60 min prior procedure. [Generic/Trade: Cream lidocaine 7% + tetracaine 7% (30, 60, 100 g).] ▶minimal absorption ♀B ▶? $$

PRAMOSONE (pramoxine—topical + hydrocortisone—topical, *★Pramox HC*) Inflammatory and pruritic manifestations of corticosteroid-responsive dermatoses: Apply three to four times per day. [Generic/Trade: 1% pramoxine/1% hydrocortisone: Cream 30, 60 g. 1% pramoxine/2.5% hydrocortisone acetate: Cream 30, 60 g. Trade only: 1% pramoxine/1% hydrocortisone: Oint 30 g. Lotion 60, 120, 240 mL. 1% pramoxine/2.5% hydrocortisone acetate: Oint 30 g. Lotion 60, 120 mL.] ▶not absorbed ♀C ▶? $$$

SELENIUM SULFIDE (*Selsun, Exsel, Versel, Tersi***)** Dandruff, seborrheic dermatitis: Apply 5 to 10 mL two times per week for

(cont.)

DERMATOLOGY

2 weeks then less frequently, thereafter. Tinea versicolor: Apply 2.5% to affected area daily for 7 days. [OTC Generic/Trade: Lotion/Shampoo 1% 120, 210, 240, 325 mL, 2.5% 120 mL. Rx Generic/Trade: Lotion/Shampoo 2.5% 120 mL. Trade only: Foam 2.25% 70 g.] ▶? ♀C ▶? $

SUNSCREEN [Many formulations available.] ▶minimal absorption ♀? ▶+ $

SYNERA (tetracaine—topical + lidocaine—topical) Prior to venipuncture or IV cannulation: Apply for 20 to 30 min prior to procedure. Prior to superficial dermatologic procedure: Apply for 30 min prior to procedure. [Trade only: Topical patch (lidocaine 70 mg + tetracaine 70 mg).] ▶minimal absorption ♀B ▶? $$

TRI-LUMA (fluocinolone—topical + hydroquinone + tretinoin—topical) Melasma of the face: Apply at bedtime for 4 to 8 weeks. [Trade only: Cream 30 g (fluocinolone 0.01% + hydroquinone 4% + tretinoin 0.05%).] ▶minimal absorption ♀C ▶? $$$$

VUSION (miconazole—topical + zinc oxide + white petrolatum) Diaper rash: Apply to affected area with each change for 7 days. [Trade only: Oint 50 g.] ▶minimal absorption ♀C ▶? $$$$$

XERESE (acyclovir—topical + hydrocortisone—topical) Recurrent herpes labialis: Apply 5 times a day, starting at the first sign of symptoms. ▶minimal absorption ♀B ▶? $$$$$

ENDOCRINE AND METABOLIC

A1C REDUCTION IN TYPE 2 DIABETES

Intervention	Expected A1C Reduction with Monotherapy
Alpha-glucosidase inhibitors	0.5–0.8%
DPP-4 inhibitors (Gliptins)	0.5–0.8%
GLP-1 agonists	0.5–1%
Insulin	1.5–3.5%
Lifestyle modifications	1–2%
Meglitinides	0.5–1.5%
Metformin	1–2%
Pramlintide	0.5–1%
Sodium–glucose cotransporter 2 (SGLT2) inhibitors	0.5–1%
Sulfonylureas	1–2%
Thiazolidinediones	0.5–1.4%

References: *Diabetes Care* 2009; 32:195. *Diabetes Care* 2015; 38: 141.

IV SOLUTIONS

Solution	Dextrose	Calories/Liter	Na*	Ca*	Lactate*	Osm*
0.9 NS	0 g/L	0	154	0	0	310
LR	0 g/L	9	130	3	28	273
D5 W	50 g/L	170	0	0	0	253
D5 0.2 NS	50 g/L	170	34	0	0	320
D5 0.45 NS	50 g/L	170	77	0	0	405
D5 0.9 NS	50 g/L	170	154	0	0	560
D5 LR	50 g/L	170	130	2.7	28	527

* All given in mEq/L

ENDOCRINE AND METABOLIC

DIABETES NUMBERS*

Criteria for diagnosis

Pre-diabetes: Fasting glucose 100–125 mg/dL
A1C 5.7–6.4% 2 h after 75 g oral glucose
load: 140–199 mg/dL

Diabetes: [†]A1C ≥ 6.5% Fasting glucose ≥ 126 mg/dL
Random glucose with symptoms ≥ 200 mg/dL
2 h after 75 g oral glucose load ≥ 200 mg/dL

Self-monitoring glucose goals (non-pregnant adults) Preprandial: 80–130
mg/dL Postprandial: < 180 mg/dL

Glucose goals in hospitalized patients

Non-critically ill: 140–180 mg/dL; may
individualize based on glycemic control
prior to hospitalization and comobidities.

Critically ill: 140–180 mg/dL; more
stringent goals (eg, 110–140 mg/dL)
may be considered in select patients
if safely achievable without
significant hypoglycemia

DIABETES NUMBERS* *(continued)*

A1C goal: < 7% for most non-pregnant adults, individualize based on patient specific factors. Consider A1C < 6.5% if goal can be achieved without significant hypoglycemia or other adverse effects. (eg, no cardiovascular disease, long life expectancy, managed with lifestyle modifications). Consider A1C < 8% if history of severe hypoglycemia, advanced microvascular or macrovascular complications, unable to achieve goal despite optimal management, complicated comorbidities, limited life expectancy. A1C goal < 7.5% for pediatric Type 1 diabetes.

Mean glucose levels by A1C:

A1C (%)	Glucose (mg/dL)
6	126
7	154
8	183
9	212
10	240

Estimated average glucose (eAG):

eAG (mg/dL) =
$(28.7 \times 46.7 \text{ A1C}) - 46.7$

(cont.)

Complications prevention & management:

ASA‡ (75–162 mg/day) in Type 1 & 2 adults for primary prevention if 10-year cardiovascular risk >10% (includes most men and women older than 50 yo with at least one other major risk factor of hypertension, smoking, dyslipidemia, albuminuria or family history of premature ASCVD) and secondary prevention (those with ASCVD) without increased bleeding risk.

ACE inhibitor or **ARB** if hypertensive or albuminuria

Statin: high-intensity therapy in those with established ASCVD or as below in other risk groups. In those age 40 or older with recent acute coronary syndrome and LDL greater than 50 mg/dL consider consider adding ezetimibe to moderate intensity statin if unable to tolertate high intensity statin therapy.

DIABETES NUMBERS* (*continued*)

Statin recommendations for those without established ASCVD

Age	ASCVD Risk Factors (hypertension, overweight/obesity, smoking, LDL ≥ 100 mg/dL)	Statin Intensity Recommendation
Less than 40 yo	No	None
	Yes	Moderate or high
40 yo or older	No	Moderate
	Yes	High, if 40–75 yo Moderate or high, if older than 75 yo

(cont.)

(cont.)

Immunizations: annual flu vaccine; hepatitis B vaccine if previously unvaccinated and 19 to 59 yo, consider if age 60 yo or older; pneumococcal vaccine: PPSV23 to all age 2 or older, if age 65 yo or older and unvaccinated give PCV13 then PPSV23 6–12 months later, if age 65 yo or older and previously vaccinated with PPSV23, give PCV13 ≥ 12 months later.

Every visit: Measure BP (goal < 140/90 mm Hg§); weight (calculate BMI & provide recommendations if overweight/obese); visual foot exam; review self-monitoring glucose record; review/adjust meds; review self-mgmt skills, dietary needs, and physical activity; smoking cessation counseling.

Twice a year: A1C in those meeting treatment goals with stable glycemia (quarterly if not); dental exam.

Annually: Screening fasting lipid profile (or q 2 years with low-risk lipid values)**; creatinine; spot urinary albumin to creatinine ratio; dilated eye exam (q2 years if no evidence of retinopathy).

DIABETES NUMBERS* *(continued)*

*See recommendations at: care.diabetesjournals.org. References: *Diabetes Care* 2016;39(Suppl 1):S1–104. Glucose values are plasma. ASCVD=atherosclerotic cardiovascular disease.

†In the absence of symptoms, confirm diagnosis with glucose testing on subsequent day.

‡Avoid ASA if younger than 21 yo due to Reye's Syndrome risk; use if younger than 30 yo has not beenstudied.

§Lower systolic targets (ie, < 130 mm Hg) may be considered on a patient-specific basis (eg, albuminuria, younger patients, additional ASCVD risk factors) if treatment goals can be met without excessive treatment burden.

**In those on statin therapy, check a fasting lipid panel as needed to monitor for adherence.

(cont.)

CORTICOSTEROIDS

CORTICOSTEROIDS	Approximate Equivalent Dose (mg)	Relative Anti-inflammatory Potency	Relative Mineralocorticoid Potency	Biological Half-life (h)
betamethasone	0.6–0.75	20–30	0	36–54
cortisone	25	0.8	2	8–12
dexamethasone	0.75	20–30	0	36–54
fludrocortisone	n/a	10	125	18–36
hydrocortisone	20	1	2	8–12
methylprednisolone	4	5	0	18–36
prednisolone	5	4	1	18–36
prednisone	5	4	1	18–36
triamcinolone	4	5	0	12–36

n/a, not available.

ENDOCRINE AND METABOLIC

Androgens / Anabolic Steroids

NOTE: *See OB/GYN section for other hormones.*

TESTOSTERONE (*Androderm, AndroGel, Axiron, Aveed, Depo-Testosterone, Natesto, Striant, Testim, Testopel, Vogelxo, ★Andriol*) Hypogonadism: Injectable enanthate or cypionate: 50 to 400 mg IM q 2 to 4 weeks. Injectable undecanoate (Aveed): 750 mg IM, repeat in 4 weeks then q 10 weeks thereafter. Testopel: 2 to 6 (150 to 450 mg testosterone) pellets SC q 3 to 6 months. Transdermal: Androderm: Start 4 mg patch to nonscrotal skin at bedtime. AndroGel 1%: Apply 5 g from gel pack or 4 pumps (5 g gel; 50 mg testosterone) from dispenser daily to shoulders/upper arms/abdomen. Androgel 1.62%: Apply 2 pumps (40.5 mg testosterone) from dispenser daily to shoulders or upper arms. Adjust based on serum testosterone concentration q 14 to 28 days. Dose range 1 to 4 pumps daily. Axiron: 60 mg (1 pump of 30 mg to each axilla) once daily. Testim: 1 tube (5 g) daily to shoulders/upper arms. Vogelxo: 50 mg (1 tube, 1 packet, or 4 pumps) once daily. Buccal: Striant: 30 mg q 12 h on upper gum above the incisor tooth; alternate sides for each application.   [Generic/Trade: Gel 1% 2.5, 5 g packet, 75 g multidose pump (AndroGel 1% 1.25 g gel containing 12.5 mg testosterone per actuation). Gel (Fortesta) 10 mg/actuation. Injection 100, 200 mg/mL (cypionate), 200 mg/mL (ethanate). Trade only: Patch 2, 4 mg/24 h (Androderm). Gel 1.62% (AndroGel 1.62%), 1.25, 2.5 g (package of 30), 75 g multidose pump (AndroGel 1.62% 20.25 mg testosterone/actuation). Gel 1%, 5 g tube (Testim). Gel (Vogelxo): 50 mg tube, 50 mg packet or multi-dose pump: 12.5 mg/actuation. Soln 90 mL multidose pump (Axiron, 30 mg/actuation). Nasal Gel (Natesto 5.5 mg/actuation pump) 7.32 g. Pellet 75 mg (Testopel). Buccal: Blister packs: 30 mg (Striant). IM injection (Aveed): 750 mg/3 mL through restricted access program.] ▶L ♀X ▶? ⊝III varies by therapy ∎

Bisphosphonates

ALENDRONATE (*Fosamax, Fosamax Plus D, Binosto, ★Fosavance*) Prevention of postmenopausal osteoporosis (Fosamax): 5 mg PO daily or 35 mg PO weekly. Treatment of postmenopausal osteoporosis (Fosamax, Fosamax Plus D, Binosto): 10 mg daily, 70 mg PO weekly, 70 mg/vitamin D3 2800 international units PO weekly, or 70 mg/vitamin D3 5600 international units PO weekly. Treatment of glucocorticoid-induced osteoporosis (Fosamax): 5 mg PO daily in men and women or 10 mg PO daily in postmenopausal women not taking estrogen. Treatment of osteoporosis in men (Fosamax, Fosamax Plus D, Binosto): 10 mg PO daily, 70 mg PO weekly, or 70 mg/vitamin D3 2800 international units PO weekly, or 70 mg/vit D3 5600 international units PO weekly. Paget's disease (Fosamax): 40 mg PO daily for 6 months. [Generic/Trade (Fosamax): Tabs 10, 70 mg. Generic only: Tabs 5, 35, 40 mg; Oral soln 70 mg/75 mL. Trade only: Fosamax Plus D: 70 mg + either 2800 or 5600 units of vitamin D3. Binosto: 70 mg effervescent tab.] ▶K ♀C ▶– $

ETIDRONATE Paget's disease: 5 to 10 mg/kg PO daily for 6 months or 11 to 20 mg/kg daily for 3 months. [Generic only: Tabs 200, 400 mg.] ▶K ♀C ▶? $$$$$

IBANDRONATE (*Boniva*) Prevention and treatment of postmenopausal osteoporosis: Oral: 150 mg PO once a month. IV: 3 mg IV q 3 months. [Generic/Trade: Tab 150 mg. IV 3 mg.] ▶K ♀C ▶? $$$$

PAMIDRONATE Hypercalcemia of malignancy: 60 to 90 mg IV over 2 to 24 h. Wait at least 7 days before considering retreatment. ▶K ♀D ▶? $$$

RISEDRONATE (*Actonel, Atelvia*) Prevention and treatment of postmenopausal osteoporosis: 5 mg PO daily, 35 mg PO weekly, or 150 mg once a month. Treatment of osteoporosis in men: 35 mg PO weekly. Prevention and treatment of glucocorticoid-induced osteoporosis: 5 mg PO daily. Paget's disease: 30 mg

(cont.)

PO daily for 2 months. [Generic/Trade: Tabs 5, 30, 35, 150 mg. Delayed-release tabs (Atelvia) 35 mg.] ▸K ♀C ▸? $$$$$

ZOLEDRONIC ACID (*Reclast, Zometa, ✦Aclasta*) Treatment of postmenopausal osteoporosis and osteoporosis in men (Reclast): 5 mg once yearly IV infusion over 15 min or longer. Prevention of postmenopausal osteoporosis: (Reclast) 5 mg IV infusion q 2 years. Prevention and treatment of glucocorticoid-induced osteoporosis (Reclast): 5 mg once a year IV infusion over 15 min or longer. Hypercalcemia (Zometa): 4 mg IV infusion over 15 min or longer. Wait at least 7 days before considering retreatment. Paget's disease (Reclast): 5 mg IV single dose infused over 15 min or longer. Multiple myeloma and metastatic bone lesions from solid tumors (Zometa): 4 mg IV infusion over 15 min or longer q 3 to 4 weeks. [Generic/Trade: 4 mg/5 mL IV (Zometa), 5 mg/100 mL IV (Reclast)] ▸K ♀D ▸? $$$$$

Corticosteroids

NOTE: *See also Dermatology, Ophthalmology.*

BETAMETHASONE (*Celestone Soluspan, ✦Betaject*) Anti-inflammatory/immunosuppressive: 0.6 to 7.2 mg/day PO divided two to four times per day; up to 9 mg/day IM. Fetal lung maturation, maternal antepartum: 12 mg IM q 24 h for 2 doses. [Generic: Syrup 0.6 mg/5 mL.] ▸L ♀C ▸– $$$$$

CORTISONE 25 to 300 mg PO daily. [Generic only: Tabs 25 mg.] ▸L ♀D ▸– $$$$$

DEXAMETHASONE (*DexPak, Dexamethasone Intensol, ✦Dexasone*) Anti-inflammatory/immunosuppressive: 0.5 to 9 mg/day PO/IV/IM, divided two to four times per day. Cerebral edema: 10 to 20 mg IV load, then 4 mg IM q 6 h (off-label IV use common) or 1 to 3 mg PO three times per day. Bronchopulmonary dysplasia in preterm infants: 0.5 mg/kg PO/IV divided q 12 h for 3 days, then taper. Croup: 0.6 mg/kg PO or IM for 1 dose. Acute asthma: age older than 2 yo: 0.6 mg/kg to max 16 mg PO

(cont.)

daily for 2 days. Fetal lung maturation, maternal antepartum: 6 mg IM q 12 h for 4 doses. Antiemetic, prophylaxis: 8 mg IV or 12 mg PO prior to chemotherapy; 8 mg PO daily for 2 to 4 days. Antiemetic, treatment: 10 to 20 mg PO/IV q 4 to 6 h. [Generic only: Tabs 0.5, 0.75, 1.0, 1.5, 2, 4, 6 mg; Elixir 0.5 mg/5 mL; Soln 0.5 mg/5 mL. Trade only: Tabs DexPak 13 day (51 total 1.5 mg tabs for a 13-day taper), DexPak 10 day (35 total 1.5 mg tabs for 10-day taper), DexPak 6 days (21 total 1.5 mg tabs for 6-day taper); Soln Dexamethasone Intensol 1 mg/1 mL (concentrate).] ▶L ♀C ▶– $

FLUDROCORTISONE Mineralocorticoid activity: 0.1 mg PO three times per week to 0.2 mg PO daily. Orthostatic hypotension: Start 0.1 mg PO daily; increase by 0.1 mg per week if needed to max 1 mg PO daily. [Generic only: Tabs 0.1 mg.] ▶L ♀C ▶? $

HYDROCORTISONE (*A-Hydrocort, Cortef, Solu-Cortef*) Adrenocortical insufficiency: 100 to 500 mg IV/IM q 2 to 6 h prn (sodium succinate) or 20 to 240 mg/day PO divided three to four times per day. Ulcerative colitis: 100 mg retention enema at bedtime (lying on side for 1 h or longer) for 21 days. [Generic/Trade: Tabs 5, 10, 20 mg; Enema 100 mg/60 mL.] ▶L ♀C ▶– $$$

METHYLPREDNISOLONE (*Solu-Medrol, Medrol, Depo-Medrol*) Anti-inflammatory/immunosuppressive: Oral (Medrol): Dose varies, 4 to 48 mg PO daily. Medrol Dosepak tapers 24 to 0 mg PO over 7 days. IM/Joints (Depo-Medrol): Dose varies, 4 to 120 mg IM q 1 to 2 weeks. Parenteral (Solu-Medrol): Dose varies, 10 to 250 mg IV/IM. Peds: 0.5 to 1.7 mg/kg PO/IV/IM divided q 6 to 12 h. [Trade only: Tabs 2 mg. Generic/Trade: Tabs 4, 8, 16, 32 mg. Medrol Dosepak (4 mg, 21 tabs).] ▶L ♀C ▶– $$

PREDNISOLONE (*Pediapred, Orapred ODT, Millipred, Veripred 20*) 5 to 60 mg PO daily. [Generic/Trade: Tabs 5 mg. Soln 5 mg/5 mL (Pediapred, raspberry flavor). Orally disintegrating tabs 10, 15, 30 mg (Orapred ODT). Trade only: Soln 10 mg/5 mL (Millipred, grape), 20mg/5 mL (Veripred). Generic only: Syrup 15 mg/5 mL. Soln 15 mg/5 mL, 25mg/5mL.] ▶L ♀C ▶+ $$$

PREDNISONE (*Deltasone, Prednisone Intensol, Rayos, ✦Winpred*) 1 to 2 mg/kg or 5 to 60 mg PO daily. [Generic only: Tabs 1, 2.5, 5, 10, 20, 50 mg. Soln 5 mg/5 mL. Dosepacks (5 mg tabs: Tapers 30 to 5 mg PO over 6 days or 30 to 10 mg over 12 days), Dosepacks Double Strength (10 mg tabs: Tapers 60 to 10 mg over 6 days, or 60 to 20 mg PO over 12 days) taper packs. Trade only: Delayed-release tabs 1, 2, 5 mg; Soln 5 mg/ mL (Prednisone Intensol).] ▶L ♀C ▶+ $

TRIAMCINOLONE (*Aristospan, Kenalog*) 4 to 48 mg PO/IM daily. Intra-articular 2.5 to 40 mg (Kenalog), 2 to 20 mg (Aristospan). [Trade only: Injection 10 mg/mL, 40 mg/mL, 5 mg/mL, 20 mg/ mL (Aristospan).] ▶L ♀C ▶– $

Diabetes-Related—Alpha-Glucosidase Inhibitors

ACARBOSE (*Precose, ✦Glucobay*) DM, Type 2: Start 25 mg PO three times per day with meals, and gradually increase as tolerated to maintenance, 50 to 100 mg three times per day. [Generic/Trade: Tabs 25, 50, 100 mg.] ▶Gut/K ♀B ▶– $$$

MIGLITOL (*Glyset*) DM, Type 2: Start 25 mg PO three times per day with meals, maintenance 50 to 100 mg three times per day. [Trade only: Tabs 25, 50, 100 mg.] ▶K ♀B ▶– $$$$$

Diabetes-Related—Combinations

NOTE: *Metformin-containing products: Assess eGFR prior to treatment and at least annually. Avoid in patients with an eGFR <30 mL/min/1.73 m^2; initiation in patients with eGFR 30 to 45 mL/min/1.73 m^2 is not recommended. In those already taking metformin if eGFR falls below 45 mL/min/1.73 m^2 reassess benefits and risks. Discontinue metformin at the time of or prior to an iodinated contrast imaging procedure and for 48 h after the procedure in those with eGFR <60 mL/min/1.73 m^2; in those with liver disease, alcoholism, or heart failure; or in those administered intra-arterial contrast. Reassess the eGFR post-procedure and reinitiate if renal function stable.*

ACTOPLUS MET (pioglitazone + metformin, *Actoplus Met XR*) DM, Type 2: 1 tab PO daily or two times per day. If inadequate control with metformin monotherapy, start 15/500 or 15/850 mg PO one to two times per day. If inadequate control with pioglitazone monotherapy, start 15/500 mg two times per day or 15/850 mg daily. Max 45/2550 mg/day. Extended-release, start 1 tab (15/1000 mg or 30/1000 mg) daily with evening meal. Max: 45/2000 mg/day. Obtain LFTs before therapy and periodically thereafter. [Generic/Trade: Tabs 15/500, 15/850 mg. Trade only: Extended-release (Actoplus Met XR) tabs: 15/1000, 30/1000 mg.] ▸KL ♀C ▸? $$$$$ ■

AVANDAMET (rosiglitazone + metformin) DM, Type 2, initial therapy (drug-naive): Start 2/500 mg PO one or two times per day. If inadequate control with metformin alone, select tab strength based on adding 4 mg/day rosiglitazone to existing metformin dose. If inadequate control with rosiglitazone alone, select tab strength based on adding 1000 mg/day metformin to existing rosiglitazone dose. Max 8/2000 mg/day. Obtain LFTs before therapy and periodically thereafter. [Trade only: Tabs 2/500, 2/1000 mg.] ▸KL ♀C ▸? $$$$ ■

DUETACT (pioglitazone + glimepiride) DM, Type 2: Start 30/2 mg PO daily. Start up to 30/4 mg PO daily if prior glimepiride therapy, or 30/2 mg PO daily if prior pioglitazone therapy; max 30/4 mg/day. Obtain LFTs before therapy and periodically thereafter. [Generic/Trade: Tabs 30/2, 30/4 mg pioglitazone/glimepiride.] ▸LK ♀C ▸— $$$$$ ■

GLUCOVANCE (glyburide + metformin) DM, Type 2, Initial therapy (drug-naive): Start 1.25/250 mg PO daily or two times per day with meals; max 10/2000 mg daily. Inadequate control with a sulfonylurea or metformin alone: Start 2.5/500 or 5/500 mg PO two times per day with meals; max 20/2000 mg daily. [Generic/Trade: Tabs 1.25/250, 2.5/500, 5/500 mg.] ▸KL ♀B ▸? $$$ ■

GLYXAMBI (empagliflozin + linagliptin) DM, Type 2: 1 tab (10 mg empagliflozin/5 mg linagliptin) PO daily in morning. May

(cont.)

increase to 25 mg empagliflozin/5 mg linagliptin PO daily. [Trade only: 10/5, 25/5 mg empagliflozin/linagliptin tabs.] ▶LK ♀C ▶? $$$$$

INVOKAMET (canagliflozin + metformin) DM, Type 2: 1 tablet PO twice daily. In patients not taking metformin, start with low dose of 500 mg metformin with gradual dose titration for GI tolerance. In patients not taking canagliflozin, start 50 mg canagliflozin. If eGFR 45 to less than 60 mL/min, max canagliflozin dose is 100 mg/day. [Trade only: 50/500, 50/1000, 150/500, 150/1000 canagliflozin/metformin tabs.] ▶KL ♀–?/X/X ▶? $$$$$ ■

JANUMET (sitagliptin + metformin, *Janumet XR*) DM, Type 2: Individualize based on patient's current therapy. Immediate-release: 1 tab PO two times per day. Extended-release: 1 tab PO daily. If inadequate control with metformin monotherapy: Immediate-release: Start 50/500 or 50/1000 mg two times per day based on current metformin dose. Extended-release: Start 100 mg sitagliptin daily plus current daily metformin. If inadequate control on sitagliptin: Immediate-release: Start 50/500 two times per day. Extended-release: Start 100/1000 daily. Max 100/2000 mg/day. Give with meals. [Trade only: Immediate-release tabs 50/500, 50/1000 mg, extended-release tabs 100/1000, 50/500, 50/1000 mg sitagliptin/metformin.] ▶K ♀B ▶? $$$$$ ■

JENTADUETO (linagliptin + metformin, *Jentadueto XR*) DM, Type 2: Immediate release: If prior metformin, start 2.5 mg linagliptin and current metformin dose PO two times per day. If no prior metformin, start 2.5/500 mg linagliptin/metformin PO two times per day. If current linagliptin/metformin, start at current doses. Extended-release: If prior metformin, start 5 mg linagliptin and current metformin dose PO daily. If no prior metformin, start 5/1000 mg linagliptin/metformin extended-release PO daily. If prior linagliptin/metformin, switch to 5 mg linagliptin and current metformin dose PO daily. Max 5/2000 mg daily. [Trade only: Immediate release tabs 2.5/500,

(cont.)

2.5/850, 2.5/1000 mg linagliptin/metformin. Extended release tabs 2.5/1000, 5/1000 linagliptin/extended-release metformin] ▶KL – ♀– ?/?/? ▶? $$$$$ ■

KAZANO **(alogliptin + metformin)** DM, Type 2: Individualize based on patient's current therapy. 1 tab PO two times per day. Max 25/2000 mg/day. Give with meals. [Trade only: 12.5/500, 12.5/1000 mg alogliptin/metformin.] ▶K – ♀B ▶ $$$$$

KOMBIGLYZE XR **(saxagliptin + metformin, ★*Komboglyze*)** DM, Type 2: If inadequately controlled on metformin alone, start 2.5 to 5 mg of saxagliptin plus current dose of metformin; give once daily with evening meal. If inadequately controlled on saxagliptin, start 5/500 mg once daily with evening meal. Max: 5/2000 mg/day. [Trade only: Tabs 5/500, 2.5/1000, 5/1000 mg.] ▶ ♀B ▶? $$$$$ ■

METAGLIP **(glipizide + metformin)** DM, Type 2, Initial therapy (drug-naive): Start 2.5/250 mg PO daily to 2.5/500 mg PO two times per day with meals; max 10/2000 mg daily. Inadequate control with a sulfonylurea or metformin alone: Start 2.5/500 or 5/500 mg PO two times per day with meals; max 20/2000 mg daily. [Generic only: Tabs 2.5/250, 2.5/500, 5/500 mg.] ▶KL ♀C ▶? $$$ ■

OSENI **(alogliptin + pioglitazone)** DM, Type 2: Individualize based on patient's current therapy. 1 tab PO daily. Max 25/45 mg/day. Obtain LFTs before therapy and periodically thereafter. [Trade only: Tabs 12.5/15, 12.5/30, 12.5/45, 25/15, 25/30, 25/45 mg alogliptin/pioglitazone.] ▶KL – ♀C ▶ $$$$$ ■

PRANDIMET **(repaglinide + metformin)** DM, Type 2, initial therapy (drug-naive): Start 1/500 mg PO daily before meals; max 10/2500 mg daily or 4/1100 mg/meal. May start higher if already taking higher coadministered doses of repaglinide and metformin. [Trade: Tabs 1/500, 2/500 mg.] ▶KL ♀C ▶? $$$$$ ■

SYNJARDY **(empagliflozin + metformin)** DM, Type 2: 1 tab PO twice daily. In patients not taking metformin, start with low dose of 500 mg metformin with gradual dose titration for GI tolerance. In patients not taking empagliflozin, start

(cont.)

5 mg empagliflozin. Titrate as tolerated for glycemic control. Max: 25/2000 mg empagliflozin/metformin per day. [Trade only: 5/500, 5/1000, 12.5/500, 12.5/1000 mg empagliflozin/metformin tabs.] ▸KL ♀C ▶? $$$$$ ■

XIGDUO XR (**dapagliflozin + metformin**) DM, Type 2: 1 tablet PO once daily in the morning with food. Individualize starting dose based on current treatment. [Trade only: 5/500, 5/1000, 10/500, 10/1000 mg dapagliflozin/metformin extended-release tabs.] ▸KL ♀C ▶? $$$$$ ■

DIABETES-RELATED—DPP-4 INHIBITORS

ALOGLIPTIN (*Nesina*)DM, Type 2: 25 mg PO daily. [Trade only: Tabs 6.25, 12.5, 25 mg.] ▸K – ♀?/?/? ▶? $$$$$

LINAGLIPTIN (*Tradjenta*, ✦ *Trajenta*) DM, Type 2: 5 mg PO once daily. [Trade only: Tab 5 mg.] ▸L – ♀B ▶? $$$$$

SAXAGLIPTIN (*Onglyza*) DM, Type 2: 2.5 or 5 mg PO daily. [Trade only: Tabs 2.5, 5 mg.] ▸LK ♀B ▶? $$$$$

SITAGLIPTIN (*Januvia*) DM, Type 2: 100 mg PO daily. [Trade only: Tabs 25, 50, 100 mg.] ▸K ♀B ▶? $$$$$

DIABETES-RELATED—GLP-1 AGONISTS

ALBIGLUTIDE (*Tanzeum*) DM, Type 2, adjunctive therapy: 30 mg SC once weekly. May increase to 50 mg SC once weekly. [Trade only: 30, 50 mg single-dose pen.] ▸proteolysis ♀C ▶? $$$$$ ■

DULAGLUTIDE (*Trulicity*) DM, Type 2: Start 0.75 mg SC once weekly. May increase to 1.5 mg SC once weekly. [Trade only: 0.75, 1.5 mg single-dose pen; 0.75, 1.5 mg single-dose prefilled syringe.] ▸proteolysis ♀C ▶? $$$$$ ■

EXENATIDE (*Byetta, Bydureon*) DM, Type 2, adjunctive therapy: Immediate-release: 5 mcg SC two times per day (within 1 h before the morning and evening meals, or 1 h before the two main meals of the day at least 6 h apart). May increase to 10 mcg SC two times per day after 1 month. Extended-release:

(cont.)

2 mg SC once weekly given any time of day without regard to meals. [Trade only: Byetta, prefilled pen (60 doses each) 5 mcg/dose, 1.2 mL; 10 mcg/dose, 2.4 mL. Bydureon (extended-release): 2 mg/vial; 2 mg/prefilled pen (single-use).] ▶ K/proteolysis ♀C ▶? $$$$$ ■

LIRAGLUTIDE (*Victoza, Saxenda*) DM, Type 2 (Victoza): Start 0.6 mg SC daily for 1 week, then increase to 1.2 mg SC daily. May increase to 1.8 mg SC daily. Chronic weight management (Saxenda): Start 0.6 mg SC daily for 1 week, then increase at weekly intervals to effective dose of 3 mg SC daily. [Trade only (Victoza): Multidose pen (18 mg/3 mL) delivers doses of 0.6, 1.2, or 1.8 mg. Trade only (Saxenda): Multidose pen (18 mg/3 mL) delivers doses of 0.6, 1.2, 1.8, 2.4, or 3 mg.] ▶proteolysis ♀C (Victoza), X (Saxenda) ▶? $$$$$ ■

Diabetes-Related—Insulins

INSULIN—INHALED SHORT-ACTING (*Afrezza*) Diabetes: Insulin naïve: Start 4 units inhaled at each meal. Switching from prandial insulin: 4 to 24 units inhaled per meal depending on prior insulin dose; round up to the nearest 4 units. Switching from premixed insulin: Estimate the mealtime dose by dividing half of the total daily injected premixed dose equally among three meals. Administer 4 to 24 units inhaled per meal depending on prior mealtime insulin dose; round up to the nearest 4 units. [Trade only: 4, 8, 12 unit cartridges.] ▶K ♀C ▶? $$$$$ ■

INSULIN—INJECTABLE, SHORT-/RAPID-ACTING (*Apidra, Novolin R, NovoLog, Humulin R, Humalog, ✦NovoRapid*) Diabetes: Doses vary, but typically total insulin 0.3 to 0.5 unit/kg/day SC in divided doses (Type 1), and 1 to 1.5 unit/kg/day SC in divided doses (Type 2). Generally, 50 to 70% of insulin requirements are provided by rapid- or short-acting insulin and the remainder from intermediate- or long-acting insulin. Administer rapid-acting insulin (Humalog, NovoLog, Apidra)

(cont.)

INJECTABLE INSULINS*

		Onset (h)	Peak (h)	Duration (h)
Rapid-/ short acting	Insulin aspart (NovoLog)	< 0.2	1–3	3–5
	Insulin glulisine (Apidra)	0.30–0.4	1	4–5
	Insulin lispro (Humalog)	0.25–0.5	0.5–2.5	3–5
	Regular (Novolin R, Humulin R)	0.5–1	2–3	5–8
Intermediate-/long acting	NPH (Novolin N, Humulin N)	2–4	4–10	10–16
	Insulin detemir (Levemir)	1–2	6–8	up to 24†
	Insulin glargine (Lantus, Toujeo, Basaglar)	2–4	peakless	24
	Insulin degludec (Tresiba)	1	peakless	>42

(cont.)

Mixtures			
Insulin aspart protamine susp/aspart (NovoLog Mix 70/30)	0.25	1–4 (biphasic)	10–16
Insulin lispro protamine susp/insulin lispro (Humalog Mix 75/25, Humalog Mix 50/50)	< 0.25	1–3 (biphasic)	10–16
NPH/Reg (Humulin 70/30, Novolin 70/30)	0.5–1	2–10 (biphasic)	10–16
Insulin degludec/aspart (Ryzodeg 70/30)	0.25	2–3	>24

*These are general guidelines, as onset, peak, and duration of activity are affected by the site of injection, physical activity, body temperature, and blood supply.

†Dose-dependent duration of action, range from 6 to 23 h.

n.a. = not available.

within 15 min before or immediately after a meal. Administer regular insulin 30 min before meals. Severe hyperkalemia: 5 to 10 units regular insulin plus concurrent dextrose IV. Profound hyperglycemia (eg, DKA): 0.1 unit regular/kg IV bolus, then initial infusion 100 units regular in 100 mL NS (1 unit/mL), at 0.1 units/kg/h. [Trade only: Injection regular 100 units/mL (Novolin R, Humulin R). Injection regular 500 units/mL (Humulin U-500, concentrated). Insulin glulisine (Apidra). Insulin lispro 100 units/mL (Humalog). Insulin aspart (NovoLog). Insulin available in pen form (100 units/mL): Novolin R InnoLet, Humulin R, Apidra SoloSTAR, Humalog KwikPen, NovoLog FlexPen. Insulin lispro 200 units/mL (Humalog U-200 KwikPen). Insulin regular 500 units/mL, concentrated (Humulin R U-500 KwikPen).] ▶LK ♀B/C ▶+ $$$$

INSULIN—INJECTABLE, INTERMEDIATE (*Novolin N, Humulin N, ReliOn Novolin N*) Diabetes: Doses vary, but typically total insulin 0.3 to 0.5 unit/kg/day SC in divided doses (Type 1), and 1 to 1.5 unit/kg/day SC in divided doses (Type 2). Generally, 50 to 70% of insulin requirements are provided by rapid- or short-acting insulin and the remainder from intermediate- or long-acting insulin. [Trade only: Injection NPH (Novolin N, Humulin N, ReliOn Novolin N). Insulin available in pen form: Humulin N KwikPen. Premixed preparations of NPH and regular insulin also available.] ▶LK ♀B/C ▶+ $$$$

INSULIN—INJECTABLE, LONG-ACTING (*Lantus, Levemir, Toujeo, Tresiba, Basaglar*) Diabetes: Doses vary, but typically total insulin 0.3 to 0.5 units/kg/day SC in divided doses (Type 1), and 1 to 1.5 units/kg/day SC in divided doses (Type 2). Generally, 50 to 70% of insulin requirements are provided by rapid- or short-acting insulin and the remainder from intermediate- or long-acting insulin. Lantus, Type 2 DM: Start 10 units or 0.2 units/kg SC daily (same time every day) in insulin-naive patients. Levemir, Type 2 DM: Start 10 units or 0.1 to 0.2 units/kg SC daily in the evening or divided twice daily in insulin-naive patients. DM, Type 1 (Lantus/Levemir): Start with

(cont.)

⅓ of total daily insulin dose; remainder of requirements from rapid- or short-acting insulin. [Trade only: Lantus (insulin glargine), Levemir (insulin detemir) 100 units/mL (U-100), 10 mL vial. Insulin available in pen form: Lantus SoloSTAR (glargine, U-100, 3 mL), Toujeo SoloSTAR (glargine, U-300, 1.5 mL), Levemir FlexTouch (detemir, U-100, 3 mL), Tresiba FlexTouch (degludec, U-100, U-200, 3 mL), Basaglar KwikPen (glargine, U-100,3 mL, avail Dec 16).] ▶LK ♀B/C ▶+ $$$$$

INSULIN—INJECTABLE COMBINATIONS (*Humalog Mix 75/25, Humalog Mix 50/50, Humulin 70/30, Novolin 70/30, NovoLog Mix 70/30), ReliOn Novolin 70/30, Ryzodeg 70/30*) Diabetes: Doses vary, but typically total insulin 0.3 to 1 unit/kg/day SC in divided doses (Type 1), and 0.5 to 1.5 unit/kg/day SC in divided doses (Type 2). Administer Humalog, NovoLog within 15 min before or immediately after a meal. Administer Ryzodeg with a meal. Administer regular insulin mixtures 30 min before meals. [Trade only: Insulin lispro protamine susp/ insulin lispro (Humalog Mix 75/25, Humalog Mix 50/50). Insulin aspart protamine/insulin aspart (NovoLog Mix 70/30). NPH and regular mixtures (Humulin 70/30, Novolin 70/30, ReliOn Novolin 70/30). Insulin degludec/insulin aspart mixture (Ryzodeg 70/30). Insulin available in pen form: NovoLog Mix 70/30 FlexPen, Humulin 70/30, Humalog Mix 75/25 KwikPen, Humalog Mix 50/50 KwikPen, Ryzodeg 70/30 FlexTouch.] ▶LK ♀B/C ▶+ $$$$$

Diabetes-Related—Meglitinides

NATEGLINIDE (*Starlix*) DM, Type 2: 120 mg PO three times per day within 30 min before meals; use 60 mg PO three times per day in patients who are near goal A1C. [Generic/Trade: Tabs 60, 120 mg.] ▶L ♀C ▶? $$$$

REPAGLINIDE (*Prandin, ✦GlucoNorm*) DM, Type 2: Start 0.5 to 2 mg PO three times per day before meals, maintenance 0.5 to 4 mg three to four times per day, max 16 mg/day. [Generic/Trade: Tabs 0.5, 1, 2 mg.] ▶L ♀C ▶? $$$

ENDOCRINE AND METABOLIC

Diabetes-Related—SGLT2 Inhibitors

CANAGLIFLOZIN (*Invokana*) DM, Type 2: 100 mg PO daily before 1st meal of the day. If tolerated and needed for glycemic control, may increase to 300 mg PO daily if eGFR greater than 60 mL/min. [Trade only: Tabs 100, 300 mg.] ▶LK – ♀– ?/X/X ▶? $$$$$

DAPAGLIFLOZIN (*Farxiga*, *Forxiga*) DM, Type 2: 5 mg PO daily in the morning, with or without food. If tolerated and needed for glycemic control, may increase to 10 mg PO daily. [Trade only: Tabs 5, 10 mg] ▶LK ♀C ▶– $$$$$

EMPAGLIFLOZIN (*Jardiance*) DM, Type 2: Start 10 mg PO daily in morning, with or without food. May increase up to 25 mg PO daily in morning, with or without food. [Trade only: 10, 25 mg.] ▶LK ♀C ▶? $$$$$

Diabetes-Related—Sulfonylureas—2nd Generation

GLICLAZIDE (*Diamicron, Diamicron MR*) Canada only. DM, Type 2, immediate-release: Start 80 to 160 mg PO daily, max 320 mg PO daily (160 mg or more per day should be in divided doses). Modified-release: Start 30 mg PO daily, max 120 mg PO daily. [Generic/Trade: Tabs 80 mg (Diamicron). Trade only: Tabs, modified-release 30 mg (Diamicron MR).] ▶KL ♀C ▶? $

GLIMEPIRIDE (*Amaryl*) DM, Type 2: Start 1 to 2 mg PO daily, usual 1 to 4 mg/day, max 8 mg/day. [Generic/Trade: Tabs 1, 2, 4 mg.] ▶LK ♀C ▶– $$

GLIPIZIDE (*Glucotrol, Glucotrol XL*) DM, Type 2: Start 5 mg PO daily, usual 10 to 20 mg/day, max 40 mg/day (divide two times per day if more than 15 mg/day). Extended-release: Start 5 mg PO daily, usual 5 to 10 mg/day, max 20 mg/day. [Generic/Trade: Tabs 5, 10 mg. Extended-release tabs 2.5, 5, 10 mg.] ▶LK ♀C ▶? $

GLYBURIDE (*DiaBeta, Glynase PresTab*, *Euglucon*) DM, Type 2: Start 1.25 to 5 mg PO daily, usual 1.25 to 20 mg daily or

(cont.)

divided two times per day, max 20 mg/day. Micronized tabs: Start 1.5 to 3 mg PO daily, usual 0.75 to 12 mg/day divided two times per day, max 12 mg/day. [Generic/Trade: Tabs (scored) 1.25, 2.5, 5 mg. Micronized tabs (scored) 1.5, 3, 6 mg.] ▶LK ♀B ▶? $

Diabetes-Related—Thiazolidinediones

PIOGLITAZONE (*Actos*) DM, Type 2: Start 15 to 30 mg PO daily, max 45 mg/day. Monitor LFTs. [Generic/Trade: Tabs 15, 30, 45 mg.] ▶L ♀C ▶– $$$$$ ■

ROSIGLITAZONE (*Avandia*) DM, Type 2 monotherapy or in combination with metformin or sulfonylurea: Start 4 mg PO daily or divided two times per day, max 8 mg/day. Obtain LFTs before therapy and periodically thereafter. [Trade only: Tabs 2, 4, 8 mg.] ▶L ♀C ▶– $$$$ ■

Diabetes-Related—Other

DEXTROSE (*Glutose, B-D Glucose, Insta-Glucose, Dex-4*) Hypoglycemia: 15 to 20 g PO once, repeat in 15 minutes if continued hypoglycemia per self-monitoring, or 0.5 to 1 g/kg (1 to 2 mL/kg) up to 25 g (50 mL) of 50% soln IV. Dilute to 25% for pediatric administration. [OTC Generic/Trade: Chewable tabs 4 g (Dex-4), 5 g (Glutose). Trade only: Oral gel 40%.] ▶L ♀C ▶? $

GLUCAGON (*GlucaGen*) Hypoglycemia: 1 mg IV/IM/SC, onset 5 to 20 min. Diagnostic aid: 1 mg IV/IM/SC. [Trade/generic: Injection 1 mg. Trade only: GlucaGen Diagnostic Kit, 1 mg; GlucaGen HypoKit 1 mg, Glucagon Emergency Kit 1 mg.] ▶LK ♀B ▶? $$$$$

METFORMIN (*Glucophage, Glucophage XR, Glumetza, Fortamet, Riomet*) DM, Type 2: Immediate-release: Start 500 mg PO one to two times per day or 850 mg PO daily with meals, may gradually increase to max 2550 mg/day. Extended-release: Glucophage XR: 500 mg PO daily with

(cont.)

evening meal; increase by 500 mg once a week to max 2000 mg/day (may divide two times per day). Glumetza: 1000 mg PO daily with evening meal; increase by 500 mg once a week to max 2000 mg/day (may divide two times per day). Fortamet: 500 to 1000 mg daily with evening meal; increase by 500 mg once a week to max 2500 mg/day. Polycystic ovary syndrome (unapproved, immediate-release): 500 mg PO three times per day. DM prevention, Type 2 (with lifestyle modifications, unapproved): 850 mg PO daily for 1 month, then increase to 850 mg PO two times per day. All products started at low doses to improve GI tolerability, gradually increase as tolerated. Avoid in patients with an eGFR less than 30 mL/min/1.73 m^2; initiation in patients with eGFR 30 to 45 mL/min/1.73 m^2 is not recommended. In those already taking metformin if eGFR falls below 45 mL/min/1.73 m^2 reassess benefits and risks. [Generic/Trade: Tabs 500, 850, 1000 mg, extended-release 500, 750 mg. Trade only, extended-release (Fortamet, Glumetza): 500, 1000 mg. Trade only (Riomet): Oral soln 500 mg/5 mL.] ▶K ♀B ▷? $$$ ■

PRAMLINTIDE (*Symlin, SymlinPen*) DM, Type 1 with mealtime insulin therapy: Initiate 15 mcg SC immediately before major meals and titrate by 15 mcg increments (if significant nausea has not occurred for at least 3 days) to maintenance 30 to 60 mcg as tolerated. DM, Type 2 with mealtime insulin therapy: Initiate 60 mcg SC immediately before major meals and increase to 120 mcg as tolerated (if significant nausea has not occurred for 3 to 7 days). Decrease initial premeal short-acting insulin doses by 50% including fixed-mix insulin (ie, 70/30). [Trade only: 1000 mcg/mL pen injector (SymlinPen) 1.5, 2.7 mL.] ▶K ♀C ▷? $$$$$ ■

Diagnostic Agents

COSYNTROPIN (*Cortrosyn, ✦Synacthen*) Rapid screen for adrenocortical insufficiency: 0.25 mg IM/IV over 2 min; measure serum cortisol before and 30 to 60 min after. ▶L ♀C ▷? $$$

Minerals

CALCIUM ACETATE (*PhosLo, Eliphos, Phoslyra*) Phosphate binder to reduce serum phosphorus in end-stage renal disease: Initially 2 tabs/caps or 10 mL of soln PO with each meal. [Generic/Trade: Gelcaps 667 mg (169 mg elem Ca). Tabs 667 mg (169 mg elem Ca). Trade only: Soln (Phoslyra): 667 mg (169 mg elemental calcium)/5 mL.] ▶K ♀C ▶? $

CALCIUM CARBONATE (*Caltrate, Mylanta Children's, Os-Cal, Oyst-Cal, Tums, Viactiv, ✶Calsan*) Supplement: 1 to 2 g elemental Ca/day or more PO with meals divided two to four times per day. Antacid: 1000 to 3000 mg PO q 2 h prn or 1 to 2 pieces gum chewed prn, max 7000 mg/day. [OTC Generic/Trade: Tabs 500, 650, 750, 1000, 1250, 1500 mg. Chewable tabs 400, 500, 750, 850, 1000, 1177, 1250 mg. Caps 1250 mg. Gum 300, 450 mg. Susp 1250 mg/5 mL. Calcium carbonate is 40% elem Ca and contains 20 mEq of elem Ca/g calcium carbonate. Not more than 500 to 600 mg elem Ca/dose. Available in combination with sodium fluoride, vitamin D, and/or vitamin K. Trade examples: Caltrate 600 + vitamin D = 600 mg elemental Ca/200 units vitamin D, Os-Cal 500 + D = 500 mg elemental Ca/200 units vitamin D, Os-Cal Extra D = 500 mg elemental Ca/400 units vitamin D, Tums (regular strength) = 200 mg elemental Ca, Tums (ultra) = 400 mg elemental Ca, Viactiv (chewable) 500 mg elemental Ca + 100 units vitamin D + 40 mcg vitamin K.] ▶K ♀+ (? 1st trimester) ▶? $

CALCIUM CHLORIDE 500 to 1000 mg slow IV q 1 to 3 days via central line or deep vein. [Generic only: Injectable 10% (1000 mg/10 mL) 10 mL ampules, vials, syringes.] ▶K ♀+ ▶+ $

CALCIUM CITRATE (*Citracal*) 1 to 2 g elemental Ca/day or more PO with meals divided two to four times per day. [OTC Trade/generic (mg elem Ca/units vitamin D): 200/250, 250/200, 315/250, 600/500 (slow release); some products available with magnesium and/or phosphorus. Chewable gummies: 250 mg with 250 units vitamin D.] ▶K ♀+ ▶+ $

CALCIUM GLUCONATE 2.25 to 14 mEq slow IV. 500 to 2000 mg PO two to four times per day. [Generic only: Injectable 10% (1000 mg/10 mL, 4.65 mEq/10 mL) 1, 10, 50, 100 mL. OTC Generic only: Tabs 500, 650, 700 mg. Chewable tabs 650 mg.] ▶K ♀+ ▶+ $

FERRIC CARBOXYMALTOSE (*Injectafer*) Iron deficiency anemia (unsatisfactory response to oral iron, non-dialysis dependent): If less than 50 kg: 15 mg/kg elemental iron IV for 2 doses, separated by at least 7 days. If 50 kg or greater: 750 mg elemental iron IV for 2 doses, separated by at least 7 days. Max: 1500 mg per course. [Trade only: 750 mg iron/15 mL vial.] ▶NA ♀C ▶? $$$$$

FERRIC GLUCONATE COMPLEX (*Ferrlecit*) 125 mg elemental iron IV over 10 min or diluted in 100 mL NS IV over 1 h. Peds age 6 yo or older: 1.5 mg/kg (max 125 mg) elemental iron diluted in 25 mL NS and administered IV over 1 h. ▶KL ♀B ▶? $$$$$

FERROUS GLUCONATE (*Fergon*) 800 to 1600 mg ferrous gluconate PO divided three times per day. [OTC Generic/Trade: Tabs (ferrous gluconate) 240 mg (27 mg elemental iron). Generic only: Tabs 324, 325 mg.] ▶K ♀+ ▶+ $

FERROUS SULFATE (*Fer-in-Sol, Feosol, Slow FE, ✦Ferodan*) 500 to 1000 mg ferrous sulfate (100 to 200 mg elemental iron) PO divided three times per day. [OTC Generic/Trade (mg ferrous sulfate): Tabs, extended-release 160 mg. Tabs 200, 324, 325 mg. OTC Generic only (mg ferrous sulfate): Soln 75 mg/0.6 mL. Elixir 220 mg/5 mL.] ▶K ♀+ ▶+ $

FERUMOXYTOL (*Feraheme*) Iron deficiency in chronic kidney disease: Give 510 mg IV infusion, followed by 510 mg IV infusion once given 3 to 8 days after initial injection. ▶KL ♀C ▶? $$$$$ ■

FLUORIDE (*Fluori-tab, ✦Fluor-A-Day*) Adult dose: 10 mL of topical rinse, swish and spit daily. Peds daily dose based on fluoride content of drinking water (table). [Generic only: Chewable tabs 0.25, 0.5, 1 mg. Gtts 0.125, 0.25, 0.5 mg/dropperful. Soln 0.2 mg/mL. Gel 0.1, 0.5, 1.23%. Rinse (sodium fluoride) 0.05, 0.1, 0.2%.] ▶K ♀? ▶? $

FLUORIDE SUPPLEMENTATION

Age	<0.3 ppm in drinking water	0.3–0.6 ppm in drinking water	>0.6 ppm in drinking water
0–6 mo	none	none	none
6 mo–3 yo	0.25 mg PO daily	none	none
3–6 yo	0.5 mg PO daily	0.25 mg PO daily	none
6–16 yo	1 mg PO daily	0.5 mg PO daily	none

JADA 2010;141:1480–1489

IRON DEXTRAN (*InFeD, DexFerrum, ✲Dexiron, Infufer*) 25 to 100 mg IM daily prn. Equations available to calculate IV dose based on wt and Hb. ▶KL ♀C ▶? $$$$$ ■

IRON POLYSACCHARIDE (*Niferex, Niferex-150, Nu-Iron 150, Ferrex 150*) 50 to 200 mg PO divided one to three times per day. [OTC Trade only: Caps 60 mg (Niferex). OTC Generic/Trade: Caps 150 mg (Niferex-150, Nu-Iron 150, Ferrex 150), Elixir 100 mg/5 mL (Niferex). 1 mg iron polysaccharide = 1 mg elemental iron.] ▶K ♀+ ▶+ $$ ■

IRON SUCROSE (*Venofer*) Iron deficiency with hemodialysis: 5 mL (100 mg elemental iron) IV over 5 min or diluted in 100 mL NS IV over 15 min or longer. Iron deficiency in nondialysis-dependent chronic kidney disease: 10 mL (200 mg elemental iron) IV over 5 min. ▶KL ♀B ▶? $$$$$ ■

MAGNESIUM CHLORIDE (*Slow-Mag*) 2 tabs PO daily. [OTC Trade only: Enteric-coated tab 64 mg. 64 mg tab Slow-Mag = 64 mg elemental magnesium.] ▶K ♀A ▶+ $

MAGNESIUM GLUCONATE (*Magtrate, Mangonate, Mag-G, ✦Maglucate*) 500 to 1000 mg PO divided three times per day. [OTC Generic only: Tabs 500 mg (27 mg elemental Mg).] ►K ♀A▶+ $

MAGNESIUM OXIDE (*Mag-200, Mag-Ox 400, Mag-Caps, Uro-Mag*) 400 to 800 mg PO daily. [OTC Generic/Trade: Caps/Tabs: 140 (84.5 mg elemental Mg); Tabs only: 200 (elemental), 250 (elemental), 400 (241 mg elemental Mg), 420 (253 mg elemental Mg), 500 mg (elemental).] ►K ♀A▶+ $

MAGNESIUM SULFATE Hypomagnesemia: 1 g of 20% soln IM q 6 h for 4 doses, or 2 g IV over 1 h (monitor for hypotension). Peds: 25 to 50 mg/kg IV/IM q 4 to 6 h for 3 to 4 doses, max single dose 2 g. Eclampsia: 4 to 6 g IV over 30 min, then 1 to 2 g/h. Drip: 5 g in 250 mL D5W (20 mg/mL), 2 g/h is a rate of 100 mL/h. Preterm labor: 6 g IV over 20 min, then 1 to 3 g/h titrated to decrease contractions. Monitor respirations and reflexes. If needed, may reverse toxic effects with calcium gluconate 1 g IV. Torsades de pointes: 1 to 2 g IV in D5W over 5 to 60 min. ►K ♀D C/D▶+ $

PHOSPHORUS (*Neutra-Phos, K-Phos*) 1 cap/packet PO four times per day. 1 to 2 tabs PO four times per day. Severe hypophosphatemia (eg, less than 1 mg/dL): 0.08 to 0.16 mmol/kg IV over 6 h. [OTC Trade only: (Neutra-Phos, Neutra-Phos K) tab/cap/packet 250 mg (8 mmol) phosphorus. Rx: Trade only: (K-Phos) tab 250 mg (8 mmol) phosphorus.] ►K ♀C ▶? $

POTASSIUM (**Cena-K**) IV infusion 10 mEq/h (diluted). 20 to 40 mEq PO one or two times per day. Use IV or immediate-release PO if rapid replacement needed. [Injectable, many different products in a variety of salt forms (ie, chloride, bicarbonate, citrate, acetate, gluconate), available in tabs, caps, liquids, effervescent tabs, packets. Potassium gluconate is available OTC. See table.] ►K ♀C ▶? $

ZINC ACETATE (*Galzin*) Dietary supplement: 8 to 12 mg (elemental) daily. Zinc deficiency: 25 to 50 mg (elemental) daily. Wilson's disease: 25 to 50 mg (elemental) PO three times per day. [Trade only: Caps 25, 50 mg elemental zinc.] ▶Minimal absorption ♀A ▶− $$$

POTASSIUM (ORAL FORMS)*

Effervescent Granules	
20 mEq	Klorvess Effervescent, K-vescent

Effervescent Tabs	
10 mEq	Effer-K
20 mEq	Effer-K
25 mEq	Effer-K, K+Care ET, K-Lyte, K-Lyte/Cl, Klor-Con/EF
50 mEq	K-Lyte DS, K-Lyte/Cl 50

Liquids	
20 mEq/15 mL	Cena-K, Kaochlor S-F, K-G Elixir, Kaochlor 10%, Kay Ciel, Kaon, Kaylixir, Kolyum, Potasalan, Twin-K
30 mEq/15 mL	Rum-K
40 mEq/15 mL	Cena-K, Kaon-Cl 20%
45 mEq/15 mL	Tri-K

Powders	
15 mEq/pack	K+Care
20 mEq/pack	Gen-K, K+Care, Kay Ciel, K-Lor, Klor-Con
25 mEq/pack	K+Care, Klor-Con 25

(cont.)

ENDOCRINE AND METABOLIC

POTASSIUM (ORAL FORMS)* (*continued*)

Tabs/Caps	
8 mEq	K+8, Klor-Con 8, Slow-K, Micro-K
10 mEq	K+10, K-Norm, Kaon-Cl 10, Klor-Con M10, Klotrix, K-Tab, K-Dur 10, Micro-K 10
20 mEq	Klor-Con M20, K-Dur 20

* Table provides examples and is not intended to be all inclusive.

ZINC SULFATE (*Orazinc*)   Dietary supplement: 8 to 12 mg (elemental) daily. Zinc deficiency: 25 to 50 mg (elemental) PO daily. [OTC Generic/Trade: Tabs 66, 110, 220 mg.] ▶Minimal absorption ♀A ▶– $

Nutritionals

BANANA BAG   Alcoholic malnutrition (example formula): Add thiamine 100 mg + folic acid 1 mg + IV multivitamins to 1 liter NS and infuse over 4 h. Magnesium sulfate 2 g may be added. "Banana bag" is jargon and not a valid drug order. Specify individual components. ▶KL ♀+ ▶+ $

LEVOCARNITINE (*Carnitor*)   10 to 20 mg/kg IV at each dialysis session. [Generic/Trade: Caps, 250, 300, 400 mg. Tabs 330, 500 mg. Oral soln 1 g/10 mL.] ▶KL ♀B ▶? $$$$$

Phosphate Binders

FERRIC CITRATE (*Auryxia*)   Treatment of hyperphosphatemia in end stage renal disease on dialysis: Start 2 tab PO three times daily with meals. Titrate by 1 to 2 tabs q week to achieve target serum phosphorous levels. Max 12 tabs/day. [Trade only (Tabs): 210 mg ferric iron (equivalent to 1 g ferric citrate).] ▶KL ♀B ▶? $$$$$ ■

LANTHANUM CARBONATE (*Fosrenol*) Hyperphosphatemia in end-stage renal disease: Start 1500 mg/day PO in divided doses with meals. Titrate dose q 2 to 3 weeks in increments of 750 mg/day until acceptable serum phosphate is reached. Most will require 1500 to 3000 mg/day to reduce phosphate to less than 6.0 mg/dL. Chew or crush tabs completely before swallowing; not to be swallowed whole. [Trade only: Chewable tabs 500, 750, 1000 mg. Oral powder 750, 1000 mg.] ▶Not absorbed ♀C ▶? $$$$$

SEVELAMER (*Renagel, Renvela*) Hyperphosphatemia: 800 to 1600 mg PO three times per day with meals. [Trade only (Renagel—sevelamer hydrochloride): Tabs 400, 800 mg. (Renvela—sevelamer carbonate): Tabs 800 mg. Powder: 800, 2400 mg packets.] ▶Not absorbed ♀C ▶? $$$$$

SUCROFERRIC OXYHYDROXIDE (*Velphoro*) Hyperphosphatemia in kidney disease on dialysis: Start 1 tab (500 mg) PO three times daily with meals, adjust weekly according to serum phosphorus concentrations. Tablets must be chewed. [Trade only: Tabs 500 mg.] ▶not absorbed ♀B ▶+ $$$$$

Thyroid Agents

LEVOTHYROXINE (*Synthroid, Tirosint, Unithroid, T4, ✦Eltroxin, Euthyrox*) Start 100 to 200 mcg PO daily (healthy adults) or 12.5 to 50 mcg PO daily (elderly or cardiovascular disease), increase by 12.5 to 25 mcg/day at 3- to 8-week intervals. Usual maintenance dose 100 to 200 mcg/day, max 300 mcg/day. [Generic/Trade: Tabs 25, 50, 75, 88, 100, 112, 125, 137, 150, 175, 200, 300 mcg. Trade only: Caps (Tirosint) 13, 25, 50, 75, 88, 100, 112, 125, 137, 150 mcg.] ▶L ♀A ▶+ $ ■

LIOTHYRONINE (*T3, Cytomel, Triostat*) Start 25 mcg PO daily, max 100 mcg/day. [Generic/Trade: Tabs 5, 25, 50 mcg.] ▶L ♀A ▶? $$ ■

METHIMAZOLE (*Tapazole*) Start 5 to 20 mg PO three times per day or 10 to 30 mg PO daily, then adjust. [Generic/Trade: Tabs 5, 10 mg.] ▶L ♀D ▶+ $$$

PROPYLTHIOURACIL (PTU, ✷*Propyl Thyracil*) Hyperthyroidism: Start 100 mg PO three times per day, then adjust. Thyroid storm: 200 to 300 mg PO four times per day, then adjust. [Generic only: Tabs 50 mg.] ▶L ♀D (but preferred over methimazole in 1st trimester) ▶+ $$$$ ■

Vitamins

ASCORBIC ACID (vitamin C, ✷*Redoxon*) 70 to 1000 mg PO daily. [OTC Generic only: Tabs 25, 50, 100, 250, 500, 1000 mg. Chewable tabs 100, 250, 500 mg. Timed-release tabs 500, 1000, 1500 mg. Timed-release caps 500 mg. Lozenges 60 mg. Liquid 35 mg/0.6 mL. Oral soln 100 mg/mL. Syrup 500 mg/5 mL.] ▶K ♀C ▶? $

CALCITRIOL (*Rocaltrol*) 0.25 to 2 mcg PO daily. Hypocalcemia and/or secondary hyperparathyroidism in chronic renal dialysis IV: 1 to 2 mcg, three times a week; increase dose by 0.5 to 1 mcg q 2 to 4 weeks. Adjust based on PTH. [Generic/Trade: Caps 0.25, 0.5 mcg. Oral soln 1 mcg/mL. Injection 1 mcg/mL.] ▶L ♀C ▶? $$

CYANOCOBALAMIN (vitamin B12, *Nascobal, B-12 Compliance Injection, Physicians EZ Use B-12*) Deficiency states: 100 to 200 mcg IM once a month or 1000 to 2000 mcg PO daily for 1 to 2 weeks followed by 1000 mcg PO daily, 500 mcg intranasal weekly. [OTC Generic only: Tabs 100, 250, 500, 1000, 5000 mcg. Extended-release Tabs 1000 mcg. SL Tabs 2500 mcg. Lozenges 50, 100, 250, 500 mcg. Rx Trade only: Nasal spray 500 mcg/spray (Nascobal 2.3 mL). Rx Trade/Generic: Injection 1000 mcg/mL.] ▶K ♀C ▶+ $

DOXERCALCIFEROL (*Hectorol*) Secondary hyperparathyroidism on dialysis: Oral: 10 mcg PO three times a week. May increase q 8 weeks by 2.5 mcg/dose; max 60 mcg/week. IV: 4 mcg IV three times a week at the end of dialysis. May increase dose q 8 weeks by 1 to 2 mcg/dose; max 18 mcg/week. Secondary hyperparathyroidism not on dialysis: Start 1 mcg PO daily, may increase by 0.5 mcg/dose q 2 weeks. Max 3.5 mcg/day. [Generic/Trade: Caps 0.5, 1, 2.5 mcg.] ▶L ♀B ▶? $$$$$

ERGOCALCIFEROL (vitamin D2, *Calciferol, Drisdol, ★OsteoForte*) Osteoporosis prevention and treatment (age 50 yo or older): 800 to 1000 units daily. Familial hypophosphatemia (vitamin D–resistant rickets): 12,000 to 500,000 units PO daily. Hypoparathyroidism: 50,000 to 200,000 units PO daily. Vitamin D deficiency: 50,000 units PO weekly or biweekly for 8 to 12 weeks. Adequate daily intake: 1 to 70 yo: 600 units (15 mcg); older than 70 yo: 800 units (20 mcg). [OTC Generic only: Caps 400, 1000, 5000 units. Soln 8000 units/mL (Calciferol). Rx Generic/Trade: Caps 50,000 units. Rx Generic only: Caps 25,000 units.] ▶L ♀A (C if exceed RDA) ▶+ $

FOLIC ACID (folate) 0.4 to 1 mg IV/IM/PO/SC daily. [OTC Brand/Generic: Tabs 0.4, 0.8 mg. Rx Generic: Tabs 1 mg.] ▶K ♀A ▶+ $

MULTIVITAMINS (MVI) Dose varies with product. Tabs come with and without iron. [OTC and Rx: Many different brands and forms available with and without iron (tabs, caps, chewable tabs, gtts, liquid).] ▶LK ♀+ ▶+ $

***NEPHRO-VITE RX* (ascorbic acid + folic acid + niacin + thiamine + riboflavin + pyridoxine + pantothenic acid + biotin + cyanocobalamin)** 1 tab PO daily. If on dialysis, take after treatment. [Generic/Trade: Vitamin C 60 mg/folic acid 1 mg/niacin 20 mg/thiamine 1.5 mg/riboflavin 1.7 mg/pyridoxine 10 mg/pantothenic acid 10 mg/biotin 300 mcg/cyanocobalamin 6 mcg.] ▶K ♀? ▶? $

***NEPHROCAP* (ascorbic acid + folic acid + niacin + thiamine + riboflavin + pyridoxine + pantothenic acid + biotin + cyanocobalamin)** 1 cap PO daily. If on dialysis, take after treatment. [Generic/Trade: Vitamin C 100 mg/folic acid 1 mg/niacin 20 mg/thiamine 1.5 mg/riboflavin 1.7 mg/pyridoxine 10 mg/pantothenic acid 5 mg/biotin 150 mcg/cyanocobalamin 6 mcg.] ▶K ♀? ▶? $$$$

NIACIN (vitamin B3, nicotinic acid, *Niacor, Slo-Niacin, Niaspan*) Niacin deficiency: 10 to 500 mg PO daily. Hyperlipidemia: Start 50 to 100 mg PO two to three times per day with meals, increase slowly, usual maintenance range

(cont.)

1.5 to 3 g/day, max 6 g/day. Extended-release (Niaspan): Start 500 mg at bedtime, increase monthly up to max 2000 mg. Extended-release formulations not listed here may have greater hepatotoxicity. Start with low doses and increase slowly to minimize flushing; 325 mg aspirin (non-EC) 30 to 60 min prior to niacin ingestion will minimize flush. [OTC Generic only: Tabs 50, 100, 250, 500 mg. Timed-release caps 250, 500 mg. Timed-release tabs 250, 500 mg. Liquid 50 mg/5 mL. Trade only: 250, 500, 750 mg (Slo-Niacin). Rx: Generic/Trade: Timed-release tabs 500, 750, 1000 mg (Niaspan, $$$$). Trade only: Tabs 500 mg (Niacor).] ▶K ♀C ▶? $

PARICALCITOL (*Zemplar*) Prevention/treatment of secondary hyperparathyroidism with renal insufficiency: 1 to 2 mcg PO daily or 2 to 4 mcg PO three times per week; increase dose by 1 mcg/day or 2 mcg/week until desired PTH level is achieved. Prevention/treatment of secondary hyperparathyroidism with renal failure (CrCl <15 mL/min): PO: To calculate initial dose divide baseline iPTH by 80 and then administer this dose in mcg three times per week. To titrate dose based on response, divide recent iPTH by 80 then administer this dose in mcg three times per week. IV: 0.04 to 0.1 mcg/kg (2.8 to 7 mcg) IV three times per week at dialysis; increase dose by 2 to 4 mcg q 2 to 4 weeks until desired PTH level is achieved. Max dose 0.24 mcg/kg (16.8 mcg). [Generic/Trade: Caps 1, 2, 4 mcg.] ▶L ♀C ▶? $$$$$

PHYTONADIONE (vitamin K, *Mephyton, AquaMephyton*) Single dose of 0.5 to 1 mg IM within 1 h after birth. Excessive oral anticoagulation: Dose varies based on INR. INR 4.5 to 10: 2012 CHEST guidelines recommend AGAINST routine vitamin K administration; INR greater than 10 with no bleeding: 2012 CHEST guidelines recommend giving vitamin K, but do not specify a dose, 2008 guidelines previously recommended 5 to 10 mg PO; serious bleeding and elevated INR: 5 to 10 mg slow IV infusion. Adequate daily intake: 120 mcg (males) and 90 mcg (females). [Trade only: Tabs 5 mg.] ▶L ♀C ▶+ $$$ ■

PYRIDOXINE (vitamin B6) 10 to 200 mg PO daily. Prevention of deficiency due to isoniazid in high-risk patients: 10 to 25 mg PO daily. Treatment of neuropathies due to isoniazid: 50 to 200 mg PO daily. Hyperemesis of pregnancy: 10 to 50 mg PO q 8 h. [OTC Generic only: Tabs 25, 50, 100, 250, 500 mg. Timed-release tab 100, 200 mg; Oral soln 200 mg/5 mL.] ▶K ♀A▶+ $

RIBOFLAVIN (vitamin B2) 5 to 25 mg PO daily. [OTC Generic only: Tabs 25, 50, 100 mg.] ▶K ♀A▶+ $

THIAMINE (vitamin B1) 10 to 100 mg IV/IM/PO daily. [OTC Generic only: Tabs 50, 100, 250, 500 mg. Enteric-coated tabs 20 mg.] ▶K ♀A▶+ $

VITAMIN A RDA: 900 mcg retinol equivalents (RE) (males), 700 mcg RE (females). Treatment of deficiency: 100,000 units IM daily for 3 days, then 50,000 units IM daily for 2 weeks. 1 RE is equivalent to 1 mcg retinol or 6 mcg beta-carotene. Max recommended daily dose 3000 mcg. [OTC Generic only: Caps 8,000, 10,000, 15,000, 25,000 units; Tabs 10,000 units. Rx: Generic: Trade only: Soln 50,000 units/mL.] ▶L ♀A (C if exceed RDA, X in high doses) ▶+ $

VITAMIN D3 (cholecalciferol) Osteoporosis prevention and treatment (age 50 or older): 800 to 1000 units daily. Familial hypophosphatemia (Vitamin D–resistant Rickets): 12,000 to 500,000 units PO daily. Hypoparathyroidism: 50,000 to 200,000 units PO daily. Adequate daily intake: 1 to 70 yo: 600 units; older than 70 yo: 800 units. [OTC Generic: 200, 400, 800, 1000, 2000, 4000, 5000 units (caps/tabs). Trade only: Soln 400, 1000, 2000, 4000 units/drop.] ▶L – ♀ ▶+ $

VITAMIN E (tocopherol, ✦Aquasol E) RDA: 22 units (natural, d-alpha-tocopherol) or 33 units (synthetic, d,l-alpha-tocopherol) or 15 mg (alpha-tocopherol). Max recommended 1000 mg alpha-tocopherol (1500 units) daily. [OTC Generic only: Tabs 200, 400 units. Caps 73.5, 100, 147, 165, 200, 330, 400, 500, 600, 1000 units. Gtts 50 mg/mL.] ▶L ♀A▶? $

Other

BROMOCRIPTINE (*Cycloset, Parlodel*) Type 2 DM: 0.8 mg PO q am (within 2 h of waking), may increase weekly by 0.8 mg to max tolerated dose of 1.6 to 4.8 mg q am. Hyperprolactinemia: Start 1.25 to 2.5 mg PO at bedtime, then increase q 3 to 7 days to usual effective dose of 2.5 to 15 mg/day, max 40 mg/day. Acromegaly: Usual effective dose is 20 to 30 mg/day, max 100 mg/day. Doses greater than 20 mg/day can be divided two times per day. Also approved for Parkinson's disease, but rarely used. Take with food to minimize dizziness and nausea. [Generic: Tabs 2.5 mg. Generic/Trade: Caps 5 mg. Trade only: Tabs 0.8 mg (Cycloset).] ▶L ♀B ▶– $$$$$

CABERGOLINE Hyperprolactinemia: 0.25 to 1 mg PO two times per week. [Generic: Tabs 0.5 mg.] ▶L ♀B ▶– $$$$$

CALCITONIN (*Miacalcin, Fortical, ✚Calcimar*) Osteoporosis: 100 units SC/IM every other day or 200 units (1 spray) intranasal daily (alternate nostrils). Paget's disease: 50 to 100 units SC/IM daily. Hypercalcemia: 4 units/kg SC/IM q 12 h. May increase after 2 days to max of 8 units/kg q 6 h. Skin test before using injectable product: 1 unit intradermally and observe for local reaction. Acute osteoporotic vertebral fracture pain (unapproved use): 100 units SC/IM daily or 200 units intranasal daily (alternate nostrils). [Generic/Trade: Nasal spray 200 units/activation in 3.7 mL bottle (minimum of 30 doses/bottle).] ▶Plasma ♀C ▶? $$$

DENOSUMAB (*Prolia*) Postmenopausal osteoporosis: 60 mg SC q 6 months. Osteoporosis in men: 60 mg SC q6 months. Increase bone mass in men receiving androgen deprivation therapy for nonmetastatic prostate cancer: 60 mg SC q 6 months. Increase bone mass in women receiving adjuvant aromatase inhibitor therapy for breast cancer at high risk of fracture: 60 mg SC q 6 months. [Trade only: 60 mg/1 mL vial (Prolia), prefilled syringe.] ▶? ♀X ▶? $$$$

DESMOPRESSIN (DDAVP, *Stimate*, ★*Minirin*, *Octostim*) Diabetes insipidus: 10 to 40 mcg intranasally daily or divided two to three times per day, 0.05 to 1.2 mg/day PO or divided two to three times per day, or 0.5 to 1 mL/day SC/IV in two divided doses. Hemophilia A, von Willebrand's disease: 0.3 mcg/kg IV over 15 to 30 min, or 150 to 300 mcg intranasally. Enuresis: 0.2 to 0.6 mg PO at bedtime. Not for children younger than 6 yo. [Trade only: Stimate nasal spray 150 mcg/0.1 mL (1 spray), 2.5 mL bottle (25 sprays). Generic/Trade (DDAVP nasal spray): 10 mcg/0.1 mL (1 spray), 5 mL bottle (50 sprays). Note difference in concentration of nasal soln. Rhinal tube: 2.5 mL bottle with 2 flexible plastic tube applicators with graduation marks for dosing. Tabs 0.1, 0.2 mg.] ▶LK ♀B ▶? $$$$$

PARATHYROID HORMONE (*Natpara*) Hypocalcemia in hypoparathyroidism: Start 50 mcg SC once daily in thigh (alternate thigh every other day). Adjust dose by 25 mcg q 4 weeks to max of 100 mcg to achieve serum calcium 8 to 9 mg/dL. [Trade only: 25, 50, 75, 100 mcg dose strength cartridges. Available through restricted-access program (NATPARA REMS).] ▶LK ♀C ▶? $$$$$ ■

PATIROMER (*Veltassa*) Hyperkalemia: 8.4 g PO daily with food. Adjust by 8.4 g daily on weekly basis as needed to achieve desired serum potassium. [Trade only: 8.4, 16.8, 22.2 g packets.] ▶not absorbed ♀− 0/0/0 ▶+ $$$$$ ■

SODIUM POLYSTYRENE SULFONATE (*Kayexalate*) Hyperkalemia: 15 g PO one to four times per day or 30 to 50 g retention enema (in sorbitol) q 6 h prn. Retain for 30 min to several hours. Irrigate with tap water after enema to prevent necrosis. [Generic only: Susp 15 g/60 mL. Powdered resin.] ▶Fecal excretion ♀C ▶? $

SOMATROPIN (human growth hormone, *Genotropin*, *Gentropin MiniQuick*, *Humatrope*, *Norditropin FlexPro*, *Nutropin AQ NuSpin*, *Nutropin AQ Pen*, *Omnitrope*, *Saizen*, *Serostim*, *Valtropin*, *Zomacton*, *Zorbitive*) Dosages vary by indication and product. [Single-dose vials (powder for injection with

(cont.)

diluent): Omnitrope: 5.8 mg vial. Saizen 5, 8.8 mg vial. Zomacton: 5, 10 mg vial. Zorbtive: 8.8 mg vial. Cartridges: Genotropin MiniQuick: 0.2, 0.4, 0.6, 0.8, 1, 1.2, 1.4, 1.6, 1.8, 2 single-use injection; 5.8, 13.8 mg cartridges. Humatrope: 6, 12, 24 mg pen cartridges; 5 mg vial (powder for injection with diluent). Pens: Norditropin FlexPro: 5, 10, 15, 30 mg. Nutropin AQ NuSpin: 5, 10, 20 mg. Omnitrope: 5, 10 mg. Saizen Click Easy 8.8 mg. Serostim: 4, 5, 6 mg single-dose vials.] ▶LK ♀B/C ▶? $$$$$

TERIPARATIDE (*Forteo*)   Treatment of postmenopausal osteoporosis, treatment of men and women with glucocorticoid-induced osteoporosis or to increase bone mass in men with primary or hypogonadal osteoporosis and high risk for fracture: 20 mcg SC daily in thigh or abdomen for no longer than 2 years. [Trade only: 28-dose pen injector (20 mcg/dose).] ▶LK ♀C ▶– $$$$$ ■

ENT

ENT COMBINATIONS (selected). Formulations and names change frequently.

	Decongestant	Antihistamine	Antitussive	Typical Adult Doses
OTC				
Benadryl-D Allergy/ Sinus Tablets	phenylephrine	diphenhydramine	–	1 tab q 4 h
Claritin-D 12-h, Alavert D-12	pseudoephedrine	loratadine	–	1 tab q 12 h
Claritin-D 24-h	pseudoephedrine	loratadine	–	1 tab daily
Dimetapp Cold & Allergy Elixir	phenylephrine	brompheniramine	–	20 mL q 4 h
Dimetapp DM Cold & Cough	phenylephrine	brompheniramine	dextromethorphan	20 mL q 4 h

(cont.)

ENT

ENT COMBINATIONS (selected). Formulations and names change frequently. (*continued*)

	Decongestant	Antihistamine	Antitussive	Typical Adult Doses
OTC				
Drixoral Cold & Allergy	pseudoephedrine	dexbrompheniramine	–	1 tab q 12 h
Mucinex-DM Extended-Release	–	–	guaifenesin, dextromethorphan	1–2 tabs q 12 h
Robitussin CF	phenylephrine	–	guaifenesin, dextromethorphan	10 mL q 4 h*
Robitussin DM, Mytussin DM	–	–	guaifenesin, dextromethorphan	10 mL q 4 h*

(cont.)

Robitussin PE, Guiatuss PE	phenylephrine	–	guaifenesin	10 mL q 4 h*B
Triaminic Cold & Allergy	phenylephrine	chlorpheniramine	–	10 mL q 4 h*
Rx Only				
Allegra-D 12-h	pseudoephedrine	fexofenadine	–	1 tab q 12 h
Allegra-D 24-h	pseudoephedrine	fexofenadine	–	1 tab daily
Bromfenex	pseudoephedrine	brompheniramine	–	1 cap q 12 h
Clarinex-D 24-h	pseudoephedrine desloratadine	desloratadine	–	1 tab daily

(cont.)

ENT

ENT COMBINATIONS (selected). Formulations and names change frequently. *(continued)*

	Decongestant	Antihistamine	Antitussive	Typical Adult Doses
Rx Only				
Deconamine	pseudoephedrine	chlorpheniramine	—	1 tab or 10 mL tid–qid
Deconamine SR, Chlordrine SR	pseudoephedrine chlorpheniramine	chlorpheniramine	—	1 tab q 12 h
Deconsal I	phenylephrine	—	guaifenesin	1–2 tabs q 12 h
Dimetane-DX	pseudoephedrine	brompheniramine	dextromethorphan	10 mL PO q 4 h

(cont.)

Duratuss	phenylephrine	—	guaifenesin	1 tab q 12 h
Duratuss HD ©II	phenylephrine	—	guaifenesin, hydrocodone	5–10 mL q 4–6 h
Entex PSE, Guaifenex PSE 120	pseudoephedrine	—	guaifenesin	1 tab q 12 h
Histussin D ©II	pseudoephedrine	—	hydrocodone	5 mL qid
Histussin HC ©II	phenylephrine	chlorpheniramine	hydrocodone	10 mL q 4 h
Humibid DM	—	—	guaifenesin, dextromethorphan	1 tab q 12 h

ENT COMBINATIONS (selected). Formulations and names change frequently. (*continued*)

	Decongestant	Antihistamine	Antitussive	Typical Adult Doses
Rx Only				
Hycotuss ©II	—	—	guaifenesin, hydrocodone	5 mL after meals & at bedtime
Phenergan/ Dextromethorphan	promethazine	promethazine	dextromethorphan	5 mL q 4–6 h
Phenergan VC	phenylephrine	promethazine	—	5 mL q 4–6 h

(cont.)

Phenergan VC w/codeine ©V	phenylephrine	promethazine	codeine	5 mL q 4–6 h
Robitussin AC ©V (generic only)	–	–	guaifenesin, codeine	10 mL q 4 h*
Robitussin DAC ©V (generic only)	pseudoephedrine	–	guaifenesin, codeine	10 mL q 4 h*
Rondec Syrup	phenylephrine	chlorpheniramine	–	5 mL qid†
Rondec DM Syrup	phenylephrine	chlorpheniramine	dextromethorphan	5 mL qid†
Rondec Oral Drops	phenylephrine	chlorpheniramine	–	0.75 to 1 mL qid

ENT COMBINATIONS (selected). Formulations and names change frequently. *(continued)*

	Decongestant	Antihistamine	Antitussive	Typical Adult Doses
Rx Only				
Rondec DM Oral Drops	phenylephrine	chlorpheniramine	dextromethorphan	0.75 to 1 mL qid
Rynatan	phenylephrine	chlorpheniramine	—	1–2 tabs q 12 h
Rynatan-P Pediatric	phenylephrine	chlorpheniramine	—	2.5–5 mL q 12 h*

(cont.)

Semprex-D	pseudoephedrine	acrivastine	—	1 c ap q 4–6 h
Tanafed (generic only)	pseudoephedrine	chlorpheniramine	—	10–20 mL q 12 h*
Tussionex ©II	—	chlorpheniramine	hydrocodone	5 mL q 12 h

tid=three times per day; qid=four times per day
*5 mL/dose if 6–11 yo. 2.5 mL if 2–5 yo.
†2.5 mL/dose if 6–11 yo. 1.25 mL if 2–5 yo.
‡Also contains acetaminophen.

Antihistamines—Non-Sedating

DESLORATADINE (*Clarinex*, ✦*Aerius*) 5 mg PO daily for age older than 12 yo. Peds: 2 mL (1 mg) PO daily for age 6 to 11 mo, ½ teaspoonful (1.25 mg) PO daily for age 12 mo to 5 yo, 1 teaspoonful (2.5 mg) or 2.5 mg ODT PO daily for age 6 to 11 yo. [Generic/Trade: Tabs 5 mg. Orally disintegrating tabs 2.5, 5 mg. Trade only: Syrup 0.5 mg/mL.] ▸LK ♀C ▸+ $

FEXOFENADINE (*Allegra*) 60 mg PO two times per day or 180 mg daily. Peds: 30 mg PO two times per day for age 2 to 11 yo. [OTC Generic/Trade: Tabs 30, 60, 180 mg. Susp 30 mg/5 mL. Trade only: Orally disintegrating tab 30 mg.] ▸LK ♀C ▸+ $

LORATADINE (*Claritin, Claritin Hives Relief, Claritin RediTabs, Alavert, Tavist ND*) 10 mg PO daily for age older than 6 yo, 5 mg PO daily for age 2 to 5 yo. [OTC Generic/Trade: Tabs 10 mg. Fast-dissolve tabs (Alavert, Claritin RediTabs) 5, 10 mg. Syrup 1 mg/mL. Rx Trade only (Claritin): Chewable tabs 5 mg; Liqui-gel caps 10 mg.] ▸LK ♀B ▸+ $

Antihistamines—Other

NOTE: *Antihistamines ineffective when treating the common cold. Contraindicated in narrow-angle glaucoma, BPH, stenosing peptic ulcer disease, and bladder obstruction. Use half the normal dose in the elderly. May cause drowsiness and/or sedation, which may be enhanced with alcohol, sedatives, and other CNS depressants. Deaths have occurred in children younger than 2 yo attributed to toxicity from cough and cold medications; the FDA does not recommend their use in this age group.*

CETIRIZINE (*Zyrtec, ✦Reactine, Aller-Relief*) Age 6 yo and older: 5 to 10 mg PO daily. Age 2 to 5 yo: initial dose 2.5 mg PO daily, max dose 2.5 mg twice a day or 5 mg once a day. Age 12 mo to < 2 yo: 2.5 mg daily with max dose of 2.5 mg twice a day. Age 6 mos to < 12 mos: 2.5 mg daily. [OTC Generic/Trade: Tabs 5, 10 mg. Syrup 5 mg/5 mL. Chewable tabs, grape

(cont.)

flavored 5, 10 mg. Trade only: oral disintegrating tab 10 mg, caps 10 mg.] ▶LK ♀B ▶– $

CHLORPHENIRAMINE (*Chlor-Trimeton, Aller-Chlor*) 4 mg PO q 4 to 6 h. Max 24 mg/day. Peds: Give 2 mg PO q 4 to 6 h for age 6 to 11 yo. Max 12 mg/day. [Generic/Trade: Tabs 4 mg. Syrup 2 mg/5 mL. Tabs, extended-release 12 mg.] ▶LK ♀B ▶– $

CLEMASTINE (*Tavist-1*) 1.34 mg PO two times per day. Max 8.04 mg/day. [OTC Generic/Trade: Tabs 1.34 mg. Rx: Generic only: Tabs 2.68 mg. Syrup 0.5 mg/5 mL.] ▶LK ♀B ▶– $

CYPROHEPTADINE (*Periactin*) Start 4 mg PO three times per day. Max 32 mg/day. [Generic only: Tabs 4 mg. Syrup 2 mg/5 mL.] ▶LK ♀B ▶– $$

DIPHENHYDRAMINE (*Benadryl, Banophen, Aller-Max, Diphen, Diphenhist, Dytan, Siladryl, Sominex, ✦Allerdryl, Nytol*) Allergic rhinitis, urticaria, hypersensitivity reactions: 25 to 50 mg IV/IM/PO q 4 to 6 h. Peds: 5 mg/kg/day divided q 4 to 6 h. EPS: 25 to 50 mg PO three to four times per day or 10 to 50 mg IV/IM three to four times per day. Insomnia: 25 to 50 mg PO at bedtime. [OTC Trade only: Tabs 25, 50 mg. Chewable tabs 12.5 mg. OTC and Rx: Generic only: Caps 25, 50 mg. Softgel cap 25 mg. OTC Generic/Trade: Soln 6.25 or 12.5 mg per 5 mL. Rx: Trade only: (Dytan) Susp 25 mg/mL. Chewable tabs 25 mg.] ▶LK ♀B ▶– $

HYDROXYZINE (*Atarax, Vistaril*) 25 to 100 mg IM/PO one to four times per day or prn. [Generic only: Tabs 10, 25, 50 mg. Caps 100 mg. Generic/Trade: Caps 25, 50 mg. Susp 25 mg/5 mL (Vistaril). Caps = Vistaril; Tabs = Atarax.] ▶L ♀C ▶– $

LEVOCETIRIZINE (*Xyzal*) 2.5 to 5 mg PO daily for age 12 yo or older. Peds: Give 2.5 mg PO daily for age 6 to 11 yo. Give 1.25 mg daily for age 6 mo to 5 yo. [Generic/Trade: Tabs, scored 5 mg. Oral soln 2.5 mg/5 mL (148 mL).] ▶K ♀B ▶– $$$

MECLIZINE (*Antivert, Bonine, Medivert, Meclicot, Meni-D*) Motion sickness: 25 to 50 mg PO 1 h prior to travel, then 25 to 50 mg PO daily. Vertigo: 25 mg PO q 6 h prn. [Rx/OTC/Generic/Trade: Tabs 12.5, 25 mg. Chewable tabs 25 mg. Rx/Trade only: Tabs 50 mg.] ▶L ♀B ▶? $

Antitussives / Expectorants

BENZONATATE (*Tessalon, Tessalon Perles, Zonatuss*)   100 to 200 mg PO three times per day. Swallow whole. Do not chew. Numbs mouth; possible choking hazard.   [Generic/Trade: Softgel caps 100, 200 mg. Trade only: Caps 150 mg (Zonatuss).] ▶L ♀C ▶? $$

DEXTROMETHORPHAN (*Benylin, Delsym, DexAlone, Robitussin Cough, Vick's 44 Cough*)   10 to 20 mg PO q 4 h or 30 mg PO q 6 to 8 h. Sustained action liquid 60 mg PO q 12 h.   [OTC Trade only: Caps 15 mg. Susp, extended-release 30 mg/5 mL (Delsym). Generic/Trade: Syrup 5, 7.5, 10, 15 mg/5 mL. Generic only: Lozenges 5, 7.5 mg.] ▶L ♀+ ▶+ $

GUAIFENESIN (*Robitussin, Hytuss, Guiatuss, Mucinex*)   100 to 400 mg PO q 4 h. 600 to 1200 mg PO q 12 h (extended-release). Peds: 50 to 100 mg/dose for age 2 to 5 yo, give 100 to 200 mg/dose for age 6 to 11 yo.   [OTC Generic/Trade: Extended-release tabs 600, 1200 mg. Liquid, Syrup 100 mg/5 mL, 200 mg/5 mL. OTC Trade only: Oral disintegrating tabs 50, 100 mg (Mucinex). OTC Generic only: Tabs 200, 400 mg.] ▶L ♀C ▶+ $

Combination Products—Rx Only

NOTE: *Decongestants in some ENT combination products can increase BP, aggravate anxiety, or cause insomnia (use caution). Some contain sedating antihistamines. Sedation can be enhanced by alcohol and other CNS depressants. Deaths have occurred in children younger than 2 yo attributed to toxicity from cough and cold medications; the FDA does not recommend their use in this age group.*

PHENERGAN WITH CODEINE (promethazine + codeine)   [Trade unavailable. Generic only: Syrup 6.25 mg promethazine/10 mg codeine/5 mL.] ▶LK ♀C ▶? ©V $ ■

REZIRA (hydrocodone + pseudoephedrine)   [Trade: Syrup 5 mg hydrocodone/60 mg pseudoephedrine/5 mL.] ▶LK – ♀C ▶– ©II $$$$

ZUTRIPRO (hydrocodone + chlorpheniramine + pseudoephedrine) [Trade: Syrup 5 mg hydrocodone/4 mg chlorpheniramine/60 mg pseudoephedrine/5 mL.] ▶LK – ♀C ▶–©Il $$$$$

Decongestants

NOTE: *See ENT—Nasal Preparations for nasal spray decongestants (oxymetazoline, phenylephrine). Deaths have occurred in children younger than 2 yo attributed to toxicity from cough and cold medications; the FDA does not recommend their use in this age group.*

PHENYLEPHRINE (*Sudafed PE*) 10 mg PO q 4 h. [OTC Trade only: Tabs 10 mg.] ▶L ♀C ▶+ $
PSEUDOEPHEDRINE (*Sudafed, Sudafed 12 Hour, Efidac/24, Dimetapp Decongestant Infant Drops, PediaCare Infants' Decongestant Drops, Triaminic Oral Infant Drops*) Adult: 60 mg PO q 4 to 6 h. Extended-release tabs: 120 mg PO two times per day or 240 mg PO daily. Peds: Give 15 mg PO q 4 to 6 h for age 2 to 5 yo, give 30 mg PO q 4 to 6 h for age 6 to 12 yo. [OTC Generic/Trade: Tabs 30, 60 mg. Tabs, extended-release 120 mg (12 h). Soln 15, 30 mg/5 mL. Trade only: Tabs, extended-release 240 mg (24 h). Rx only in some states.] ▶L ♀C ▶+ $

Ear Preparations

AURALGAN (benzocaine—otic + antipyrine) 2 to 4 gtts in ear(s) three to four times per day prn. [Generic only: Otic soln 10, 15 mL.] ▶Not absorbed ♀C ▶? $
CARBAMIDE PEROXIDE (*Debrox, Murine Ear*) 5 to 10 gtts in ear(s) two times per day for up to 4 days. [OTC Generic/Trade: Otic soln 6.5%, 15 mL.] ▶Not absorbed ♀? ▶? $
CIPRO HC OTIC (ciprofloxacin—otic + hydrocortisone—otic) 3 gtts in ear(s) two times per day for 7 days for age 1 yo to adult. [Trade only: Otic susp 10 mL.] ▶Not absorbed ♀C ▶– $$$$$

***CIPRODEX OTIC* (ciprofloxacin—otic + dexamethasone—otic)** 4 gtts in ear(s) two times per day for 7 days for age 6 mo to adult. [Trade only: Otic susp 7.5 mL.] ▶Not absorbed ♀C ▶— $$$$$

CIPROFLOXACIN—OTIC (*Cetraxal*) 1 single-use container in ear(s) two times per day for 7 days for age 1 yo to adult. [Trade only: 0.25 mL single-use containers with 0.2% ciprofloxacin soln, #14. Otic Suspension 1 mL vial of 60 mg/mL.] ▶Not absorbed ♀C ▶— $$$

***CORTISPORIN OTIC* (hydrocortisone—otic + polymyxin—otic + neomycin—otic)** 4 gtts in ear(s) three to four times per day up to 10 days of soln or susp. Peds: 3 gtts in ear(s) three to four times per day up to 10 days. Caution with perforated TMs or tympanostomy tubes as this increases the risk of neomycin ototoxicity, especially if use prolonged or repeated. Use susp rather than acidic soln. [Generic/Trade: Otic soln 10 mL. Generic only: Otic susp 10 mL.] ▶Not absorbed ♀? ▶? $$

***CORTISPORIN TC OTIC* (hydrocortisone—otic + neomycin—otic + thonzonium + colistin)** 4 to 5 gtts in ear(s) three to four times per day up to 10 days. [Generic only: Otic susp, 5 mL. Trade only: Otic susp, 10 mL.] ▶Not absorbed ♀? ▶? $$$

***DOMEBORO OTIC* (acetic acid + aluminum acetate)** 4 to 6 gtts in ear(s) q 2 to 3 h. Peds: 2 to 3 gtts in ear(s) q 3 to 4 h. [Generic only: Otic soln 60 mL.] ▶Not absorbed ♀? ▶? $$$

FLUOCINOLONE—OTIC (*DermOtic*) 5 gtts in affected ear(s) two times per day for 7 to 14 days for age 2 yo to adult. [Generic/Trade: Otic oil 0.01% 20 mL.] ▶L ♀C ▶? $$$$$

OFLOXACIN—OTIC (*Floxin Otic*) Otitis externa: 5 gtts in ear(s) daily for age 1 to 12 yo, 10 gtts in ear(s) daily for age 12 yo or older. [Generic/Trade: Otic soln 0.3% 5, 10 mL. Trade only: "Singles": Single-dispensing containers 0.25 mL (5 gtts), 2 per foil pouch.] ▶Not absorbed ♀C ▶— $$$

***SWIM-EAR* (isopropyl alcohol + anhydrous glycerins)** 4 to 5 gtts in ears after swimming. [OTC Trade only: Otic soln 30 mL.] ▶Not absorbed ♀? ▶? $

Mouth and Lip Preparations

CEVIMELINE (*Evoxac*) Dry mouth due to Sjögren's syndrome: 30 mg PO three times per day. [Generic/Trade: Caps 30 mg.] ▶L ♀C ▶– $$$$$

CHLORHEXIDINE GLUCONATE (*Peridex, Periogard*) Rinse with 15 mL of undiluted soln for 30 sec two times per day. Do not swallow. Spit after rinsing. [Generic/Trade: Oral rinse 0.12% 15 mL, 118 mL, and 473 mL bottles.] ▶Fecal excretion ♀B ▶? $

DEBACTEROL **(sulfuric acid + sulfonated phenolics)** Aphthous stomatitis, mucositis: Apply to dry ulcer. Rinse with water. [Trade only: 1 mL prefilled, single-use applicator.] ▶Not absorbed ♀C ▶+ $$

GELCLAIR **(maltodextrin + propylene glycol)** Aphthous ulcers, mucositis, stomatitis: Rinse mouth with 1 packet three times per day or prn. Do not eat or drink for 1 h after treatment. [Trade only: 15, 90 packets/box.] ▶Not absorbed ♀+ ▶+ $$$$$

LIDOCAINE—VISCOUS (*Xylocaine*) Mouth or lip pain in adults only: 15 to 20 mL topically or swish and spit q 3 h. [Generic/Trade: Soln 2%, 15 mL unit dose, 100 mL bottle. Soln 4%, 50 mL.] ▶LK ♀B ▶+ $

MAGIC MOUTHWASH **(diphenhydramine + Mylanta + sucralfate)** 5 mL PO swish and spit or swish and swallow three times per day before meals and prn. [Compounded susp. A standard mixture is 30 mL diphenhydramine liquid (12.5 mg/5 mL)/60 mL Mylanta or Maalox/4 g Carafate.] ▶LK ♀ ▶– $$$

PILOCARPINE (*Salagen*) Dry mouth due to radiation of head and neck or Sjögren's syndrome: 5 mg PO three to four times per day. [Generic/Trade: Tabs 5, 7.5 mg.] ▶L ♀C ▶– $$$$

Nasal Preparations—Corticosteroids

BECLOMETHASONE—NASAL (*Beconase AQ, Qnasl*) Beconase AQ: 1 to 2 spray(s) per nostril two times per day. Qnasl: 1 to 2 spray(s) per nostril daily. [Trade only: Beconase AQ

(cont.)

42 mcg/spray, 200 sprays/bottle. Qnasl: 40 mcg/spray, 60 or 120 sprays/bottle. Qnasl: 80 mcg/spray, 120 sprays/bottle.] ▶L ♀C ▶? $$$$

BUDESONIDE—NASAL (*Rhinocort Allergy Spray, Rhinocort Aqua*) 1 to 4 sprays per nostril daily. [Generic/Trade: Nasal inhaler 120 sprays/bottle. Trade only: Rhinocort Allergy Spray available OTC ($).] ▶L ♀B ▶? $$$$

CICLESONIDE—NASAL (*Omnaris, Zetonna*) Omnaris: 2 sprays per nostril daily. Zetonna: 1 actuation per nostril daily. [Trade only: Nasal spray, 50 mcg/spray, 120 sprays/bottle (Omnaris). Nasal aerosol, 37 mcg/actuation, 60 actuations/canister (Zetonna).] ▶L ♀C ▶? $$$$$

FLUNISOLIDE—NASAL (*Nasalide, ✦Rhinalar*) Start 2 sprays per nostril two times per day. Max 8 sprays/nostril/day. [Generic only: Nasal soln 0.025%.] ▶L ♀C ▶? $$$

FLUTICASONE—NASAL (*Flonase, Veramyst*) 2 sprays per nostril daily. [Generic: fluticasone Rx nasal spray 0.05% 15.8 mL 120 sprays/bottle. Brand: Flonase OTC nasal spray 0.05% 9.9 mL 60 sprays/bottle and 15.8 mL 120 sprays/bottle] ▶L ♀C ▶? $

MOMETASONE—NASAL (*Nasonex*) Adult: 2 sprays/nostril daily. Peds 2 to 11 yo: 1 spray/nostril daily. [Generic/Trade: Nasal spray, 120 sprays/bottle.] ▶L ♀C ▶? $$$$$

TRIAMCINOLONE—NASAL (*Nasacort AQ, Nasacort HFA, Tri-Nasal, AllerNaze*) Allergic rhinitis: 1 to 2 sprays per nostril daily. [Trade only: OTC: Nasal spray, 55 mcg/spray, 120 sprays/bottle (Nasacort Allergy 24HR) . Generic only: Rx: Nasal spray, 55 mcg/spray, 120 sprays/bottle.] ▶L ♀C ▶– $

Nasal Preparations—Other

AZELASTINE—NASAL (*Astelin, Astepro*) 1 to 2 sprays per nostril two times per day. [Generic/Trade: Astepro 0.15% nasal spray 200 sprays/bottle. Generic only: 0.1% nasal spray 200 sprays/bottle.] ▶L ♀C ▶? $$$$

CETACAINE (benzocaine + tetracaine + butamben) Topical anesthesia of mucous membranes: Spray: Apply for no more than 1 sec. Liquid or gel: Apply with cotton applicator directly to site. [Trade only: (14%/2%/2%) Spray 56 mL. Topical liquid 56 mL. Topical gel 5, 29 g.] ▶LK ♀C ▶? $$

CROMOLYN—NASAL (*NasalCrom*) 1 spray per nostril three to four times per day. [OTC Generic/Trade: Nasal inhaler 200 sprays/bottle 13, 26 mL.] ▶LK ♀B ▶+ $

DYMISTA (azelastine—nasal + fluticasone—nasal) 1 spray per nostril 2 times per day. [Trade only: Nasal spray: 137 mcg azelastine/50 mcg fluticasone/spray, 120 sprays/bottle.] ▶L – ♀C ▶? $$$$$

IPRATROPIUM—NASAL (*Atrovent Nasal Spray*) 2 sprays per nostril two to four times per day. [Generic/Trade: Nasal spray 0.03%, 30 mL (345 sprays)/bottle, 0.06%, 15 mL (165 sprays)/bottle.] ▶L ♀B ▶? $$

LEVOCABASTINE—NASAL (✦*Livostin*) Canada only. 2 sprays per nostril two times per day, increase prn to three to four times per day. [Trade only: Nasal spray 0.5 mg/mL, plastic bottles of 15 mL. 50 mcg/spray.] ▶L (but minimal absorption) ♀C ▶– $$

OLOPATADINE—NASAL (*Patanase*) 2 sprays per nostril two times per day. [Generic/Trade: Nasal spray 0.6% soln, 240 sprays/bottle.] ▶L ♀C ▶? $$$$$

OXYMETAZOLINE (*Afrin, Dristan 12 Hr Nasal, Nostrilla, Vicks Sinex 12 Hr*) 2 to 3 gtts/sprays per nostril two times per day prn nasal congestion for no more than 3 days. [OTC Generic/Trade: Nasal spray 0.05% 15, 30 mL; Nose gtts 0.05% 20 mL with dropper.] ▶L ♀C ▶? $

PHENYLEPHRINE—NASAL (*Neo-Synephrine*) 2 to 3 sprays or gtts per nostril q 4 h prn for no more than 3 days. [OTC Generic/Trade: Nasal gtts/spray 0.25, 0.5, 1% (15 mL).] ▶L ♀C ▶? $

SALINE NASAL SPRAY (*SeaMist, Entsol, Pretz, NaSal, Ocean, ✦hydraSense*) Nasal dryness: 1 to 3 sprays or gtts per nostril prn. [Generic/Trade (OTC): Nasal spray 0.4, 0.5, 0.65, 0.75%. Nasal gtts 0.4, 0.65%. Trade only: Preservative-free nasal spray 3% (Entsol).] ▶Not metabolized ♀A ▶+ $

GASTROENTEROLOGY

HELICOBACTER PYLORI THERAPY

- Triple therapy PO for 10 to 14 days: clarithromycin 500 mg two times per day plus amoxicillin 1 g two times per day (or metronidazole 500 mg two times per day) plus PPI*
- Quadruple therapy PO for 14 days: bismuth subsalicylate 525 mg (or 30 mL) four times per day plus metronidazole four times per day plus tetracycline 500 mg four times per day plus a PPI* or an H2 blocker†
- PPI or H2 blocker may need to be continued past 14 days to heal the ulcer.

*PPIs include esomeprazole 40 mg daily, lansoprazole 30 mg two times per day, omeprazole 20 mg two times per day, pantoprazole 40 mg two times per day, rabeprazole 20 mg two times per day, pantoprazole 40 mg two times per day, rabeprazole 20 mg two times per day.
†H2 blockers include cimetidine 400 mg two times per day, famotidine 20 mg two times per day, nizatidine 150 mg two times per day, ranitidine 150 mg two times per day. Adapted from *Treat Guidel Med Lett* 2008:55.

Antidiarrheals

BISMUTH SUBSALICYLATE (*Pepto-Bismol, Kaopectate*) 2 tabs or caplets or 30 mL (262 mg/15 mL) PO q 30 min to 1 h up to 8 doses per day for up to 2 days. Peds: 5 mL (262 mg/15 mL) or $^1/_3$ tab, chew tab, or cap PO for age 3 to 6 yo, 10 mL (262 mg/15 mL) or $^2/_3$ tab, chew tab, or cap PO for age 6 to 9 yo. Risk

(cont.)

of Reye's syndrome in children. [OTC Generic/Trade: Chewable tabs 262 mg. Susp 262, 525, 750 mg/15 mL. Caplets 262 mg (Pepto-Bismol). OTC Trade only: Susp 87 mg/5 mL (Kaopectate Children's Liquid).] ▶K ♀D ▶? $

IMODIUM MULTI-SYMPTOM RELIEF **(loperamide + simethicone)** 2 tabs or caplets PO initially, then 1 tab or caplet PO after each unformed stool to a max of 4 tabs/caplets per day. Peds: 1 tab or caplet PO initially, then ½ caplet PO after each unformed stool (up to 2 tabs or caplets PO per day for age 6 to 8 yo or wt 48 to 59 lbs or up to 3 tabs or caplets PO per day for age 9 to 11 yo or wt 60 to 95 lbs). [OTC Generic/Trade: Caplets, Chewable tabs 2 mg loperamide/125 mg simethicone.] ▶L ♀C ▶+ $

LOMOTIL **(diphenoxylate + atropine)** 2 tabs or 10 mL PO four times per day. [Generic/Trade: Oral soln or tab 2.5 mg/0.025 mg diphenoxylate/atropine per 5 mL or tab.] ▶L ♀C ▶– ⊚V $

LOPERAMIDE (*Imodium, Imodium AD, ✦Loperacap, Diarr-Eze*) 4 mg PO initially, then 2 mg PO after each unformed stool to max 16 mg per day. Peds: 1 mg PO three times per day for wt 13 to 20 kg, 2 mg PO two times per day for wt 21 to 30 kg, 2 mg PO three times per day for wt greater than 30 kg. [OTC Generic/Trade: Tabs 2 mg. Oral soln 1 mg/5 mL. Oral soln 1 mg/7.5 mL.] ▶L ♀C ▶+ $

MOTOFEN **(difenoxin + atropine)** 2 tabs PO initially, then 1 tab after each loose stool q 3 to 4 h prn (up to 8 tabs per day). [Trade only: Tabs difenoxin 1 mg + atropine 0.025 mg.] ▶L ♀C ▶– ⊚IV $$$$$

OPIUM (*opium tincture, paregoric*) Paregoric: 5 to 10 mL PO daily (up to four times). Opium tincture: 0.6 mL (range 0.3 to 1 mL) PO q 2 to 6 h, prn, to a max of 6 mL per day. Opium tincture contains 25 times more morphine than paregoric. [Trade only: Opium tincture 10% (deodorized opium tincture, 10 mg morphine equivalent/mL). Generic only: Paregoric (camphorated opium tincture, 2 mg morphine equivalent/5 mL).] ▶L ♀C ▶? ⊚II $$$

Antiemetics—5-HT3 Receptor Antagonists

AKYNZEO (palonosetron + netupitant) Nausea with chemo: 1 capsule PO 1 h prior to chemo. [Trade only: Capsule (0.5 mg palonosetron + 300 mg netupitant).] ▶L ♀C ▶ $$$$$

DOLASETRON (Anzemet) Nausea with chemo: 100 mg PO single dose. Prevention/treatment of post-op N/V: 12.5 mg IV 15 min before end of anesthesia (prevention) or at onset of N/V (treatment). [Trade only: Tabs 50, 100 mg. Injectable no longer available in Canada.] ▶LK ♀B ▶? $$$$

GRANISETRON (Sancuso) Nausea with chemo: Transdermal (Sancuso): 1 patch to upper outer arm at least 24 h (but up to 48 h) before chemotherapy. Remove 24 h after completion of chemotherapy. Can be worn up to 7 days depending on the duration of chemo. 10 mcg /kg IV within 30 min of chemo. 2 mg once daily PO or 1 mg twice daily PO to start up to 1 hour before chemotherapy. Prevention of N/V with radiation: 2 mg PO within 1 hour of radiation. [Trade only: Transdermal patch (Sancuso) 34.3 mg of granisetron delivering 3.1 mg/24 h. Generic only: Tablet 1 mg.] ▶L ♀B ▶? $$$$

ONDANSETRON (Zofran, Zuplenz) Nausea with chemo: IV: 0.15 mg/kg dose (max 16 mg) 30 min prior to chemo and repeated at 4 h and 8 h after 1st dose for age 6 mo or older. PO: 4 mg PO 30 min prior to chemo and repeat at 4 h and 8 h for age 4 to 11 yo, 8 mg PO and repeated 8 h later for age 12 yo or older. Prevention of post-op N/V: 4 mg IV over 2 to 5 min or 4 mg IM 30 min before end of surgery or 16 mg PO 1 h before anesthesia. Give 0.1 mg/kg IV over 2 min to 5 min as a single dose for age 1 mo to 12 yo if wt 40 kg or less; 4 mg IV over 2 min to 5 min as a single dose if wt greater than 40 kg. Prevention of N/V associated with radiotherapy: 8 mg PO three times per day. [Generic/Trade: Tabs 4, 8, 24 mg. Orally disintegrating tabs 4, 8 mg. Oral soln 4 mg/5 mL. Trade only: Oral film (Zuplenz) 4, 8 mg.] ▶L ♀B ▶? $$$$$

PALONOSETRON (Aloxi) Nausea with chemo: 0.25 mg IV over 30 sec, 30 min prior to chemo. Children 1 mo to 17 yo: 20 mcg/kg

(cont.)

(max 1.5 mg) IV over 15 min, 30 min prior to chemo. Prevention of postop N/V: 0.075 mg IV over 10 sec just prior to anesthesia. [Trade only: Injectable.] ▶L ♀B ▶? $$$$$

Antiemetics—Other

APREPITANT (*Emend, fosaprepitant*) Prevention of nausea with moderately to highly emetogenic chemo, in combination with a corticosteroid and a 5-HT3 antagonist: 125 mg PO on day 1 (1 h prior to chemo), then 80 mg PO q am on days 2 and 3. Alternatively, single dose of 150 mg IV (fosaprepitant) over 20 to 30 min, with a corticosteroid and a 5-HT3 antagonist. In children 6 months and older, 3 mg/kg (max 125 mg) on day 1, then 2 mg/kg (max 80 mg) PO on days 2 and 3. Prevention of postop N/V: 40 mg PO within 3 h prior to anesthesia. [Trade only (aprepitant): Caps 40, 80, 125 mg. Susp 125 mg. IV form is fosaprepitant.] ▶L ♀B ▶? $$$$$

DICLEGIS (doxylamine + pyridoxine, *✦Diclectin*) N/V due to pregnancy: 2 tabs PO at bedtime. If not controlled, can increase to max 4 tabs daily (1 tab PO q am, 1 tab PO mid-afternoon, 2 tabs PO at bedtime). [Trade: Tabs doxylamine 10 mg and pyridoxine 10 mg.] ▶LK –♀A ▶– $$$$$

DIMENHYDRINATE (*Dramamine, ✦Gravol*) 50 to 100 mg PO/IM/IV q 4 to 6 h prn (max 400 mg/24 h PO, 600 mg/day IV/IM). Canada only: 50 to 100 mg/dose PR q 6 to 8 h prn. [OTC Generic/Trade: Tabs 50 mg. Trade only: Chewable tabs 25, 50 mg. Canada only: Supps 25, 50, 100 mg.] ▶LK ♀B ▶– $

✦DOMPERIDONE Canada only. Postprandial dyspepsia: 10 to 20 mg PO three to four times per day, 30 min before a meal. N/V: 20 mg PO three to four times per day. [Canada only. Trade/Generic: Tabs 10, 20 mg.] ▶L ♀? ▶ $$

DOXYLAMINE (*Unisom Nighttime Sleep Aid SleepTabs, others*) N/V associated with pregnancy: 12.5 mg PO two to four times per day; often used in combination with pyridoxine. Do not use in children younger than 12 yo. Some Unisom products contain

(cont.)

diphenhydramine instead of doxylamine. [OTC, Generic/Trade: Tabs 25 mg. Chewable tab 5 mg (Aldex-N).] ▶L ♀A ▷? $

DRONABINOL (*Syndros, Marinol*) Nausea with chemo: 5 mg/m^2 PO 1 to 3 h before chemo then 5 mg/m^2/dose q 2 to 4 h after chemo for 4 to 6 doses/day. Syndros: 4.2 mg/m^2 PO 1 to 3 hours before chemo, on an empty stomach, then every 2 to 4 hours after chemotherapy for up to 4 to 6 doses daily. Anorexia associated with AIDS: Initially 2.5 mg PO two times per day before lunch and dinner. If indicated and tolerated, increase to 20 mg/day. Syndros: 2.1 mg PO twice daily, 1 hour before luch and dinner. [Generic/Trade: Caps 2.5, 5, 10 mg. Oral soln (Syndros) 5 mg/mL.] ▶L ♀C ▷– ⊚III $$$$$

DROPERIDOL (*Inapsine*) 0.625 to 2.5 mg IV or 2.5 mg IM. May cause fatal QT prolongation, even in patients with no risk factors. Monitor ECG before. ▶L ♀C ▷? $

METOCLOPRAMIDE (*Reglan, Metozolv ODT, ✦Maxeran*) GERD/diabetic gastroparesis: 10 mg IV/IM q 2 to 3 h prn. 10 to 15 mg PO four times per day, 30 min before meals and at bedtime. Caution with long-term (more than 3 months) use. Prevention of postop nausea: 10 to 20 mg IM/IV near end of surgical procedure, may repeat q 3 to 4 h prn. [Generic/Trade: Tabs 5, 10 mg. Trade: Orally disintegrating tabs 5, 10 mg (Metozolv). Generic only: Oral soln 5 mg/5 mL.] ▶K ♀B ▷? $

NABILONE (*Cesamet*) 1 to 2 mg PO two times per day, 1 to 3 h before chemotherapy. [Trade only: Caps 1 mg.] ▶L ♀C ▷– ⊚II $$$$$

PHOSPHORATED CARBOHYDRATES (*Emetrol*) 15 to 30 mL PO q 15 min prn, max 5 doses. Peds: 5 to 10 mL per dose. [OTC Generic/Trade: Soln containing dextrose, fructose, and phosphoric acid.] ▶L ♀A ▷+ $

PROCHLORPERAZINE (*Compazine, ✦Stemetil*) 5 to 10 mg IV over at least 2 min. 5 to 10 mg PO/IM three to four times per day. 25 mg PR q 12 h. Sustained-release: 15 mg PO q am or 10 mg PO q 12 h. Peds: 0.1 mg/kg/dose PO/PR three to four times per day or 0.1 to 0.15 mg/kg/dose IM three to four times per

(cont.)

day. Brand name Compazine no longer available. [Generic only: Tabs 5, 10, 25 mg. Generic/Trade: Supp 25 mg.] ▶LK ♀C ▶? $

PROMETHAZINE (*Phenergan*) Adults: 12.5 to 25 mg PO/IM/ PR q 4 to 6 h. Peds: 0.25 to 1 mg/kg PO/IM/PR q 4 to 6 h. Contraindicated if age younger than 2 yo; caution in older children. IV use common but not approved. Brand name Phenergan no longer available. [Generic only: Tabs 12.5, 25, 50 mg. Syrup 6.25 mg/5 mL. Generic/Trade: Supp 12.5, 25, 50 mg.] ▶LK ♀C ▶– $

SCOPOLAMINE (*Transderm-Scop*, ✱*Transderm-V*) Motion sickness: Apply 1 disc (1.5 mg) behind ear 4 h prior to event; replace q 3 days. [Trade only: Topical disc 1.5 mg/72 h, box of 4. Injectable soln.] ▶L ♀C ▶+ $$$

TRIMETHOBENZAMIDE (*Tigan*) 300 mg PO q 6 to 8 h, 200 mg IM q 6 to 8 h. [Generic/Trade: Caps 300 mg.] ▶LK ♀C ▶? $$

Antiulcer—Antacids

ALKA-SELTZER (**acetylsalicylic acid + citrate + bicarbonate**) 2 regular-strength tabs in 4 oz water q 4 h PO prn (up to 8 tabs daily for age younger than 60 yo, up to 4 tabs daily for age 60 yo or older) or 2 extra-strength tabs in 4 oz water q 6 h PO prn (up to 7 tabs daily for age younger than 60 yo, up to 3 tabs daily for age 60 yo or older). [OTC Generic/Trade: Regular-strength, original: Aspirin 325 mg + citric acid 1000 mg + sodium bicarbonate 1916 mg. Regular-strength lemon-lime and cherry: 325 mg + 1000 mg + 1700 mg. Extra-strength: 500 mg + 1000 mg + 1985 mg. Not all forms of Alka-Seltzer contain aspirin (eg, Alka-Seltzer Heartburn Relief).] ▶LK ♀? (– 3rd trimester) ▶? $

ALUMINUM HYDROXIDE (*Alternagel, Amphojel, Alu-Tab, Alu-Cap, ✱Basaljel, Mucaine*) 5 to 10 mL or 300 to 600 mg PO up to 6 times per day. Constipating. [OTC Generic/Trade: Susp 320, 600 mg/ 5 mL.] ▶K ♀C ▶? $

GAVISCON (**aluminum hydroxide + magnesium carbonate**) 15 to 30 mL (regular-strength) or 10 mL (extra-strength) PO four

(cont.)

times per day prn. [OTC Trade only: Tabs: Extra-strength (Al hydroxide 160 mg + Mg carbonate 105 mg). Liquid: Regular-strength (Al hydroxide 95 mg + Mg carbonate 358 mg per 15 mL), extra-strength (Al hydroxide 254 mg + Mg carbonate 237.5 mg per 5 mL).] ▶K♀? ▶? $

MAALOX (**aluminum hydroxide + magnesium hydroxide**) 10 mL to 20 mL PO prn. [OTC Generic/Trade: Susp (225/200 mg per 5 mL). Other strengths available.] ▶K♀C▶? $

MYLANTA (**aluminum hydroxide + magnesium hydroxide + simethicone**) 10 to 20 mL PO between meals and at bedtime prn. [OTC Generic/Trade: Liquid (various concentrations, eg, regular-strength, maximum-strength, supreme).] ▶K♀C▶? $

ROLAIDS (**calcium carbonate + magnesium hydroxide**) 2 to 4 tabs PO q 1 h prn, max 12 tabs/day (regular-strength) or 10 tabs/day (extra-strength). [OTC Trade only: Tabs, regular-strength (Ca carbonate 550 mg, Mg hydroxide 110 mg), extra-strength (Ca carbonate 675 mg, Mg hydroxide 135 mg).] ▶K ♀? ▶? $

Antiulcer—H2 Antagonists

CIMETIDINE (**Tagamet, Tagamet HB**) 300 mg IV/IM/PO q 6 to 8 h, 400 mg PO two times per day, or 400 to 800 mg PO at bedtime. Erosive esophagitis: 800 mg PO two times per day or 400 mg PO four times per day. Continuous IV infusion 37.5 to 50 mg/h (900 to 1200 mg/day). [Tabs 200, 300, 400, 800 mg. Rx Generic only: Oral soln 300 mg/5 mL. OTC Generic/Trade: Tabs 200 mg.] ▶LK♀B▶+ $

FAMOTIDINE (**Pepcid, Pepcid AC, Maximum Strength Pepcid AC**) 20 mg IV q 12 h, 20 to 40 mg PO at bedtime, or 20 mg PO two times per day. [Generic/Trade: Tabs 10 mg (OTC, Pepcid AC Acid Controller), 20 mg (Rx and OTC, Maximum Strength Pepcid AC), 40 mg. Rx Generic/Trade: Susp 40 mg/5 mL.] ▶LK ♀B▶? $

NIZATIDINE (**Axid**) 150 to 300 mg PO at bedtime, or 150 mg PO two times per day. [Generic only: Caps 150, 300 mg. Oral soln 15 mg/mL (120, 480 mL).] ▶K ♀B▶? $$$$

PEPCID COMPLETE (famotidine + calcium carbonate + magnesium hydroxide) 1 tab PO prn. Max 2 tabs/day. [OTC trade/generic: Chewable tabs, famotidine 10 mg with Ca carbonate 800 mg and Mg hydroxide 165 mg.] ▶LK ♀B ▷? $

RANITIDINE (*Zantac, Zantac EFFERdose, Zantac 75, Zantac 150, Peptic Relief*) 150 mg PO two times per day or 300 mg PO at bedtime. 50 mg IV/IM q 8 h, or continuous infusion 6.25 mg/h (150 mg/day). [Generic/Trade: Tabs 75 mg (OTC: Zantac 75), 150 mg (OTC and Rx: Zantac 150), 300 mg. Syrup 75 mg/5 mL. Rx Generic only: Caps 150, 300 mg.] ▶K ♀B ▷? $

Antiulcer—Helicobacter pylori Treatment

PREVPAC (lansoprazole + amoxicillin + clarithromycin, ✚*HP-Pac*) 1 dose PO two times per day for 10 to 14 days. [Generic/Trade: Each dose consists of lansoprazole 30 mg cap + amoxicillin 1 g (two 500 mg caps), + clarithromycin 500 mg tab.] ▶LK ♀C ▷ $$$$$

PYLERA (bismuth subcitrate potassium + metronidazole + tetracycline) 3 caps PO four times per day (after meals and at bedtime) for 10 days. Use with omeprazole 20 mg PO two times per day. [Trade only: Each cap contains bismuth subcitrate potassium 140 mg + metronidazole 125 mg + tetracycline 125 mg.] ▶LK ♀D ▷– $$$$$

Antiulcer—Proton Pump Inhibitors

DEXLANSOPRAZOLE (*Dexilant, Dexilant SoluTab*) Take without regard to meals. Healing of erosive esophagitis: 60 mg PO once daily for up to 8 weeks. Maintenance of erosive esophagitis: 30 mg PO once daily for up to 6 months. Symptomatic nonerosive GERD: 30 mg PO once daily for 4 weeks. [Trade only: Cap 30, 60 mg. Orally-disintegrating tablet 30 mg (Dexilant SoluTab).] ▶L ♀B ▷– $$$$$

ESOMEPRAZOLE (*Nexium*) Erosive esophagitis: 20 to 40 mg PO daily for 4 to 8 weeks. Maintenance of erosive esophagitis: 20 mg

(cont.)

PO daily. Zollinger-Ellison: 40 mg PO two times per day. GERD: 20 mg PO daily for 4 weeks. Prevention of NSAID-associated gastric ulcer: 20 to 40 mg PO daily for up to 6 months. H. pylori eradication: 40 mg PO daily with amoxicillin 1000 mg PO two times per day and clarithromycin 500 mg PO two times per day for 10 days. [Rx Generic/Trade: Caps, delayed-release 20, 40 mg. Trade only: Delayed-release granules for oral susp 2.5, 5, 10, 20, 40 mg per packet. OTC/Trade: Caps, delayed-release 20 mg.] ▶L ♀B ▶? $

LANSOPRAZOLE (Prevacid) Heartburn: 15 mg PO daily. Duodenal ulcer: 15 mg PO daily for 4 weeks. Maintenance therapy after healing of duodenal ulcer: 15 mg PO daily for up to 12 months. NSAID-induced gastric ulcer: 30 mg PO daily for 8 weeks (treatment), 15 mg PO daily for up to 12 weeks (prevention). GERD: 15 mg PO daily for up to 8 weeks. Gastric ulcer: 30 mg PO daily for up to 8 weeks. Erosive esophagitis: 30 mg PO daily for up to 8 weeks or 30 mg IV daily for 7 days or until taking PO. [OTC Generic/Trade: Caps 15 mg. Rx Generic/Trade: 15, 30 mg. Orally disintegrating tabs 15, 30 mg.] ▶L ♀B ▶? $$$

OMEPRAZOLE (Prilosec, ✸Losec) GERD, duodenal ulcer, erosive esophagitis: 20 mg PO daily. Heartburn (OTC): 20 mg PO daily for 14 days. Gastric ulcer: 40 mg PO daily. Hypersecretory conditions: 60 mg PO daily. [Rx Generic/Trade: Caps 10, 20, 40 mg. Trade only: Granules for oral susp 2.5 mg, 10 mg. OTC Trade only: Cap 20 mg.] ▶L ♀C ▶? $

PANTOPRAZOLE (Protonix, ✸Pantoloc, Tecta) Treatment of erosive esophagitis associated with GERD: 40 mg PO daily for 8 to 16 weeks. Maintenance of erosive esophagitis: 40 mg PO once daily. Zollinger-Ellison syndrome and other hypersecretory conditions: 40 mg PO twice daily or 80 mg IV q 8 to 12 h for 7 days until taking PO. [Generic/Trade: Tabs 20, 40 mg. Trade only: Granules for susp 40 mg/packet.] ▶L ♀B ▶? $

RABEPRAZOLE (AcipHex, ✸Pariet) GERD, duodenal ulcer, erosive esophagitis: 20 mg PO daily. [Generic/Trade: Tabs

(cont.)

20 mg. Trade only: Sprinkle caps (open and sprinkle on soft food or liquid) 5, 10 mg.] ▶L ♀C ▶? $$$$$

ZEGERID (**omeprazole + bicarbonate**)   Duodenal ulcer, GERD, erosive esophagitis: 20 mg PO daily for 4 to 8 weeks. Maintenance of erosive esophagitis: 20 mg PO daily. Gastric ulcer: 40 mg PO once daily for 4 to 8 weeks. Reduction of risk of upper GI bleed in critically ill (susp only): 40 mg PO, then 40 mg 6 to 8 h later, then 40 mg once daily thereafter for up to 14 days. [OTC Trade only ($): Omeprazole/sodium bicarbonate caps 20 mg/1.1 g. Rx Generic/Trade ($$$$$): Caps 20 mg/1.1 g and 40 mg/1.1 g. Trade only: Powder packets for susp 20 mg/1.68 g and 40 mg/1.68 g.] ▶L ♀C ▶? $

Antiulcer—Other

DICYCLOMINE (*Bentyl*, *❄Bentylol*)   10 to 20 mg PO/IM four times per day up to 40 mg PO four times per day. [Generic/Trade: Tabs 20 mg. Caps 10 mg.] ▶LK ♀B ▶– $

DONNATAL (**phenobarbital + hyoscyamine + atropine + scopolamine**)   1 to 2 tabs/caps or 5 to 10 mL PO three to four times per day. 1 extended-release tab PO q 8 to 12 h. [Generic/trade: Phenobarbital 16.2 mg + hyoscyamine 0.1 mg + atropine 0.02 mg + scopolamine 6.5 mcg in each tab or 5 mL. Trade only: Extended-release tabs, 48.6 + 0.3111 + 0.0582 + 0.0195 mg.] ▶LK ♀C ▶– $$$

HYOSCINE (*❄Buscopan*)   Canada only: GI or bladder spasm: 10 to 20 mg PO/IV up to 60 mg daily (PO) or 100 mg daily (IV). [Canada Trade only: Tabs 10 mg.] ▶LK ♀C ▶? $$

HYOSCYAMINE (*Anaspaz, A-spaz, Cystospaz, ED Spaz, Hyosol, Hyospaz, Levbid, Levsin, Medispaz, NuLev, Spacol, Spasdel, Symax*)   Bladder spasm, control gastric secretion, GI hypermotility, irritable bowel syndrome: 0.125 to 0.25 mg PO/SL q 4 h or prn. Extended-release: 0.375 to 0.75 mg PO q 12 h. Max 1.5 mg/day. [Generic/Trade: Tabs 0.125. SL tabs 0.125 mg. Chewable tabs 0.125 mg. Extended-release tabs 0.375 mg. Elixir 0.125 mg/5 mL. Gtts 0.125 mg/1 mL.] ▶LK ♀C ▶– $

MISOPROSTOL (*PGE1, Cytotec*) Prevention of NSAID-induced gastric ulcers: 100 mcg PO two times per day, then titrate as tolerated up to 200 mcg PO four times per day. Cervical ripening: 25 mcg intravaginally q 3 to 6 h (or 50 mcg q 6 h). First trimester pregnancy failure: 800 mcg intravaginally, repeat on day 3 if expulsion incomplete. [Generic/Trade: Oral tabs 100, 200 mcg.] ▶LK ♀X ▶— $$$$

PROPANTHELINE (*Pro-Banthine*) 7.5 to 15 mg PO 30 min before meals and 30 mg at bedtime. [Generic only: Tabs 15 mg.] ▶LK ♀C ▶— $$$$

SIMETHICONE (*Mylicon, Gas-X, Phazyme, ✚Ovol*) 40 to 360 mg PO four times per day prn, max 500 mg/day. Infants: 20 mg PO four times per day prn. [OTC Generic/Trade: Chewable tabs 80, 125 mg. Gtts 40 mg/0.6 mL. Trade only: Softgels 166 mg (Gas-X), 180 mg (Phazyme). Strips, oral (Gas-X) 62.5 mg (adults), 40 mg (children).] ▶not absorbed ♀C but + ▶? $

SUCRALFATE (*Carafate, ✚Sulcrate*) 1 g PO 1 h before meals (2 h before other medications) and at bedtime. [Generic/Trade: Tabs 1 g. Susp 1 g/10 mL.] ▶not absorbed ♀B ▶? $$

Laxatives—Bulk-Forming

METHYLCELLULOSE (*Citrucel*) 1 heaping tablespoon in 8 oz water or 2 caplets PO daily (up to six doses per day). [OTC Trade only: Regular and sugar-free packets and multiple-use canisters, Clear-mix soln, Caplets 500 mg.] ▶not absorbed ♀+ ▶? $

POLYCARBOPHIL (*FiberCon, Konsyl Fiber, Equalactin*) Laxative: 2 tabs (1250 mg) PO four times per day prn. Diarrhea: 2 tabs (1250 mg) PO q 30 min. Max daily dose 6 g. [OTC Generic/Trade: Tabs/Caps 625 mg. OTC Trade only: Chewable tabs 625 mg (Equalactin).] ▶not absorbed ♀+ ▶? $

PSYLLIUM (*Metamucil, Fiberall, Konsyl, Hydrocil*) 1 teaspoon in liquid, 1 packet in liquid, or 1 to 2 wafers with liquid PO daily (up to three times per day). [OTC Generic/Trade: Regular and sugar-free powder, granules, caps, wafers, including various flavors and various amounts of psyllium.] ▶not absorbed ♀+ ▶? $

Laxatives—Osmotic

GLYCERIN (*Fleet*) 1 adult or infant supp or 5 to 15 mL as an enema PR prn. [OTC Generic/Trade: Supp, infant and adult. Soln (Fleet Babylax) 4 mL/applicator.] ▶not absorbed ♀C ▶ $

LACTULOSE (*Enulose, Kristalose*) Constipation: 15 to 30 mL (syrup) or 10 to 20 g (powder for oral soln) PO daily. Hepatic encephalopathy: 30 to 45 mL (syrup) PO three to four times per day, or 300 mL retention enema. [Generic/Trade: Syrup 10 g/15 mL. Trade only (Kristalose): 10, 20 g packets for oral soln.] ▶absorbed ♀B ▶? $$

MAGNESIUM CITRATE 150 to 300 mL PO once or in divided doses. 2 to 4 mL/kg/day once or in divided doses for age younger than 6 yo. [OTC Generic only: Soln 300 mL/bottle. Low-sodium and sugar-free available.] ▶K ♀B ▶? $

MAGNESIUM HYDROXIDE (*Milk of Magnesia*) Laxative: 30 to 60 mL regular-strength (400 mg per 5 mL) liquid PO. Antacid: 5 to 15 mL regular-strength liquid or 622 to 1244 mg PO four times per day prn. [OTC Generic/Trade: Susp 400 mg/5 mL. Trade only: Chewable tabs 311, 400 mg. Generic only: Susp 800 mg/5 mL, (concentrated) 1200 mg/5 mL, sugar-free 400 mg/5 mL.] ▶K ♀+ ▶? $

POLYETHYLENE GLYCOL (*MiraLax, GlycoLax, ✦Lax-A-Day, Restoralax*) 17 g (1 heaping tablespoon) in 4 to 8 oz water, juice, soda, coffee, or tea PO daily. [OTC Generic/Trade: Powder for oral soln 17 g/scoop, 17 g packets. Rx Generic/Trade: Powder for oral soln 17 g/scoop.] ▶not absorbed ♀C ▶ $

POLYETHYLENE GLYCOL WITH ELECTROLYTES (*GoLYTELY, Colyte, Suclear, Suprep, TriLyte, NuLYTELY, MoviPrep, HalfLytely, ✦Klean-Prep, Electropeg, Peg-Lyte*) Bowel prep: 240 mL q 10 min PO or 20 to 30 mL/min per NG until 4 L are consumed. MoviPrep, Suclear, Suprep: Follow specific instructions. [Generic/Trade: Powder for oral soln in disposable jug 4 L or 2 L (MoviPrep). Trade only: GoLYTELY Packet for oral soln to make 3.785 L. Suclear: Dose 1 (16 oz) and dose 2 (2 L bottle) for reconstitution. Suprep: Two 6 oz bottles.] ▶not absorbed ♀C ▶? $

PREPOPIK (**sodium picosulfate**) Preferred method: 1 packet (diluted in 5 oz water) evening before the colonoscopy and second packet (diluted in 5 oz water) morning prior to colonoscopy. Alternatively, first dose during afternoon or early evening before the colonoscopy and second dose 6 h later in evening before colonoscopy. Additional clear liquids should be consumed. [Trade: 2 packets of 16 g powder for reconstitution.] ▶minimal absorption ♀B ▶? $

SODIUM PHOSPHATE (*Fleet enema, Fleet EZ-Prep, Accu-Prep, OsmoPrep, Visicol, ✱Enemol, Phoslax*) Constipation: 1 adult or pediatric enema PR or 20 to 30 mL of oral soln PO prn (max 45 mL/24 h). Prep prior to colonoscopy: Visicol: Evening before colonoscopy: 3 tabs with 8 oz clear liquid q 15 min until 20 tabs are consumed. Day of colonoscopy: Starting 3 to 5 h before procedure, 3 tabs with 8 oz clear liquid q 15 min until 20 tabs are consumed. OsmoPrep: 32 tabs PO with total of 2 quarts clear liquids as follows: evening before procedure: 4 tabs PO with 8 oz of clear liquids q 15 min for a total of 20 tabs; day of procedure: 3 to 5 h before procedure, 4 tabs with 8 oz of clear liquids q 15 min for a total of 12 tabs. [OTC Generic/Trade: Adult enema, oral soln. OTC Trade only: Pediatric enema, bowel prep. Rx Trade only: Visicol, OsmoPrep tabs ($$$$) 1.5 g.] ▶not absorbed ♀C ▶? $ ■

SORBITOL 30 to 150 mL (of 70% soln) PO or 120 mL (of 25 to 30% soln) PR as a single dose. Cathartic: 4.3 mL/kg PO. [Generic only: Soln 70%.] ▶not absorbed ♀C ▶? $

SUPREP (**sodium sulfate + potassium sulfate + magnesium sulfate**) Evening before colonoscopy: Dilute 1 bottle to 16 oz with water and drink, then drink 32 oz water over next hour. Next morning, repeat both steps. Complete 1 h before colonoscopy. [Trade: Two 6 oz bottles for dilution.] ▶not absorbed ♀C ▶? $$$

Laxatives—Stimulant

BISACODYL (*Correctol, Dulcolax, Feen-a-Mint, Fleet*) 5 to 15 mg PO once daily prn, 10 mg PR once daily prn, 5 to 10 mg PR once daily prn if 2 to 11 yo. [OTC Generic/Trade: Tabs 5 mg; Supp 10 mg. OTC Trade only: Enema, 10 mg/30 mL.] ▶L ♀C ▶? $

CASCARA 5 mL of aromatic fluid extract PO at bedtime prn. [Rx Generic only: Liquid aromatic fluid extract.] ▶L ♀C ▶+ $

CASTOR OIL Children: 5 to 15 mL/dose of castor oil PO or 7.5 to 30 mL emulsified castor oil PO once a day. Adult: 15 to 60 mL castor oil or 30 to 60 mL emulsified castor oil PO once a day. [OTC Generic only: Oil 60, 120, 180, 480 mL.] ▶not absorbed ♀X ▶? $

SENNA (*Senokot, SenokotXTRA, Ex-Lax, Fletcher's Castoria*) 2 tabs or 10 to 15 mL syrup PO. Max 8 tabs, 30 mL syrup/day. [OTC Generic/Trade (all dosing is based on sennosides content; 1 mg sennosides is equivalent to 21.7 mg standardized senna concentrate): Syrup 8.8 mg/5 mL. Liquid 33.3 mg senna concentrate/mL (Fletcher's Castoria). Tabs 8.6, 15, 17, 25 mg. Chewable tabs 10, 15 mg.] ▶L ♀C ▶+ $

Laxatives—Stool Softener

DOCUSATE (*Colace, Docu-Soft, DOK, Dulcolax, Docu-Liquid, Enemeez, Fleet Sof-Lax, Octycine, Silace*) Constipation: Docusate calcium: 240 mg PO daily. Docusate sodium: 50 to 500 mg/day PO divided in 1 to 4 doses. Peds: 10 to 40 mg/day for age younger than 3 yo, give 20 to 60 mg/day for age 3 to 6 yo, give 40 to 150 mg/day for age 6 to 12 yo. In all cases, doses are divided up to four times per day. Cerumen impaction: 1 mL in affected ear. [Docusate calcium OTC Generic/Trade: Caps 240 mg. Docusate sodium OTC Generic/Trade: Caps 50, 100, 250 mg. Liquid 50 mg/5 mL. Syrup 20 mg/5 mL. Docusate sodium OTC Trade only (Enemeez): Enema, rectal 283 mg/5 mL.] ▶L ♀A ▶? $

Laxatives—Other or Combinations

LUBIPROSTONE (*Amitiza*) Chronic idiopathic constipation: 24 mcg PO two times per day with food and water. Irritable bowel syndrome with constipation in women age 18 yo or older: 8 mcg PO two times per day. Opioid-induced constipation in adults

(cont.)

with chronic, non-cancer pain: 24 mcg PO two times per day with food and water. [Trade only: Caps 8, 24 mcg.] ▶gut ♀C ▶? $$$$$

MINERAL OIL (*Kondremul, Fleet Mineral Oil Enema, Liqui-Doss, ✚Lansoÿl*) 15 to 45 mL PO. Peds: 5 to 15 mL/dose PO. Mineral oil enema: 60 to 150 mL PR. Peds: 30 to 60 mL PR. [OTC Generic/Trade: Oil (30, 480 mL), Enema (Fleet). OTC Trade only: Oral liquid (Liqui-Doss) 13.5 mg/15 mL. Oral microemulsion (Kondremul) 2.5 mg/5 mL.] ▶not absorbed ♀C ▶? $

PERI-COLACE (**docusate + sennosides**) 2 to 4 tabs PO once daily or in divided doses prn. [OTC Generic/Trade: Tabs 50 mg docusate + 8.6 mg sennosides.] ▶L ♀C ▶? $

SENOKOT-S (**senna + docusate**) 2 tabs PO daily. [OTC Generic/ Trade: Tabs 8.6 mg senna concentrate + 50 mg docusate.] ▶L ♀C ▶+ $

Ulcerative Colitis

BALSALAZIDE (*Colazal, Giazo*) Active mild to moderate ulcerative colitis: 2.25 g PO three times per day (Colazal) for 8 to 12 weeks or three 1.1 g (3.3 g) tabs PO twice per day for 8 weeks (Giazo). Giazo is for males only, not approved for use in females. [Generic/Trade (Colazal): Caps 750 mg. Trade (Giazo): Tabs 1.1 g.] ▶minimal absorption ♀B ▶? $$$$$

MESALAMINE (*5-aminosalicylic acid, Apriso, 5-Aspirin, Lialda, Pentasa, Canasa, Rowasa, Delzicol, Asacol HD, ✚Mesasal, Salofalk*) Apriso: 1.5 g (4 caps) PO q am. Delzicol: 800 mg PO three times a day (treatment) or 800 mg PO twice a day (maintenance). Pentasa: 1000 mg PO four times daily or two 800 mg tablets three times daily (4.8 g/day) with or without food for 6 weeks. Lialda: 2.4 to 4.8 g PO daily with a meal. Canasa: 500 mg PR two to three times per day or 1000 mg PR at bedtime. Susp: 4 g enema PR at bedtime (retain 8 h) for 3 to 6 weeks. Asacol HD: 1.6 g PO three times a day for 6 weeks. [Trade only: Delayed-release caps (Delzicol) 400 mg. Controlled-release

(cont.)

caps 250, 500 mg (Pentasa). Delayed-release tabs 800 mg (Asacol HD), 1200 mg (Lialda). Rectal supp 1000 mg (Canasa). Controlled-release caps 0.375 g (Apriso). Generic/Trade: Rectal susp 4 g/60 mL (Rowasa).] ▶gut ♀C ▶? $$$$$

OLSALAZINE (*Dipentum*) Ulcerative colitis: 500 mg PO two times per day with food. [Trade only: Caps 250 mg.] ▶L ♀C ▶− $$$$$

SULFASALAZINE—GASTROENTEROLOGY (*Azulfidine, Azulfidine EN-tabs, ✦Salazo-pyrin En-tabs*) Ulcerative colitis: 500 to 1000 mg PO four times per day. Peds, age 6 yo and older: 30 to 60 mg/kg/day PO divided q 4 to 6 h. May turn body fluids, contact lenses, or skin orange-yellow. [Generic/Trade: Tabs 500 mg, scored. Enteric-coated, delayed-release (EN-tabs) 500 mg.] ▶L ♀B ▶? $$

VEDOLIZUMAB (*Entyvio*) ▶? ♀B ▶? $$$$$ Active ulcerative colitis or Crohn's disease, moderate to severe: 300 mg IV infused over 30 minutes at weeks 0, 2, 6, and then q 8 weeks. Discontinue if no benefit by week 14. Indicated for patients intolerant or unresponsive to TNF-blockers, or corticosteroid-dependent or -intolerant.

Other GI Agents

ALOSETRON (*Lotronex*) Prescribers should complete REMs training prior to prescribing. Diarrhea-predominant irritable bowel syndrome in women who have failed conventional therapy: 0.5 mg PO two times per day for 4 weeks; discontinue in patients who become constipated. If well tolerated and symptoms not controlled after 4 weeks, may increase to 1 mg PO two times per day. Discontinue if symptoms not controlled in 4 weeks on 1 mg PO two times per day. [Generic/Trade: Tabs 0.5, 1 mg.] ▶L ♀B ▶? $$$$$ ■

ALPHA-GALACTOSIDASE (*Beano*) 1 tab per ½ cup gassy food, 2 to 3 tabs PO (chew, swallow, crumble) or 1 melt-away tab per typical meal. [OTC Trade only: Tabs, melt-away tabs.] ▶minimal absorption ♀? ▶? $

ALVIMOPAN (*Entereg*) Short-term (up to 15 doses) in hospitalized patients undergoing partial large or small bowel resection surgery with primary anastomosis: 12 mg PO 30 min to 5 h prior to surgery, then 12 mg PO two times per day starting the day after surgery for up to 7 days. [Trade only: Caps 12 mg.] ▶intestinal flora ♀B ▶? $$$$$ ■

BUDESONIDE (*Entocort EC, Uceris*) Mild to moderate Crohn's, induction of remission: 9 mg PO daily for up to 8 weeks. May repeat 8-week course for recurring episodes. 1 metered dose applied to rectal area twice daily for 2 weeks followed by 1 metered dose once daily for 4 weeks (Uceris foam). Maintenance: 6 mg PO daily for 3 months (Entocort only). Mild to moderate ulcerative colitis, induction of remission: 9 mg PO q am for up to 8 weeks. [Generic/Trade: Caps 3 mg. Trade only: Extended-release tabs (Uceris) 9 mg. (Uceris for ulcerative colitis, only).Rectal foam (Uceris) 2 mg/metered dose, 14 actuations/canister.] ▶L ♀C ▶? $$$$$

CHLORDIAZEPOXIDE—CLIDINIUM 1 to 2 caps PO three to four times per day. [Generic: Caps, chlordiazepoxide 5 mg + clidinium 2.5 mg.] ▶K ♀D ▶– $$$$

***CONTRAVE* (naltrexone + bupropion)** 1 tab PO daily for 1 week, then 1 tab PO twice daily for 1 week, then 2 tabs PO q am and 1 tab PO q pm for 1 week, then 2 tabs PO twice daily. [Trade only: Tabs (naltrexone 8 mg + bupropion 90 mg).] ▶LK ♀X ▶? $$$$$ ■

CROFELEMER (*Fulyzaq*) Noninfectious AIDS diarrhea: 125 mg PO twice daily. [Trade: Delayed-release tab 125 mg.] ▶minimal absorption ♀C ▶? $$$$$

ELUXADOLINE (*Viberzi*) Diarrhea-predominant IBS: 100 mg PO twice daily. Reduce dose to 75 mg PO twice daily in patients who cannot tolerate the higher dose, those who do not have a gallbladder, those with mild to moderate heaptic impairment, and patients who are receiving OATP1B1 inhibitors such as cyclosporine, alfentanil, ergotamine, fentanyl, sirolimus, tacrolimus, others. [Rx, Trade: tabs 75 mg, 100 mg.] ▶glucuronidation ♀? ?/?/?/? ▶ ⊚IV $$$$$

GLYCOPYRROLATE (*Robinul, Robinul Forte, Cuvposa*) Peptic ulcer disease: 1 to 2 mg PO two to three times per day. Chronic drooling in children (Cuvposa): 0.02 mg/kg PO three times per day. Preop/intraoperative respiratory antisecretory effect: 4 mcg/kg IV 30-60 minutes before anesthesia or at the time the preanesthetic narcotic or sedative is administered. [Trade: Soln 1 mg/5 mL (480 mL, Cuvposa). Generic/Trade: Tabs 1, 2 mg.] ▶K ♀B ▶? $$$$

LACTASE (*Lactaid*) Swallow or chew 3 caplets (Original-strength), 2 tabs/caplets (Extra-strength), 1 caplet (Ultra) with 1st bite of dairy foods. Adjust dose based on response. [OTC Generic/Trade: Caps, Chewable tabs.] ▶not absorbed ♀+ ▶+ $

LINACLOTIDE (*Linzess, ✦Constella*) Irritable bowel syndrome: 290 mcg PO daily. Chronic idiopathic constipation: 145 mcg PO once daily. Contraindicated in children 6 years or younger. [Trade: Caps 145, 290 mcg.] ▶gut – ♀C ▶? $$$$$ ■

LORCASERIN (*Belviq*) Obesity or overweight with comorbidities: 10 mg PO twice a day. [Trade: Tabs 10 mg.] ▶L ♀X ▶ $$$$$

METHYLNALTREXONE (*Relistor*) Opioid-induced constipation with chronic non-cancer pain:12 mcg SC once daily or 450 mg PO once daily in the morning. Opioid induced constiaption in pateints with advanced illness who are receiving palliative care: Less than 38 kg: 0.15 mg/kg SC every other day; 38 kg to 61 kg: 8 mg SC every other day; 62 kg to 114 kg: 12 mg SC every other day; 115 kg or greater: 0.15 mg/kg SC every other day. [Rx, Trade: Single-use vial 12 mg/0.6 mL soln for SC injection; single-use prefilled syringe 8 mg/0.4 mL and 12 mg/0.6 mL soln for SC injection. Tabs 150 mg.] ▶unchanged ♀B ▶? $$$$$

NALOXEGOL (*Movantik*) Opioid-induced constipation: 25 mg PO once daily; if not tolerated, reduce dose to 12.5 mg. [Trade only: Tabs 12.5, 25 mg.] ▶L ♀C ▶– $$$$$

NEOMYCIN—ORAL (*Neo-Fradin*) Hepatic encephalopathy: 4 to 12 g/day PO divided q 4 to 6 h. Peds: 50 to 100 mg/kg/day PO divided q 6 to 8 h. [Generic only: Tabs 500 mg. Trade only: Soln 125 mg/5 mL.] ▶minimal absorption ♀D ▶? $$$

OBETICHOLIC ACID (*Ocaliva*) Primary biliary cholangitis, with ursodiol if no response to ursodiol for at least year or without ursodiol in those intolerant to ursodiol: 5 mg PO daily. Can be increased to 10 mg once daily in 3 months if inadequate response. [Trade only: Tabs 5, 10 mg.] ▶L bile ♀? ?/?/? ▶? $$$$$

OCTREOTIDE (*Sandostatin, Sandostatin LAR*) Variceal bleeding: Bolus 25 to 50 mcg IV followed by infusion 25 to 50 mcg/h. AIDS diarrhea: 25 to 250 mcg SC three times per day. [Generic/Trade: Injection vials 0.05, 0.1, 0.2, 0.5, 1 mg. Trade only: Long-acting injectable susp (Sandostatin LAR) 10, 20, 30 mg.] ▶LK ♀B ▶? $$$$$

ORLISTAT (*Alli, Xenical*) Weight loss: 60 to 120 mg PO three times per day with meals. [OTC Trade only (Alli): Caps 60 mg. Rx Trade only (Xenical): Caps 120 mg.] ▶gut ♀X ▶? $$$

PANCREATIN (*Creon, Ku-Zyme, ✦Entozyme*) 8000 to 24,000 units lipase (1 to 2 tabs/caps) PO with meals and snacks. [Tabs, Caps with varying amounts of lipase, amylase, and protease.] ▶gut ♀C ▶? $$$

PANCRELIPASE (*Creon, Pancreaze, Pancrecarb, Cotazym, Ku-Zyme HP, Ultresa, Viokace, Zenpep*) Varies by wt. Initial infant dose 2000 to 4000 lipase units PO per 120 mL formula or breastmilk. 12 mo or older to younger than 4 yo: 1000 lipase units/kg PO. 4 yo or older: 500 lipase units/kg per meal PO, max 2500 lipase units/kg per meal. [Tabs, Caps, Powder with varying amounts of lipase, amylase, and protease.] ▶gut ♀C ▶? $$$

PINAVERIUM (*Dicetel*) Canada only. 50 to 100 mg PO three times per day. [Trade only: Tabs 50, 100 mg.] ▶? ♀C ▶— $$$

QSYMIA (phentermine + topiramate) Obesity or overweight with comorbidities: 3.75 mg/23 mg PO once daily for 14 days, then increase to 7.5 mg/46 mg PO once daily. Max dose 15 mg/92 mg PO daily. Taper over 1 week when discontinuing. [Trade: Tabs 3.75/23, 7.5/46, 11.25/69, 15/92 mg (phentermine/topiramate).] ▶KL ♀X ▶— ©IV $$$$$

RECTIV (*nitroglycerin—rectal*) Painful chronic anal fissures: Apply 1 inch intra-anally q 12 for up to 3 weeks. [Trade only: Oint 0.4% 30 g.] ▸L ♀C▸? $$$$$

SECRETIN (*SecreFlo, ChiRhoStim*) Test dose 0.2 mcg IV. If tolerated, 0.2 to 0.4 mcg/kg IV over 1 min. ▸serum ♀C▸? $$$$$

TEDUGLUTIDE (*Gattex*) Short bowel syndrome patients receiving IV TPN: 0.05 mg/kg (max 3.8 mg) SC daily. [Trade only: 5 mg/vial, powder for reconstitution.] ▸endogenous ♀B▸? $$$$$

URSODIOL (*Actigall, URSO, URSO Forte*) Gallstone solution (Actigall): 8 to 10 mg/kg/day PO divided two to three times per day. Prevention of gallstones associated with rapid wt loss (Actigall): 300 mg PO two times per day. Primary biliary cirrhosis (URSO): 13 to 15 mg/kg/day PO divided in 2 to 4 doses. [Generic/Trade: Caps 300 mg, Tabs 250, 500 mg.] ▸bile ♀B▸? $$$

HEMATOLOGY/ANTICOAGULANTS

Anticoagulants - Direct Thrombin Inhibitors

ARGATROBAN HIT: Start 2 mcg/kg/min IV infusion. Get PTT at baseline and 2 h after starting infusion. Adjust dose (max dose: 10 mcg/kg/min) until PTT is 1.5 to 3 times baseline (not more than 100 sec). ACCP recommends starting at max of 2 mcg/kg/min with lower doses of 0.5 to 1.2 mcg/kg/min in patients with heart failure, multi-organ failure, anasarca, or post-cardiac surgery. ▶L ♀B ▶– $$$$$

BIVALIRUDIN (*Angiomax*) Anticoagulation during PCI (patients with HIT or with HIT and thrombosis syndrome): 0.75 mg/kg IV bolus prior to intervention, then 1.75 mg/kg/h for duration of procedure. May continue infusion up to 4 h post-procedure (should be considered post-STEMI to reduce risk of stent thrombosis), then may additionally infuse 0.2 mg/kg/h for up to 20 h more. For CrCl less than 30 mL/min, reduce infusion dose to 1 mg/kg/h after bolus. For patients on dialysis, reduce infusion to 0.25 mg/kg/h after bolus. Use with aspirin 300 to 325 mg PO daily. ▶proteolysis/K ♀B ▶? $$$$$

DABIGATRAN (*Pradaxa*) Stroke prevention in atrial fibrillation: CrCl greater than 30 mL/min: 150 mg PO two times per day; CrCl between 15 and 30 mL/min: 75 mg PO two times per day; CrCl less than 15 mL/min: contraindicated. Per ACCP CHEST guidelines, not recommended if CrCl is less than 30 mL/min. Treatment of DVT/PE: CrCl greater than 30 mL/min: 150 mg PO two times per day after 5 to 10 days of parenteral anticoagulation. Reduction in risk of DVT/PE: CrCl greater than 30 mL/min: 150 mg PO two times per day after previous treatment. VTE prevention in hip replacement surgery: CrCl greater than 30 mL/min: 110 mg orally one dose given 1 to 4 h after surgery or start 220 mg once if started on postop day 1, then 220 mg daily for 28 to 35 days. [Trade only: Caps 75, 110, 150 mg.] ▶K ♀C ▶? $$$$$ ■

DESIRUDIN (*Iprivask*) DVT prophylaxis (hip replacement surgery): 15 mg SC q 12 h. (If CrCl is 31 to 60 mL/min, give

(cont.)

5 mg SC q 12 h; if CrCl less than 31 mL/min, give 1.7 mg SC q 12 h.) ▶K ♀C ▶? $$$$$ ■

Anticoagulants-Factor Xa Inhibitors

APIXABAN (*Eliquis*) Nonvalvular atrial fibrillation: 5 mg PO two times per day. If at least two of the following characteristics: age 80 yo or older, wt 60 kg or less, serum creatinine 1.5 mg/dL or greater, then decrease dose to 2.5 mg PO two times daily. DVT prophylaxis in hip or knee replacement: 2.5 mg PO two times per day. Treatment of DVT/PE: 10 mg PO two times daily for 7 days, then 5 mg PO two times daily. Reduction in risk of recurrence of DVT/PE: 2.5 mg PO two times daily after initial therapy for treatment. [Trade only: Tabs 2.5, 5 mg.] ▶LK ♀B ▶? $$$$$ ■

EDOXABAN (*Savaysa*) Nonvalvular atrial fibrillation: CrCl greater than 50 up to and including 95 mL/min: 60 mg PO daily. CrCl 15 to 50 mL/min: 30 mg PO daily. Treatment of DVT/PE: 60 mg PO daily after 5 to 10 days of parenteral anticoagulation. CrCl 15 to 50 mL/min or body weight 60 kg or less or certain P-gp inhibitors: 30 mg PO daily after 5 to 10 days of parenteral anticoagulation. [Trade only: 15, 30, 60 mg tabs.] ▶K ♀C ▶? $$$$$ ■

FONDAPARINUX (*Arixtra*) DVT prophylaxis, hip/knee replacement or hip fracture surgery, abdominal surgery: 2.5 mg SC daily starting 6 to 8 h postop. DVT/PE treatment based on wt: wt less than 50 kg: 5 mg SC daily; wt between 50 and 100 kg: 7.5 mg SC daily; wt greater than 100 kg: 10 mg SC daily for at least 5 days and therapeutic oral anticoagulation. [Generic/Trade: Prefilled syringes 2.5 mg/0.5 mL, 5 mg/0.4 mL, 7.5 mg/0.6 mL, 10 mg/0.8 mL.] ▶K ♀B ▶? $$$$$ ■

RIVAROXABAN (*Xarelto*) DVT prophylaxis in knee or hip replacement: 10 mg PO daily, if CrCl less than 30 mL/min avoid use. Nonvalvular atrial fibrillation: 20 mg PO daily if CrCl greater than 50 mL/min; reduce dose to 15 mg PO daily if CrCl 15 to 50 mL/min, avoid use if CrCl less than 15 mL/min. DVT/PE treatment and to reduce risk of DVT/PE recurrence:

(cont.)

15 mg PO two times daily with food for 21 days, then 20 mg PO daily with food. If CrCl 30 to 49 mL/min: 15 mg PO twice daily with food for 3 weeks, then 15 mg PO daily with food. [Trade only: Tabs 10, 15, 20 mg.] ▸K – ♀C ▸? $$$$$ ■

Anticoagulants—Low Molecular Weight Heparins (LMWH)

DALTEPARIN (*Fragmin*) DVT prophylaxis, acute medical illness with restricted mobility: 5000 units SC daily. DVT prophylaxis, abdominal surgery: 2500 units SC 1 to 2 h preop and daily postop. DVT prophylaxis, abdominal surgery in patients with malignancy: 5000 units SC evening before surgery and daily postop, or 2500 units 1 to 2 h preop and 12 h later, then 5000 units daily. DVT prophylaxis, hip replacement: Preop start (day of surgery): 2500 units SC given 2 h preop, 4 to 8 h postop, then 5000 units daily starting at least 6 h after 2nd dose, or 5000 units 10 to 14 h preop, 4 to 8 h postop, then daily (approximately 24 h between doses). Preop start (evening before surgery): 5000 units SC given evening before surgery then 5000 units daily starting at least 4 to 8 h postop (approximately 24 h between doses). Postop start: 2500 units 4 to 8 h postop, then 5000 units daily starting at least 6 h after 1st dose. Treatment of DVT/PE in cancer: 200 units/kg SC daily for 1 month, then 150 units/kg SC daily for 5 months; max 18,000 units/day. Unstable angina or non-Q-wave MI: 120 units/kg up to 10,000 units SC q 12 h with aspirin (75 to 165 mg/day PO) until clinically stable. [Trade only: Single-dose syringes 2500, 5000 units/0.2 mL, 7500 units/0.3 mL, 10,000 units/1 mL, 12,500 units/0.5 mL, 15,000 units/0.6 mL, 18,000 units/0.72 mL; Multidose vial 10,000 units/mL, 9.5 mL and 25,000 units/mL, 3.8 mL.] ▸KL ♀B ▸+ $$$$$ ■

ENOXAPARIN (*Lovenox*) See table. [Generic/Trade: Syringes 30, 40 mg; graduated syringes 60, 80, 100, 120, 150 mg. Concentration is 100 mg/mL except for 120, 150 mg, which are 150 mg/mL. All syringes also available preservative free. Available as Multidose vial 300 mg.] ▸KL ♀B ▸+ $$$$$ ■

ENOXAPARIN ADULT DOSING

Indication	Dose	Dosing in Renal Impairment (CrCl <30 mL/min)*
DVT prophylaxis		
Abdominal surgery	40 mg SC once daily	30 mg SC once daily
Knee replacement	30 mg SC q 12 h	30 mg SC once daily
Hip replacement	30 mg SC q 12 h or 40 mg SC once daily	30 mg SC once daily
Medical patients	40 mg SC once daily	30 mg SC once daily
Acute DVT		
Inpatient treatment with or without PE	1 mg/kg SC q 12 h or 1.5 mg/kg SC once daily	1 mg/kg SC once daily
Outpatient treatment without PE	1 mg/kg SC q 12 h	1 mg/kg SC once daily

(cont.)

Acute coronary syndrome		
Unstable angina and non-Q-wave MI with aspirin	1 mg/kg SC q 12 h with aspirin	1 mg/kg SC once daily
Acute STEMI in patients younger than 75 yo with aspirin†	30 mg IV bolus with 1 mg/kg SC dose, then 1 mg/kg SC q 12 h (max 100 mg/dose for the 1st two doses)	30 mg IV bolus with 1 mg/kg SC dose, then 1 mg/kg SC once daily
Acute STEMI in patients 75 yo or older with aspirin†	No IV bolus, 0.75 mg/kg SC q 12 h (max 75 mg/dose for the 1st two doses)	No IV bolus, 1 mg/kg SC once daily

DVT = Deep vein thrombosis. PE = pulmonary embolism.

*Not FDA-approved in dialysis.

†If used with thrombolytics, SC dose should be started between 15 min before and 30 min after thrombolytic dose.

(cont.)

HEPARIN DOSING FOR ACUTE CORONARY SYNDROME (ACS)

ST elevation myocardial infarction (STEMI)	Adjunct to thrombolytics: For use with alteplase, reteplase, or tenecteplase: Bolus 60 units/kg IV load (max 4000 units), then initial infusion 12 units/kg/h (max 1000 units/h) adjusted to achieve target PTT 1.5 to 2 times control.
Unstable angina/non-ST elevation myocardial infarction (UA/NSTEMI)	Initial treatment: Bolus 60 units/kg IV load (max 4000 units), then initiate infusion at 12 to 15 units/kg/h (max 1000 units) and adjusted to achieve target PTT 1.5 to 2.5 times control.

Percutaneous coronary intervention (PCI)	With prior anticoagulant therapy but *without* concurrent GPIIb/IIIa inhibitor planned: Additional heparin as needed (2000 to 5000 units) to achieve target ACT 250–300 seconds for HemoTec or 300–350 seconds for Hemochron.
	With prior anticoagulant therapy but *with* planned concurrent GPIIb/IIIa inhibitor: Additional heparin as needed (2000 to 5000 units) to achieve target 200–250 seconds.
	Without prior anticoagulant therapy but *without* concurrent GPIIb/IIIa inhibitor planned: Bolus 70–100 units/kg with target ACT 250–300 seconds for HemoTec or 300–350 seconds for Hemochron.
	Without prior anticoagulant therapy but *with* planned concurrent GPIIb/IIIa inhibitor: Bolus 50–70 units/kg with target ACT 200–250 seconds.

WEIGHT-BASED HEPARIN DOSING FOR DVT/PE*

Initial dose	80 units/kg IV bolus, then 18 units/kg/h; check PTT in 6 h
PTT less than 35 sec (less than 1.2 × control)	80 units/kg IV bolus, then increase infusion rate by 4 units/kg/h
PTT 35–45 sec (1.2–1.5 × control)	40 units/kg IV bolus, then increase infusion by 2 units/kg/h
PTT 46–70 sec (1.5–2.3 × control)	No change
PTT 71–90 sec (2.3–3 × control)	Decrease infusion rate by 2 units/kg/h
PTT greater than 90 sec (greater than 3 × control)	Hold infusion for 1 h, then decrease infusion rate by 3 units/kg/h

Adapted from *Ann Intern Med* 1993;119;874. *Chest* 2012;141:e28S, e154S. *Circulation* 2001;103:2994.

*PTT = Activated partial thromboplastin time. Reagent-specific target PTT may differ; use institutional nomogram when available. Consider establishing a max bolus dose/max initial infusion rate or use an adjusted body in obesity. Monitor PTT 6 h after heparin initiation and 6 h after each dosage adjustment. When PTT is stable within therapeutic range, monitor every morning. Therapeutic PTT range corresponds to anti-factor Xa activity of 0.3–0.7 units/mL. Check platelets between days 3 and 5. Can begin warfarin on 1 day of heparin; continue heparin for at least 4–5 days of combined therapy.

Anticoagulants—Other

HEPARIN Venous thrombosis/pulmonary embolus treatment: Load 80 units/kg IV, then initiate infusion at 18 units/kg/h. Adjust based on coagulation testing (PTT)—see Table. DVT prophylaxis: 5000 units SC q 8 to 12 h. Acute coronary syndromes with or without PCI: 60 units/kg IV, then 12 units/kg/h infusion, adjust according to aPTT or antiXa. See Table. Peds: Load 50 units/kg IV, then infuse 25 units/kg/h. [Generic only: 1000, 5000, 10,000, 20,000 units/mL in various vial and syringe sizes.] ▶Reticuloendothelial system ♀C but + ▶+ $$ ■

WARFARIN (*Coumadin, Jantoven*) Individualize dosing. Start 2 to 5 mg PO daily for 1 to 2 days, then adjust dose to maintain therapeutic INR. For healthy outpatients, 2012 ACCP CHEST guidelines recommend starting at 10 mg PO daily for 2 days, then adjust dose to maintain therapeutic INR. See product information if CYP2C9 or VKOR1C genotypes are known. [Generic/Trade: Tabs 1, 2, 2.5, 3, 4, 5, 6, 7.5, 10 mg.] ▶L ♀X, (D for mechanical heart valve replacement) ▶+ $ ■

THERAPEUTIC GOALS FOR ANTICOAGULATION WITH WARFARIN

INR Range*	Indication
2.0–3.0	Atrial fibrillation, deep venous thrombosis, pulmonary embolism, bioprosthetic heart valve (mitral position), mechanical prosthetic heart valve (aortic position)
2.5–3.5	Mechanical prosthetic heart valve (mitral position)

Adapted from: *Chest* 2012; 141:e422S, e425S, e533S, e578S; see these guidelines for additional information and other indications.
*Aim for an INR in the middle of the INR range (eg, 2.5 for range of 2 to 3 and 3.0 for range of 2.5 to 3.5).

WARFARIN—SELECTED DRUG INTERACTIONS

Assume possible interactions with any medication. When starting/stopping a chronic medication, the INR should be checked at least weekly for 2 to 3 weeks and dose adjusted accordingly. When starting an interacting anti-infective agent, the National Quality Forum recommends checking the INR within 3 to 7 days. Similarly, monitor if significant change in diet (including supplements) or illness resulting in decreased oral intake. For further information regarding mechanism or management, refer to the *Tarascon Pocket Pharmacopoeia* drug interactions database (mobile or Web edition).

Increased anticoagulant effect of warfarin / Increased risk of bleeding

Monitor INR when agents below started, stopped, or dosage changed. Consider alternative agent. Acetaminophen ≥ 2 g/day for ≥ 3 to 4 days, allopurinol, amiodarone*, anabolic steroids, ASA¶, cefixime, cefoperazone, cefotetan, celecoxib, chloramphenicol, cimetidine†, corticosteroids, danazol, danshen, disulfiram, dong quai, erlotinib, etravirine, fibrates, fish oil, fluconazole, fluoroquinolones, fluorouracil, fluvoxamine, fosphenytoin (acute), garlic supplements, gemcitabine, gemfibrozil, glucosamine-chondroitin, ginkgo, ifosfamide, imatinib, isoniazid, itraconazole, ketoconazole, leflunomide, lepirudin, levothyroxine#, macrolides‡, metronidazole, miconazole (intravaginal), neomycin (PO for >1 to 2 days), NSAIDs¶, olsalazine, omeprazole,

(cont.)

WARFARIN—SELECTED DRUG INTERACTIONS (*continued*)

paroxetine, penicillin (high-dose IV), pentoxifylline, phenytoin (acute), propafenone, quinidine, quinine, statins§, sulfinpyrazone (with later inhibition), sulfonamides, tamoxifen, testosterones tetracyclines, tramadol, tigecycline, tipranavir, TCAs, valproate, voriconazole, vorinostat, vitamin A (high-dose), vitamin E, zafirlukast, zileuton

Decreased anticoagulant effect of warfarin / Increased risk of thrombosis

Monitor INR when agents below started, stopped, or dosage changed. Consider alternative agent. Aprepitant, cefotetan, azathioprine, barbiturates, bosentan, carbamazepine, coenzyme Q-10, dicloxacillin, fosphenytoin (chronic), ginseng (American), griseofulvin, mercaptopurine, mesalamine, methimazole$^{#}$, mitotane, nafcillin, oral contraceptives**, phenytoin (chronic), primidone, propylthiouracil$^{#}$, raloxifene, ribavirin, rifabutin, rifampin, rifapentine, ritonavir, St. John's wort, vitamin C (high-dose). *Use alternative to agents below. Or give at different times of day and monitor INR when agent started, stopped, or dose/dosing schedule changed.* Cholestyramine, colestipol††, sucralfate

*Interaction may be delayed; monitor INR for several weeks after starting and several months after stopping amiodarone. May need to decrease warfarin dose by 33 to 50%.
†Famotidine, nizatidine, or ranitidine, are alternatives.
‡Azithromycin appears to have lower risk of interaction than clarithromycin or erythromycin.

(cont.)

HEMATOLOGY/ANTICOAGULANTS

WARFARIN—SELECTED DRUG INTERACTIONS (*continued*)

§Pravastatin appears to have lower risk of interaction.
#Hyperthyroidism/thyroid replacement increases metabolism of clotting factors, increasing response to warfarin therapy, and increased bleed risk (typically requires lowering warfarin dose). Reversal of hyperthyroidism (as with methimazole, propylthiouracil) will decrease metabolism of clotting factors and decrease response to warfarin (typically requires increasing warfarin dose).
¶ Does not necessarily increase INR, but increases bleeding risk. Check INR frequently and monitor for GI bleeding.
**Does not necessarily decrease INR, but may induce hypercoagulability.
††Likely lower risk than cholestyramine. Adapted from: Coumadin product information; *Am Fam Phys* 1999; 59:635; *Chest* 2004;126:204S; *Hansten and Horn's Drug Interactions Analysis and Management*; *Ann Intern Med* 2004; 141:23; *Arch Intern Med* 2005;165:1095. *Tarascon Pocket Pharmacopoeia* drug interactions database (Mobile or Web edition). National Quality Forum http://www.qualityforum.org.

Colony-Stimulating Factors

FILGRASTIM (filgrastim-Sndz, Tbo-filgrastim, G-CSF **Neupogen, Granix, Zarxio**) Neutropenia: 5 mcg/kg SC/IV daily. Bone marrow transplant: 10 mcg/kg/day SC/IV infusion. Concomitant myelosuppressive doses of radiation: 10 mcg/kg SC daily. [Trade: Single-dose vials (Neupogen): 300 mcg/1 mL, 480 mcg/1.6 mL. Biosimilars, Single-dose syringes: Granix, tbo-filgrastim: 300 mcg/0.5 mL, 480 mcg/0.8 mL; Zarxio, filgrastim-sndz: 300 mcg/0.5 mL, 480 mcg/0.8 mL.] ▶L ♀C ▶? $$$$$

PEGFILGRASTIM (**Neulasta, Neulasta Onpro**) Myelosuppressive chemo: 6 mg SC once each chemo cycle. Myelosuppresive

(cont.)

radiation: 6 mg SC for two doses administered one week apart. [Trade only: Single-dose syringe (Neulasta, Neulasta Onpro) or syringe kit (Neulasta Onpro) 6 mg/0.6 mL] ▶Plasma ♀C ▷? $$$$$
SARGRAMOSTIM (GM-CSF, *Leukine*) Specialized dosing for bone marrow transplant. ▶L ♀C ▷? $$$$$

Erythropoiesis Stimulating Agents

DARBEPOETIN (*Aranesp*) Anemia of chronic renal failure: 0.45 mcg/kg IV/SC once a week, or 0.75 mcg/kg q 2 weeks in some nondialysis patients. Cancer chemo anemia: 2.25 mcg/kg SC weekly, or 500 mcg SC q 3 weeks. Adjust dose based on Hb. [Trade only: Single-dose vials: 25, 40, 60, 100, 200, 300, 500 mcg/1 mL, and 150 mcg/0.75 mL. Single-dose prefilled syringes or autoinjectors: 10 mcg/0.4mL, 25 mcg/0.42 mL, 40 mcg/0.4 mL, 60 mcg/0.3 mL, 100 mcg/0.5 mL, 150 mcg/0.3 mL, 200 mcg/0.4 mL, 300 mcg/0.6 mL, 500 mcg/1 mL.] ▶cellular sialidases, L ♀C ▷? $$$$$ ■
EPOETIN ALFA (*Epogen, Procrit*, erythropoietin alpha, ✦*Eprex*) Anemia: 1 dose IV/SC 3 times a week. Initial dose if renal failure is 50 to 100 units/kg, Zidovudine-induced anemia is 100 units/kg, or chemo-associated anemia is 150 units/kg. Alternate for chemo-associated anemia: 40,000 units SC once a week. Adjust dose based on Hb. [Trade only: Single-dose 1-mL vials 2000, 3000, 4000, 10,000, 40,000 units/mL. Multidose vials 10,000 units/mL, 2 mL; 20,000 units/mL, 1 mL.] ▶L ♀C ▷? $$$$$ ■
METHOXY POLYETHYLENE GLYCOL-EPOETIN BETA (*Mircera*) Anemia of chronic renal failure: Initial dose 0.6 mcg/kg IV/SC q2weeks. Adjust dose based on Hb. [Trade only: Single-dose pre-filled syringe 30, 50, 75, 100, 120, 150, 200, 250, 360 mcg.] ▶L ♀C ▷? $$$$ ■

Other Hematological Agents

AMINOCAPROIC ACID (*Amicar*) Hemostasis: 4 to 5 g PO/IV over 1 h, then 1 g/h prn. [Trade only: Tabs 500, 1000 mg. Syrup 250 mg/mL] ▶K ♀D ▷? $ IV $$$$$ Oral

ANAGRELIDE (*Agrylin*) Thrombocythemia due to myeloproliferative disorders: Start 0.5 mg PO four times per day or 1 mg PO two times per day, then after 1 week adjust to lowest effective dose. Max 10 mg/day. [Generic/Trade: Caps 0.5 mg. Generic only: Caps 1 mg.] ▶LK ♀C ▶? $$$$$

DEFERASIROX (*Exjade, Jadenu*) Chronic iron overload due to blood transfusions: Exjade: 20 mg/kg PO daily; adjust dose q 3 to 6 months based on ferritin trends. Max 40 mg/kg/day. Jadenu: 14 mg/kg PO daily; adjust dose monthly based on ferritin trends. Max 28 mg/kg/day. Chronic iron overload in non-transfusion-dependent thalassemia syndromes: Exjade: 10 mg/kg PO daily; adjust dose based on ferritin and liver iron concentration. Max 20 mg/kg/day. Jadenu: 7 mg/kg PO daily; adjust dose based on ferritin and liver iron concentration. Max 14 mg/kg/day. [Trade only: Exjade: 125, 250, 500 mg tabs for dissolving into oral susp; Jadenu: 90, 180, 360 mg tabs.] ▶L ♀– ?/?/? ▶? $$$$$ ■

HYDROXYUREA (*Hydrea, Droxia*) Sickle cell anemia (Droxia): Start 15 mg/kg PO daily while monitoring CBC q 2 weeks. If no marrow depression, then increase dose q 12 weeks by 5 mg/kg/day (max 35 mg/kg/day). Head and neck cancer with radiation (Hydrea): 15mg/kg PO daily. Resistant chronic myeloid leukemia: 15 mg/kg PO daily. Give concomitant folic acid. [Generic/Trade: Caps 500 mg. Trade only: (Droxia) Caps 200, 300, 400 mg.] ▶LK ♀ X/X/X ▶– $$$ ■

IDARUCIZUMAB (*Praxbind*) Reversal of dabigatran anticoagulation for emergency surgery/procedures or life-threatening/uncontrolled bleeding: 5 g IV. [Trade only: 2.5 g/50 mL vial.] ▶? Biodegradation ♀?/?/? ▶? $$$$$

PROTAMINE Reversal of heparin: Within 30 minutes of IV heparin: 1 mg antagonizes about 100 units heparin. If greater than 30 minutes since IV heparin: 0.5 mg antagonizes about 100 units heparin. Due to short half-life of heparin (60 to 90 min), use IV heparin doses only from last several hours to calculate dose of protamine. SC heparin may require prolonged

(cont.)

administration of protamine. Reversal of low-molecular-weight heparin: If within 8 h of LMWH dose: Give 1 mg protamine per 100 anti-Xa units of dalteparin or 1 mg protamine per 1 mg enoxaparin. Smaller doses advised if greater than 8 h since LMWH administration. Give IV (max 50 mg) over 10 min. May cause allergy/anaphylaxis. ▶Plasma ♀C ▶? $ ■

PROTHROMBIN COMPLEX CONCENTRATE (*Kcentra*) Vitamin K antagonist reversal for acute major bleed or urgent surgery/invasive procedure: Individualized dosing based on pre-treatment INR and body weight. INR 2 to less than 4: 25 units of Factor IX/kg body weight (max: 2500 units); INR 4 to 6: 35 units of Factor IX/kg body weight (max: 3500 units); INR greater than 6: 50 units of Factor IX/kg body weight (max 5000 units). [Brand: 500, 1000 unit vial.] ▶N/A ♀C ▶? $$$$$ ■

HERBAL AND ALTERNATIVE THERAPIES

NOTE: *In the United States, herbal and alternative therapies are regulated as dietary supplements, not drugs. Premarketing evaluation and FDA approval are not required unless specific therapeutic claims are made. Because these products are not required to demonstrate safety and efficacy, it is unclear whether many of them have any health benefit and some can cause harm. In addition, the actual ingredients may vary considerably from the ingredients on the label, and may be adulterated.*

ALOE VERA (acemannan, burn plant) Topical: Efficacy unclear for seborrheic dermatitis, psoriasis, genital herpes, skin burns. Do not apply to surgical incisions; impaired healing reported. Oral: Efficacy unclear for mild to moderate active ulcerative colitis, type 2 diabetes. OTC laxatives containing aloe latex were removed from US market due to possible increased risk of colon cancer. [Not by prescription.] ▶LK ♀ oral − topical + ? ▶ oral − topical + ? $

ALPHA LIPOIC ACID (lipoic acid, thioctic acid, ALA) Peripheral neuropathy (possibly effective): Usual dose is 600 mg PO daily. [Not by prescription] ▶intracellular ♀C ▶? $

ARTICHOKE LEAF EXTRACT (*Cynara scolymus*) May reduce total cholesterol, but clinical significance is unclear. Possibly effective for functional dyspepsia. [Not by prescription.] ▶? ♀? ▶? $

ASTRAGALUS (*Astragalus membranaceus, huang qi, Jin Fu Kang*) Used with other herbs in traditional Chinese medicine for CAD, CHF, chronic liver disease, kidney disease, viral infections, and upper respiratory tract infection. Possibly effective for improving survival and performance status with platinum-based chemotherapy for non-small-cell lung cancer. But astragalus-based herbal formula (Jin Fu Kang) did not affect survival in phase II study of non-small-cell lung cancer. [Not by prescription.] ▶? ♀? ▶? $

BUTTERBUR (*Petasites hybridus, Petadolex*) Migraine prophylaxis (effective): Petadolex 50 to 75 mg PO two times per day. Allergic rhinitis prophylaxis (possibly effective): Petadolex 50 mg PO two times per day. Efficacy unclear for asthma. [Not by prescription. Standardized pyrrolizidine-free extracts: Petadolex tabs 50, 75 mg.] ▶? ♀– ▶– $$

CHAMOMILE (*Matricaria recutita*—German chamomile, *Anthemis nobilis*—Roman chamomile) Oral extract: Modest benefit for generalized anxiety disorder, but little to no benefit for primary chronic insomnia. Topical: Efficacy unclear for skin infections or inflammation. [Not by prescription.] ▶? ♀– ▶? $

CHASTEBERRY (*Vitex agnus castus* fruit extract, *Femaprin*) Premenstrual syndrome (possibly effective): 20 mg PO daily of extract ZE 440 (Femaprin) [Not by prescription.] ▶? ♀– ▶– $

CHONDROITIN Does not appear effective for relief of OA pain overall. Chondroitin 400 mg PO three times per day + glucosamine may improve pain in subgroup of patients with moderate to severe knee OA. [Not by prescription.] ▶K ♀? ▶? $

COENZYME Q10 (CoQ-10, ubiquinone) Heart failure: 100 to 300 mg/day PO divided two to three times per day (conflicting clinical trials; AHA/ACC does not recommend). Statin-induced myalgia: 100 to 200 mg PO daily (efficacy unclear; conflicting clinical trials). Prevention of migraine (possibly effective): 100 mg PO three times per day. May be considered for migraine prevention per American Academy of Neurology and American Headache Society. Efficacy unclear for hypertension and improving athletic performance. Appears ineffective for diabetes. Did not improve cancer-related fatigue or quality of life in RCT of women with breast cancer. Does not slow functional decline in early Parkinson disease. [Not by prescription.] ▶Bile ♀– ▶– $$

CRANBERRY (*CranActin, Vaccinium macrocarpon*) Prevention of UTI (possibly ineffective): 300 mL/day PO cranberry juice cocktail. Usual dose of cranberry juice extract caps/tabs is 300 to 400 mg PO two times per day. Insufficient data to assess efficacy for treatment of UTI. Potential increase in

(cont.)

INR with warfarin. [Not by prescription.] ▶? ♀ + in food, − in supplements ▶+ in food, − in supplements $

CREATINE Promoted to enhance athletic performance. No benefit for endurance exercise; modest benefit for intense anaerobic tasks lasting less than 30 sec. Usual loading dose of 10 to 20 g/day PO for 4 to 7 days, then 2 to 5 g/day divided two times per day. Can slightly increase serum creatinine in young adults. [Not by prescription.] ▶LK ♀− ▶− $

DEHYDROEPIANDROSTERONE (DHEA, _Aslera, Fidelin, prasterone_) To improve well-being in women with adrenal insufficiency: 50 mg PO daily (possibly effective; conflicting clinical trials). Does not improve cognition, quality of life, or sexual function in elderly. Not recommended as androgen replacement in late-onset male hypogonadism. [Not by prescription.] ▶Peripheral conversion to estrogens and androgens ♀− ▶− $

DEVIL'S CLAW (_Harpagophytum procumbens, Doloteffin, Harpadol_) OA, acute exacerbation of chronic low-back pain (possibly effective): 2400 mg extract/day (50 to 100 mg harpagoside/day) PO divided two to three times per day. [Not by prescription. Extracts standardized to harpagoside content.] ▶? ♀− ▶− $

ECHINACEA (_E. purpurea, E. angustifolia, E. pallida, EchinaGuard, Echinacin Madaus_) Conflicting clinical trials for prevention or treatment of upper respiratory infections. Does not appear effective for treatment of common cold in adults. [Not by prescription.] ▶L ♀− ▶− $

ELDERBERRY (_Sambucus nigra, Sambucol_) Efficacy unclear for influenza, sinusitis, and bronchitis. [Not by prescription.] ▶LK ♀− ▶− $

FENUGREEK (_Trigonella foenum-graecum_) Efficacy unclear for diabetes and hyperlipidemia. [Not by prescription.] ▶? ♀− ▶? $$

FEVERFEW (_Chrysanthemum parthenium, MigreLief, Tanacetum parthenium L._) Prevention of migraine (probably effective): 50 to 100 mg extract PO daily. Response may take 1 to 2 months. [Not by prescription.] ▶? ♀− ▶− $

FLAVOCOXID (*Limbrel*) OA (efficacy unclear): 250 to 500 mg PO two times per day. Case of hepatotoxicity and hypersensitivity pneumonitis. [Caps 250, 500 mg. (Marketed as prescription-only medical food).] ▶L♀− ▶− $$$

GARLIC SUPPLEMENTS (*Allium sativum, Kwai, Kyolic*) Ineffective for hyperlipidemia. Small reductions in BP, but efficacy for HTN unclear. Does not appear effective for diabetes. Efficacy unclear for common cold. Significantly decreases saquinavir levels. May increase bleeding risk with warfarin with/without increase in INR. [Not by prescription.] ▶LK♀− ▶− $

GINGER (*Zingiber officinale*) Acute chemotherapy-induced nausea (efficacy unclear as adjunct to standard antiemetics): 250 to 500 mg PO two times per day for 6 days, starting 3 days before chemo. Possibly ineffective for prevention of motion sickness. Does not appear effective for postop N/V. American Congress of Obstetricians and Gynecologists considers ginger 250 mg PO four times per day a nonpharmacologic option for N/V in pregnancy. Some experts advise pregnant women to limit dose to usual dietary amount (no more than 1 g/day). Some European countries advise pregnant women to avoid ginger supplements because it is cytotoxic in vitro. Benefit appears modest for OA pain, minimal for dysmenorrhea. [Not by prescription.] ▶bile ♀? ▶? $

GINKGO BILOBA (EGb 761, *Ginkgold, Ginkoba*) Dementia (efficacy unclear): 40 mg PO three times per day of standardized extract (24% ginkgo flavone glycosides, 6% terpene lactones). American Psychiatric Association and others find evidence too weak to recommend for Alzheimer's or other dementias. Does not prevent dementia in elderly or improve memory in people with normal cognitive function. Does not appear to prevent acute altitude sickness. Ineffective for intermittent claudication, tinnitus. Possible risk of stroke. [Not by prescription.] ▶K♀− ▶− $

GINSENG—AMERICAN (*Panax quinquefolius L., Cold-FX, Cold-FX Extra*) Prevention of colds/flu (possible modest

(cont.)

efficacy): 1 to 2 caps Cold-FX PO two times per day or 1 cap Cold-FX Extra PO two times per day during flu season. Ineffective for cold treatment. Cancer-related fatigue (possibly effective; conflicting data): 1000 mg PO two times per day in am and midafternoon. Postprandial hyperglycemia in type 2 diabetes (possibly effective): 3 g PO taken with or up to 2 h before meal. [Not by prescription.] ▶K ♀– ▶– $

GINSENG—ASIAN (*Panax ginseng, Ginsana,* **Korean red ginseng**) Promoted to improve vitality and well being: 200 mg PO daily. Ginsana: 2 caps PO daily or 1 cap PO two times per day. Preliminary evidence of efficacy for erectile dysfunction. Efficacy unclear for improving physical or psychomotor performance, diabetes, herpes simplex infections, or cognitive or immune function. American Congress of Obstetricians and Gynecologists and North American Menopause Society recommend against use for postmenopausal hot flashes. [Not by prescription.] ▶? ♀– ▶– $

GINSENG—SIBERIAN (*Eleutherococcus senticosus,* **Ci-wu-jia**) Does not appear effective for improving athletic endurance or chronic fatigue syndrome. May interfere with some digoxin assays. [Not by prescription.] ▶? ♀– ▶– $

GLUCOSAMINE (*Cosamin DS, Dona*) OA: Glucosamine HCl 500 mg PO three times per day or glucosamine sulfate (Dona $$) 1500 mg PO once daily. Appears ineffective overall for OA pain, but glucosamine plus chondroitin may improve pain in moderate to severe knee OA. [Not by prescription.] ▶L ♀– ▶– $

GREEN TEA (*Camellia sinensis, Polyphenon E*) Minimal efficacy for short-term weight loss, hyperlipidemia. Large doses may decrease INR with warfarin due to vitamin K content. Can decrease nadolol exposure; avoid coadministration. May contain caffeine. [Not by prescription. Green tea extract available in caps standardized to polyphenol content.] ▶LK ♀+ in moderate amount in food, – in supplements ▶+ in moderate amount in food, – in supplements $

HAWTHORN (*Crataegus, Crataegutt, HeartCare*) Mild heart failure (possibly effective): 80 mg PO two times per day to 160 mg PO three times per day (HeartCare 80 mg tabs), but American College of Cardiology does not recommend. [Not by prescription.] ▸? ♀– ▸– $

HONEY (*Medihoney*) Topical for burn/wound (including diabetic foot, stasis leg ulcers, pressure ulcers, 1st- and 2nd-degree partial thickness burns): Apply Medihoney for 12 to 24 h/day. Oral for nocturnal cough due to upper respiratory tract infection in children (effective): Give PO within 30 min before sleep. Dose is ½ tsp for 2 to 5 yo, 1 tsp for 6 to 11 yo, 2 tsp for 12 to 18 yo. Not for children younger than 1 yo due to risk of infant botulism. [Mostly not by prescription. Medihoney is FDA approved.] ▸? ♀+ ▸+ $ for oral $$$ for Medihoney

HORSE CHESTNUT SEED EXTRACT (*Aesculus hippocastanum, Venastat*) Chronic venous insufficiency (effective): 1 cap Venastat PO two times per day with water before meals. American College of Cardiology found evidence insufficient to recommend for peripheral arterial disease. [Not by prescription. Venastat (standardized to 16.7% escin) Caps 600 mg.] ▸? ♀– ▸– $

LICORICE (*CankerMelt, Glycyrrhiza*) Chronic high doses can cause pseudoprimary aldosteronism (with HTN, edema, hypokalemia). Prevention of postop sore throat (possibly effective): Licorice 0.5 g in 30 mL water gargled 5 minutes before anesthesia. Aphthous ulcers (efficacy unclear): Apply CankerMelt oral patch to ulcer for 16 h/day until healed. [Not by prescription.] ▸bile ♀– ▸– $

MELATONIN To reduce jet lag after flights over more than 5 time zones (effective): 0.5 to 5 mg PO at bedtime for 3 to 6 nights starting on day of arrival. [Not by prescription.] ▸L ♀– ▸– $

MILK THISTLE (*Silybum marianum, Legalon*, silymarin, *Thisilyn*) Hepatic cirrhosis (efficacy unclear): 100 to 200 mg PO three times per day of standardized extract (70 to 80% silymarin). Appears ineffective for hepatitis C. [Not by prescription.] ▸LK ♀– ▸– $

NONI (*Morinda citrifolia*) Promoted for many medical disorders; but insufficient data to assess efficacy. Potassium content comparable to orange juice; hyperkalemia reported in chronic renal failure. Cases of hepatotoxicity. [Not by prescription.] ▶? ♀− ▶− $$$

PEPPERMINT OIL (*Colpermin, IBGard*) Irritable bowel syndrome (possibly effective), age 15 yo or older: 1 to 2 enteric-coated caps PO three times per day before meals. Do not crush or chew caps. Avoid products that are not enteric-coated. [Not by prescription. Enteric-coated capsules: Colpermin (187 mg peppermint oil/0.2 mL), IBGard (90 mg ultra-purified peppermint oil/cap; marketed as medical food).] ▶LK ♀+ in food, ? in supplements ▶+ in food, ? in supplements $

PROBIOTICS (*Acidophilus, Align, Bacid, Bifantis, Bifidobacteria, BioGaia, Culturelle, Florastor, Gerber Soothe Colic drops, Lactobacillus, Power-Dophilus, Primadophilus, Saccharomyces boulardii, VSL#3*) Ulcerative colitis (effective): VSL#3 take 4 to 8 caps/day, or 1 to 2 sachets/day, or 0.5 to 1 DS sachet/day. Active ulcerative colitis unresponsive to conventional therapy:VSL #3 take 4 to 8 sachets/day or 2 to 4 DS sachets/day. Pouchitis(effective): VSL #3 take 2 to 4 sachets/day or 1 to 2 DS sachets/day. Irritable bowel syndrome:VSL #3 take 0.5 to 1 sachet/day or 2 to 4 caps/day. Mix VSL #3 with cold non-carbonated beverage or cold food before ingesting immediately; caps can be swallowed whole. Prevention of antibiotic-associated diarrhea (effective): *Saccharomyces boulardii* 500 mg PO two times per day (Florastor 2 caps PO two times per day) for adults; 250 mg PO two times per day (Floraster 1 cap/packet PO two times per day) for peds. For peds: *Lactobacillus* GG (Culturelle) 10 to 20 billion cells/day PO given 2 h before/after antibiotic. IDSA recommends against probiotics for prevention of *C. difficile*–associated diarrhea; safety and efficacy are unclear. Peds, acute gastroenteritis, adjunct to rehydration (effective): *Lactobacillus* GG at least 10 billion cells per day PO for 5 to 7 days or *Saccharomyces boulardii* 250 to

(cont.)

750 mg per day PO for 5 to 7 days. Infant colic (efficacy unclear; conflicting study results): 5 drops of *L. reuteri* DSM 17938 (Gerber Soothe Colic drops) PO once daily for 21 days. Align: 1 cap PO once daily to relieve abdominal pain/bloating. [Mostly not by prescription. Culturelle contains Lactobacillus GG 5 billion CFU per powder packet/chewable tab of Culturelle Kids, 10 billion CFU per cap/chewable tab of Culturelle Digestive Health, 15 billion CFU per cap of Culturelle Health & Wellness, 20 billion CFU per cap of Culturelle Extra Strength Digestive Health. Florastor and Florastor Kids contain *Saccharomyces boulardii* 250 mg per cap/powder packet (contains lactose). VSL#3 (medical food) contains 450 billion CFA/sachet (non-prescription), 900 billion CFU/DS sachet (Rx only), 225 billion cells/2 caps (non-prescription). VSL#3 contains *Bifidobacterium breve, B. longum, B. infantis, Lactobacillus acidophilus, L. plantarum, L. casei, L. bulgaricus, Streptococcus thermophilus*. Align contains *Bifidobacterium infantis* 35624, 1 billion cells/cap. Gerber Soothe Colic drops contains *Lactobacillus reuteri* DSM 17938, 100 million cells per 5 drops. BioGaia ProTectis contains *Lactobacillus reuteri* DSM 17938, 100 million cells per chewable tab/straw.] ▶? ♀+ ▶+ $

PYGEUM AFRICANUM (African plum tree) BPH (may have modest efficacy): 50 to 100 mg PO two times per day or 100 mg PO daily of standardized extract containing 14% triterpenes. [Not by prescription.] ▶? ♀− ▶− $

RED CLOVER (red clover isoflavone extract, *Trifolium pratense, Promensil, Trinovin*) Postmenopausal vasomotor symptoms (conflicting evidence; does not appear effective overall, but may have modest benefit for severe symptoms): Promensil 1 tab PO daily to two times per day with meals. [Not by prescription. Isoflavone content (genistein, daidzein, biochanin, formononetin) is 40 mg/tab in Promensil and Trinovin.] ▶Gut, L, K♀− ▶− $$

RED YEAST RICE (*Monascus purpureus, Xuezhikang, Zhibituo, Hypocol*) Hyperlipidemia: Usual dose is 1200 mg PO two times per day. Efficacy depends on whether formulation

(cont.)

contains lovastatin or other statins. In the US, red yeast rice should not contain more than trace amounts of statins, but some products contain up to 10 mg lovastatin per cap. Some clinicians consider red yeast rice an alternative for patients who develop myalgia with prescription statins. Can cause myopathy. Some formulations may contain citrinin, a potential nephrotoxin. [Not by prescription. Xuezhikang marketed in Asia, Norway (HypoCol).] ▶L♀– ▶– $$

S-ADENOSYLMETHIONINE (SAM-e) Mild to moderate depression (effective): 800 to 1600 mg/day PO in divided doses with meals. Efficacy unclear for OA. [Not by prescription.] ▶L♀? ▶? $$$

SOUR CHERRY (Prunus cerasus, Montmorency cherry) OA (efficacy unclear): 240 mL juice PO two times per day. Prevention of gout (efficacy unclear): 15 mL concentrate PO two times per day. Insomnia (possibly effective): 240 mL juice or 30 mL concentrate PO two times per day. Prevention of exercise-induced muscle damage/pain after strenuous exercise (efficacy unclear): 240 or 360 mL juice or 30 mL concentrate PO two times per day. Dilute concentrate before drinking. [Not by prescription.] ▶LK ♀ + for moderate amount in food, – in supplements ▶ + for moderate amount in food, – in supplements $$

SOY (Genisoy, Healthy Woman, Novasoy, Phyto soya) Postmenopausal vasomotor symptoms (modest benefit): Per North American Menopause Society, consider 50 mg/day or more of soy isoflavones for at least 12 weeks. Conflicting clinical trials for postmenopausal bone loss. Per American Cancer Society and other experts, breast cancer survivors (including tamoxifen-treated women) can consume up to 2 servings/day of soy foods, but should avoid supplements (including soy powder). [Not by prescription.] ▶Gut, L, K♀+ for food, ? for supplements ▶+ for food, ? for supplements $

ST. JOHN'S WORT (Hypericum perforatum) Mild to moderate depression (effective): 300 mg PO three times per day of standardized extract (0.3% hypericin). Does not appear

(cont.)

effective for ADHD. May decrease efficacy of other drugs (eg, ritonavir, oral contraceptives) by inducing CYPs and p-glycoprotein. May cause serotonin syndrome; caution with SSRI/SNRI and avoid MAOI. [Not by prescription.] ▶L ♀– ▶– $

TEA TREE OIL (melaleuca oil, *Melaleuca alternifolia*) Not for oral use; CNS toxicity reported. Limited evidence for topical treatment of onychomycosis, tinea pedis, acne vulgaris, dandruff, pediculosis. [Not by prescription.] ▶? ♀– ▶– $

VALERIAN (*Valeriana officinalis, Alluna*) Insomnia (possibly modestly effective; conflicting clinical trials): 400 to 900 mg of standardized extract PO 30 min before bedtime. Alluna: 2 tabs PO 1 h before bedtime. [Not by prescription.] ▶? ♀– ▶– $

WILLOW BARK EXTRACT (*Salicis cortex,* salicin) OA, low-back pain (possibly effcctive): 60 to 240 mg/day salicin PO divided two to three times per day. [Not by prescription. Some products standardized to 15% salicin content.] ▶K ♀– ▶– $

IMMUNOLOGY

ADULT IMMUNIZATION SCHEDULE (for more information see CDC website at cdc.gov)

ADULT IMMUNIZATION SCHEDULE*

Tetanus, diphtheria (Td): For all ages, 1 dose booster q 10 years.

Pertussis: Single dose of pertussis in adults younger than 65 yo (as part of Tdap), at least 10 years since last tetanus dose. Boostrix is approved age 10 or older; Adacel is approved age 10 to 64 yo. Administer 1 dose Tdap during each pregnancy.

Influenza: 1 yearly dose (trivalent or quadrivalent) if age 50 yo or older. If younger than 50 yo, then 1 yearly dose if healthcare worker, pregnant, chronic underlying illness, household contact of person with chronic underlying illness or household contact with children younger than 5 yo, or those who request vaccination. Intranasal vaccine indicated for healthy adults younger than 50 yo. Fluzone HD or Fluad vaccine indicated for 65 yrs or older.

(cont.)

ADULT IMMUNIZATION SCHEDULE (for more information see CDC website at cdc.gov) (continued)

ADULT IMMUNIZATION SCHEDULE*

*Pneumococcal (polysaccharide):*Pneumococcal Polysaccharide Vaccine (PPSV23, Pneumovax 23) and Pneumococcal Conjugate Vaccine (PCV13, Prevnar 13)

1 lifetime dose PCV13 plus 1-3 lifetime doses PPSV23; final dose PPSV23 should in every case be administered > age 65:

- Healthy adults: 1 dose PCV13 and 1 dose PPSV23, both administered > age 65
- In chronic heart, lung, liver disease, diabetes, alcoholism, active smoking, CSF leak or cochlear implant: 1 dose PPSV23 age 19-64, 1 dose PCV13 > age 65 and 1 dose PPSV23 > age 65 at least 5 years since last received PPSV23 dose.
- In immunocompromising conditions, hemoglobinopathies, or anatomical or functional asplenia, 1 dose PCV13 age >19, 2 doses PPSV23 age 19-64 with interval of at least 5 years between doses, and 1 dose PPSV23 > age 65 at least 5 years since last received PPSV23 dose.

In vaccine naive patients where both PCV13 and PPSV23 are indicated, it is preferable to administer PCV13 first.

In most cases, allow 1 year interval between PCV13 and PPSV23 (see CDC schedule for exceptions).

(cont.)

Hepatitis A: For previously unvaccinated at any adolescent/adult age with clotting factor disorders, chronic liver disease, or travel to endemic areas, illegal drug use, men having sex with men, regular babysitters and household contacts of international adoptees (travel to endemic areas, illegal drug use, men having sex with men), 2 doses (0, 6 to 12 months). Twinrix (hepatitis A + B) requires 3-dose series.

Hepatitis B: For all ages with medical (hemodialysis, clotting factor recipients, chronic liver disease diabetes < age 60 [diabetes ≥60 is discretionary]), occupational (healthcare or public safety workers with blood exposure), behavioral (illegal drug use, multiple sex partners, those seeking evaluation or treatment of sexually transmitted disease, men having sex with men), or other (household/sex contacts of those with chronic HBV or HIV infections, clients/staff of developmentally disabled, more than 6 months of travel to high-risk areas, inmates of correctional facilities) indications, 3 doses (0, 1–2, 4–6 months). Hemodialysis patients require 4 doses and higher dose (40 mcg).

Measles, mumps, rubella (MMR): If born during or after 1957 and immunity in doubt, see www.cdc.gov.

Varicella: For all ages if immunity in doubt, age 13 yo or older, 2 doses separated by 4 to 8 weeks.

CHILDHOOD IMMUNIZATION SCHEDULE*

Age	Birth	1	2	4	6	12	15	18	2	4-6	11-12
					Months					Years	
Hepatitis B	HB	HB				HB					
Rotavirus			Rota	Rota	Rota@						
DTP			DTaP	DTaP	DTaP		DTaP	DTaP		DTaP	
H influenzae b			Hib	Hib	Hib^x	Hib^x					
Pneumococcal**			PCV	PCV	PCV	PCV			(PPSV if indicated*)		
Polio			IPV	IPV		IPV				IPV#	

(cont.)

	Influenza (yearly)† ≥6 months			
Influenza†				
MMR		MMR	MMR	MMR
Varicella		Varicella	Varicella	Varicella
Hepatitis A¶		Hep A × 2¶		
Papillomavirus§,¶				HPV × 3§
Meningococcal^				MCV^

*2016 schedule from the CDC, ACIP, AAP, & AAFP, see CDC website (www.cdc.gov).

**Administer 1 dose Prevnar 13 to all healthy children 24 to 59 mo having an incomplete schedule.

***When immunizing adolescents 10 yo or older, consider Tdap if patient has never received a pertussis booster. (Boostrix if 10 yo or older, Adacel if 11 to 64 yo).

@If using Rotarix, give at 2 and 4 mo (no earlier than 6 weeks). Give at 2, 4, and 6 mo if using Rotateq. Max age for final dose is 8 mo.

(cont.)

CHILDHOOD IMMUNIZATION SCHEDULE* (continued)

Last IPV on or after 4th birthday, and at least 6 months since last dose.

✕ If using PedvaxHib or Comvax, dose at 6 mo not necessary, but booster at 12 to 15 mo indicated.

† For healthy patients age 2 yo or older can use intranasal form. If age younger than 9 yo and receiving for first time, administer 2 doses 4 or more weeks apart for injected form and 6 or more weeks apart for intranasal form. FluLaval, Fluarix, and single-dose Fluzone syringe not indicated in younger than 3 years. Fluvirin not indicated in younger than 4 years. Do not use Afluria in younger than 9 years. Do not use Flucelvax, Fluzone ID or Fluzone HD in children.

¶ Two doses 6 to 18 months apart. Twinrix (hep A + hep B) requires 3 doses.

§ Second and third doses 2 and 6 months after 1st dose. Also approved (Gardasil only) for males 9 to 26 yo to reduce risk of genital warts. Either the quadrivalent or 9-valent or 2-valent (females only) vaccine can be used. Vaccination may begin as early as 9 years of age.

^ Vaccinate all children at age 11 to 12 years with a single dose of Menactra or Menveo, with a booster dose at age 16. For high-risk younger children, refer to CDC for recommendations. Consider Trumendat or Bexero in children 10 years or older who are at risk for meningococcal disease.

TETANUS WOUND CARE (www.cdc.gov)

Cell Paragraph	Unknown or less than 3 prior tetanus immunizations	3 or more prior tetanus immunizations
Non-tetanus-prone wound (eg, clean and minor)	DTaP if < 7 yo, Td if 7-10 yo, Tdap if 11 yo or older and no previous Tdap and Td if previously received Tdap.	Td if more than 10 years since last dose
Tetanus-prone wound (eg, dirt, contamination, punctures, crush components)	DTaP if < 7 yo, Td if 7-10 yo, Tdap if 11 yo or older and no previous Tdap and Td if previously received Tdap. Tetanus immune globulin 250 units IM at different site.	Td if more than 5 years since last dose

If patient age 10 yo or older has never received a pertussis booster consider DTaP (Boostrix if 10 yo or older, Adacel if 11–64 yo).

Immunizations

NOTE: *For vaccine info see CDC website (www.cdc.gov).*

BCG VACCINE 0.2 to 0.3 mL percutaneously. ▶immune system ♀C ▶? $$$$ ■

COMVAX (haemophilus B vaccine + hepatitis B vaccine) Infants born of HBsAg (negative) mothers: 0.5 mL IM for 3 doses, given at 2, 4, and 12 to 15 months. ▸immune system ♀C▶? $$$

DIPHTHERIA, TETANUS, AND ACELLULAR PERTUSSIS VACCINE (*DTaP, Tdap, Infanrix, Daptacel, Boostrix, Adacel, ✚TripacelEE*) 0.5 mL IM. Do not use Boostrix or Adacel for primary childhood vaccination series. ACIP recommends TDAP in every pregnancy, preferably between 27 and 35 weeks' gestation. ▸immune system ♀C▶− $$

DIPHTHERIA-TETANUS TOXOID (*Td, DT, ✚D2T5*) 0.5 mL IM. [Injection DT (Peds: 6 weeks to 6 yo).] Td (adult and children at least 7 yo).] ▸immune system ♀C▶? $

HAEMOPHILUS B VACCINE (*ActHIB, Hiberix, PedvaxHIB*) 0.5 mL IM. Dosing schedule varies depending on formulation used and age of child at 1st dose. ▸immune system ♀C▶? $$

HEPATITIS A VACCINE (*Havrix, Vaqta, ✚Avaxim*) Adult formulation 1 mL IM, repeat in 6 to 12 months. Peds: 0.5 mL IM for age 1 yo or older, repeat 6 to 18 months later. [Single-dose vial (specify pediatric or adult).] ▸immune system ♀C▶+ $$$

HEPATITIS B VACCINE (*Engerix-B, Recombivax HB*) Adults: 1 mL IM, repeat 1 and 6 months later. ACIP recommends hepatitis B vaccine for all previously unvaccinated diabetics age 19 through 59 years; vaccinate as soon as possible after diabetes diagnosis. Children: Dosing based on age and maternal HBsAg status. ▸immune system ♀C▶+ $$$

HUMAN PAPILLOMAVIRUS RECOMBINANT VACCINE (*Cervarix, Gardasil*) 0.5 mL IM at time 0, 2, and 6 months. ▸immune system ♀B▶? $$$$$

INFLUENZA VACCINE—INACTIVATED INJECTION (*Fluad, Afluria, Fluarix, FluLaval, Fluzone, Fluvirin, Flucelvax, Flublok, ✚Influvac, Agriflu, Flulaval Tetra, Fluviral, Vaxigrip*) 0.5 mL IM or ID (Fluzone ID). Fluarix, FluLaval not indicated in children younger than 3 yo. Fluvirin not indicated in children younger than 4 yo. Afluria not indicated in children younger than 9 yo.

(cont.)

Flublok for 18 to 49 yo. Flucelvax for 18 yo and older. Fluzone ID for 18 to 64 yo. Fluzone HD and Fluad for 65 yo and older. ▶immune system ♀C ▶+ $

INFLUENZA VACCINE—LIVE INTRANASAL (*FluMist*) The CDC recommends against the use of FluMist for the 2016-17 season. 1 dose (0.2 mL) intranasally. Use only if 2 to 49 yo. If available, live, intranasal vaccine should be preferentially used for healthy children age 2 through 8 yo who have no contraindications or precautions. ▶immune system ♀C ▶+ $

JAPANESE ENCEPHALITIS VACCINE (*Ixiaro*) 1 mL SC for 3 doses on day 0, 7, and 30. ▶immune system ♀C ▶? $$$$

MEASLES, MUMPS, AND RUBELLA VACCINE (*M-M-R II*, ✚*Priorix*) 0.5 mL (1 vial) SC. ▶immune system ♀C ▶+ $$$

MENINGOCOCCAL VACCINE (*Bexsero, Menveo, Menomune-A/C/Y/W-135, Menactra, Trumenba,* ✚*Menjugate*) 0.5 mL SC or IM (depending on product) to high-risk individuals (asplenia, etc), repeat in 2 months. Menveo: Four-dose series starting at 2 mo at 2, 4, 6, and 12 months. Menactra: Vaccinate all children 11 to 12 yo, and 16 yo. One dose only if between 13 and 18 yo and previously unvaccinated. Trumenba: Three-dose series (0.5 mL) starting at 0, 2, and 6 months in those 10 to 25 years. Bexsero: 2 doses (0.5 mL) at 0 and 1 month in those 10 to 25 years. Although Trumenba and Bexsero are approved for use in ages 10 to 25 yo, ACIP gives no upper age limit. ▶immune system ♀C ▶? $$$$

PEDIARIX (**diphtheria tetanus and acellular pertussis vaccine + hepatitis B vaccine + polio vaccine**) 0.5 mL IM at 2, 4, 6 mo. ▶immune system ♀C ▶? $$$

PNEUMOCOCCAL 13-VALENT CONJUGATE VACCINE (*Prevnar 13*) 0.5 mL IM for 3 doses at 2 mo, 4 mo, and 6 mo, followed by a 4th dose at 12 to 15 mo. Indicated for some high-risk adolescents and adults (immunocompromised adults, asplenic state, sickle cell/hemoglobinopathy, renal failure, CSF leak, Cochlear implant) as an adjunct to the 23-valent pneumococcal vaccine. All adults 65 years or older should receive one dose.

(cont.)

Delay 13-valent vaccine at least 1 year after 23-valent vaccine or delay 23-valent vaccine 8 weeks after 13-valent vaccine. ▶immune system ♀C ▶? $$$

PNEUMOCOCCAL 23-VALENT VACCINEPPSV23 (*Pneumovax, ✦Pneumo 23*) 0.5 mL IM or SC. ▶immune system ♀C ▶+ $$

POLIO VACCINE (*IPOL*) 0.5 mL IM or SC. ▶immune system ♀C ▶? $$

PROQUAD (measles, mumps, and rubella vaccine + varicella vaccine) 0.5 mL (1 vial) SC for age 12 mo to 12 yo. ▶immune system ♀C ▶? $$$$

RABIES VACCINE (*RabAvert, Imovax Rabies, BioRab*) 1 mL IM in deltoid region on days 0, 3, 7, 14, 28. ▶immune system ♀C ▶? $$$$$

ROTAVIRUS VACCINE (*RotaTeq, Rotarix*) RotaTeq: 1st dose (2 mL PO) between 6 and 12 weeks of age, and then 2nd and 3rd doses at 4- to 10-week intervals thereafter (last dose no later than 32 weeks). Rotarix: 1st dose (1 mL) at 6 weeks of age, 2nd dose (1 mL) at least 4 weeks later, and last dose prior to 24 weeks of age. [Trade only: Oral susp 2 mL (RotaTeq), 1 mL (Rotarix).] ▶immune system ♀– ▶? $$$$$

TETANUS TOXOID 0.5 mL IM or SC. ▶immune system ♀C ▶+ $$

TWINRIX (hepatitis A vaccine + hepatitis B vaccine) Adults: 1 mL IM in deltoid, repeat 1 and 6 months later. All 3 doses required for hepatitis A immunity. Accelerated dosing schedule: 0, 7, 21, and 30 days and booster dose at 12 months. ▶immune system ♀C ▶? $$$$

TYPHOID VACCINE—INACTIVATED INJECTION (*Typhim Vi, ✦Typherix*) 0.5 mL IM single dose. May revaccinate q 2 to 5 years if high risk. ▶immune system ♀C ▶? $$

TYPHOID VACCINE—LIVE ORAL (*Vivotif Berna*) 1 cap every other day for 4 doses. May revaccinate every 2 to 5 years if high risk. [Trade only: Caps.] ▶immune system ♀C ▶? $$

VARICELLA VACCINE (*Varivax, ✦Varilrix*) Children 1 to 12 yo: 0.5 mL SC. Repeat dose at ages 4 to 6 yo. Age 13 yo or older: 0.5 mL SC, repeat 4 to 8 weeks later. ▶immune system ♀C ▶+ $$$$

YELLOW FEVER VACCINE (*YF-Vax*) 0.5 mL SC. ▶immune system ♀C ▶+ $$$

ZOSTER VACCINE—LIVE (*Zostavax*) 0.65 mL SC single dose for age 50 yo or older. However, ACIP recommends immunizing those 60 yo and older. ▶immune system ♀C ▶? $$$$

Immunoglobulins

BOTULISM IMMUNE GLOBULIN (*BabyBIG*) Infant botulism: Give 1 mL/kg (50 mg/kg) IV for age younger than 1 yo. ▶L ♀? ▶? $$$$$

HEPATITIS B IMMUNE GLOBULIN (*H-BIG, HyperHep B, HepaGam B, NABI-HB*) 0.06 mL/kg IM within 24 h of needlestick, ocular, or mucosal exposure to hepatitis B, repeat in 1 month. ▶L ♀C ▶? $$$

IMMUNE GLOBULIN—INTRAMUSCULAR (*Baygam, ✱Gamastan*) Hepatitis A prophylaxis: 0.02 to 0.06 mL/kg IM depending on length of travel to endemic area. Measles (within 6 days postexposure): 0.2 to 0.25 mL/kg IM. ▶L ♀C ▶? $$$$ ■

IMMUNE GLOBULIN—INTRAVENOUS (*Carimune, Flebogamma, Gammagard, Gammaplex, Gamunex, Octagam, Privigen*) IV dosage varies by indication and product. ▶L ♀C ▶? $$$$$ ■

IMMUNE GLOBULIN—SUBCUTANEOUS (*Vivaglobulin, Hizentra*) 100 to 200 mg/kg SC weekly. ▶L ♀C ▶? $$$$$ ■

LYMPHOCYTE IMMUNE GLOBULIN (*Atgam*) Specialized dosing. ▶L ♀C ▶? $$$$$

RABIES IMMUNE GLOBULIN HUMAN (*Imogam Rabies-HT, HyperRAB S/D*) 20 units/kg, as much as possible infiltrated around bite, the rest IM. ▶L ♀C ▶? $$$$$

RSV IMMUNE GLOBULIN (*RespiGam*) IV infusion for prevention of respiratory syncytial virus. ▶plasma ♀C ▶? $$$$$

Immunosuppression

BASILIXIMAB (*Simulect*) Specialized dosing for organ transplantation. ▶plasma ♀B ▶? $$$$$

BELATACEPT (*Nulojix*) Specialized dosing for organ transplantation. ▸serum ♀C ▸– $$$$$ ■

CYCLOSPORINE (*Sandimmune, Neoral, Gengraf*) Specialized dosing for organ transplantation, RA, and psoriasis. [Generic/Trade: Microemulsion Caps 25, 100 mg. Generic/Trade: Caps (Sandimmune) 25, 100 mg. Soln (Sandimmune) 100 mg/mL. Microemulsion soln (Neoral, Gengraf) 100 mg/mL.] ▸L ♀C ▸– $$$$$

EVEROLIMUS (*Zortress*) Specialized dosing for organ transplantation. [Trade: Tabs 0.25, 0.5, 0.75 mg.] ▸L – ♀C ▸– $$$$$

MYCOPHENOLATE MOFETIL (*CellCept, Myfortic*) Specialized dosing for organ transplantation. [Generic/Trade: Caps 250 mg. Tabs 500 mg. Tabs, extended-release (Myfortic): 180, 360 mg. Trade only (CellCept): Susp 200 mg/mL (160 mL).] ▸? ♀D ▸– $$ ■

SIROLIMUS (*Rapamune*) Specialized dosing for organ transplantation. [Generic/Trade: Tabs 0.5, 1, 2 mg. Trade only: Soln 1 mg/mL (60 mL).] ▸L ♀C ▸– $$$$$

TACROLIMUS (*Astagraf XL, Hecoria, Prograf, FK 506, Envarsus XR, ✦Advagraf*) Specialized dosing for organ transplantation. [Generic/Trade: Caps 0.5, 1, 5 mg. Trade only: Extended-release caps (Astagraf XL) 0.5, 1, 5 mg. (Envarsus XR) 0.75, 1, 4 mg.] ▸L ♀C ▸– $$$$$

Other

TUBERCULIN PPD (*Aplisol, Tubersol, Mantoux, PPD*) 5 tuberculin units (0.1 mL) intradermally, read 48 to 72 h later. Consider two-step testing initially in those who are going to be retested periodically (e.g., health care workers, nursing home residents). ▸L ♀C ▸+ $

NEUROLOGY

MOTOR FUNCTION BY NERVE ROOTS

Level	Motor Function
C3/C4/C5	Diaphragm
C5/C6	Deltoid/biceps
C7/C8	Triceps
C8/T1	Finger flexion/intrinsics
T1–T12	Intercostal/abd muscles
L2/L3	Hip flexion
L2/L3/L4	Hip adductor/quads
L4/L5	Ankle dorsiflexion
S1/S2	Ankle plantarflexion
S2/S3/S4	Rectal tone

Dermatomes

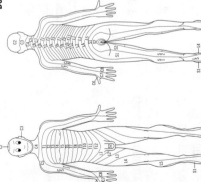

(cont.)

NEUROLOGY

Dermatomes (continued)

LUMBOSACRAL NERVE ROOT COMPRESSIONS	_Root_	_Motor_	_Sensory_	_Reflex_
	L4	quadriceps	medial foot	knee-jerk
	L5	dorsiflexors	dorsum of foot	medial hamstring
	S1	plantarflexors	lateral foot	ankle-jerk

GLASGOW COMA SCALE

Eye Opening
4. Spontaneous
3. To command
2. To pain
1. None

Verbal Activity
5. Oriented
4. Confused
3. Inappropriate
2. Incomprehensible
1. None

Motor Activity
6. Obeys commands
5. Localizes pain
4. Withdraws to pain
3. Flexion to pain
2. Extension to pain
1. None

Alzheimer's Disease—Cholinesterase Inhibitors

DONEPEZIL (*Aricept*) Start 5 mg PO at bedtime. May increase to 10 mg PO at bedtime in 4 to 6 weeks. Max 10 mg/day for mild to moderate disease. For moderate to severe disease (MMSE 10 or less): May increase after 3 months to 23 mg/day. ODT form should be dissolved on the top of the tongue. [Generic/Trade: Tabs 5, 10, 23 mg. Orally disintegrating tabs 5, 10 mg.] ▶LK ♀C ▶? $

GALANTAMINE (*Razadyne, Razadyne ER, ✦Reminyl*) Immediate-release: Start 4 mg PO two times per day with food; increase to 8 mg two times per day after at least 4 weeks. May increase to 12 mg two times per day after another 4 weeks or more. Extended-release: Start 8 mg PO every am with food; increase to 16 mg after at least 4 weeks. May increase to 24 mg after another 4 weeks or more. [Generic/Trade: Tabs 4, 8, 12 mg. Extended-release caps 8, 16, 24 mg. Oral soln 4 mg/mL.] ▶LK ♀C ▶? $$$$

RIVASTIGMINE (*Exelon, Exelon Patch*) Alzheimer's disease (mild to moderate): Start 1.5 mg PO two times per day with food. Increase to 3 mg two times per day after 2 weeks. May increase to 4.5 mg twice daily and then 6 mg twice daily at two-week intervals. Usual effective range 6 to 12 mg/day. Max 12 mg/day. Patch: Start 4.6 mg/24 h once daily; may increase after 1 month or more to recommended dose of 9.5 mg/24 h, max 13.3 mg/24 h. Rotate sites. Dementia in Parkinson's disease (mild to moderate): Start 1.5 mg PO twice daily with food. Increase by 3 mg/day at intervals of 4 weeks or more to max 12 mg/day. May increase to 4.5 mg twice daily then 6 mg twice daily at 4 week intervals. Max 12 mg/day. Patch: Use dosing for Alzheimer's disease. [Generic/Trade: Caps 1.5, 3, 4.5, 6 mg. Trade only: Transdermal patch: 4.6 mg/24 h, 9.5 mg/24 h, 13.3 mg/24 h. Oral solution 2 mg/mL.] ▶L cholinesterase-mediated hydrolysis ♀B ▶? $$$$$

Alzheimer's Disease—NMDA Receptor Antagonists

MEMANTINE (*Namenda, Namenda XR, ✦Ebixa*) Start 5 mg PO daily. Increase by 5 mg/day at weekly intervals to max 20 mg/day. Doses greater than 5 mg/day should be divided two times per day. Reduce dose to 5 mg twice daily with severe renal impairment. Extended-release: start 7 mg once daily. Increase at weekly intervals to target dose of 28 mg/day. Reduce to 14 mg/day in severe renal impairment. [Generic/Trade: Tabs 5, 10 mg. Oral soln 2 mg/mL. Trade only: Extended-release caps 7, 14, 21, 28 mg.] ▶KL ♀B ▷? $$$

NAMZARIC (**memantine extended-release + donepezil**) For patients stabilized on donepezil 10 mg alone start Namzaric 7 mg/10 mg PO once daily in the evening. Increase weekly by 7 mg/day of memantine to recommended dose of 28 mg/10 mg. For patients already stabilized on memantine 10 mg twice daily or 28 mg/day of extended-release, start recommended dose of Namzaric 28 mg/10 mg PO once daily in the evening. Reduce maintenance dose to 14/10 mg for severe renal insufficiency (ClCr 5 to 29 mL/min). [Trade only: Caps, extended-release memantine + donepezil 7 mg/10 mg, 14/10, 21 mg/10 mg, 28/10 mg.] ▶KL ♀C ▷?

Anticonvulsants

NOTE: *Avoid rapid discontinuation of anticonvulsants because this can precipitate seizures or other withdrawal symptoms. Increased risk of suicidal ideation or behaviors with antiepileptic drugs. Monitor closely for signs of depression, anxiety, hostility, hypomania/mania, or suicidality. Symptoms may develop within 1 week of initiation, and risk continues for at least 24 weeks.*

BIVARACETAM (*Briviact*) Start 50 mg PO/IV twice daily. May reduce to 25 mg PO/IV twice daily or increase to 100 mg PO/IV twice daily based on efficacy and tolerability. Reserve IV use

(cont.)

for when PO not possible. For all stages of hepatic impairment reduce initial dose to 25 mg twice daily with a max dose of 75 mg twice daily. [Trade only: Tabs 10, 25, 50, 75, 100 mg. Oral soln 10 mg/mL.] ▶L Primarily hydrolyzed, some by CYP2C19 ♀C Consider enrolling in registry ▶? ©V

CARBAMAZEPINE (*Tegretol, Tegretol XR, Carbatrol, Epitol, Equetro*) Epilepsy: Ages 13 yo and older: 200 mg PO twice daily, then increase by 200 mg/day at weekly intervals divided into three or four doses (immediate-release tabs) or two times per day (extended-release). Usual max 1000 mg/day but doses up to 1600 mg/day have been used. Age 6 to 12 yo: Start 100 mg PO twice daily (immediate-release or extended-release) or ½ teaspoon (50 mg) susp four times daily. Increase by 100 mg/day at weekly intervals divided into three or four daily doses (immediate-release tabs or susp) or two times per day (extended-release). Max 1,000 mg/day. Age younger than 6 yo: Start 10 to 20 mg/kg/day PO divided into two to three doses per day (immediate-release tabs) or four times per day (susp). Increase weekly prn. Max 35 mg/kg/day. Bipolar disorder, acute manic/mixed episodes (Equetro): Start 200 mg PO two times per day; increase by 200 mg/day to max 1600 mg/day. Trigeminal neuralgia: Start 100 mg PO two times per day (regular and XR tabs) or 50 mg PO four times daily (susp). May increase by 200 mg/day until pain relieved or max 1200 mg/day. Usual range 400 to 800 mg/day. Aplastic anemia, agranulocytosis, many drug interactions. [Generic/Trade: Tabs 200 mg, Chewable tabs 100 mg, Susp 100 mg/5 mL. Extended-release tabs (Tegretol XR) 100, 200, 400 mg. Extended-release caps (Carbatrol) 100, 200, 300 mg. Trade only: Extended-release caps (Equetro) 100, 200, 300 mg.] ▶LK ♀D ▶+ $$ ∎

CLOBAZAM (*ONFI, ✦Frisium*) US, adults and children 2 yo and older, weight greater than 30 kg: Start 5 mg PO twice per day. Increase to 10 mg PO twice daily after 1 week, then to 20 mg PO twice daily after 2 weeks. Wt 30 kg or less: Start 5 mg PO daily. Increase to 5 mg PO twice per day after 1 week, then 10 mg

(cont.)

PO twice per day after 2 weeks. Canada, adults: Start 5 to 15 mg PO daily. Increase prn to max 80 mg/day. Children younger than 2 yo: 0.5 to 1 mg/kg PO daily. Children age 2 to 16 yo: Start 5 mg PO daily. May increase prn to max 40 mg/day. Geriatric dosing: Start 5 mg PO daily. Titrate according to weight to 10 mg to 20 mg per day as tolerated and required. Max 40 mg/day. [Trade only: Tabs 10, 20 mg. Oral susp 2.5 mg/mL.] ▸L ♀C ▸─ ⊙IV $$$$$

ESLICARBAZEPINE (*Aptiom*) Start 400 mg PO once daily. May start 800 mg PO once daily if the need for seizure control outweighs risks of side effects. Increase dose weekly by 400 mg to 600 mg to recommended dose of 800 mg to 1600 mg once daily based on response and tolerability. [Trade only: Tabs 200, 400, 600, 800 mg.] ▸L ♀C ▸? Enters breastmilk $$$$$

ETHOSUXIMIDE (*Zarontin*) Age 3 to 6 yo: Start 250 mg PO daily (or divided two times per day). Age older than 6 yo: Start 500 mg PO daily (or divided two times per day). Max 1.5 g/day. The optimal dose for most pediatric patients is 20 mg/kg/day. [Generic/Trade: Caps 250 mg. Syrup 250 mg/5 mL.] ▸LK ♀?/?/?. Briggs assigned a "C" rating. ▸+ $$$$

EZOGABINE (*POTIGA*) Start 100 mg PO three times per day. Increase weekly by no more than 150 mg three times daily to usual maintenance dose of 200 to 400 mg PO three times daily or max of 250 mg three times daily if older than 65 yo. Reduce dose for moderate to severe renal or hepatic impairment. [Trade: Tabs 50, 200, 300, 400 mg.] ▸KL ─ ♀C ▸? $$$$$ ■

FOSPHENYTOIN (*Cerebyx*) Status epilepticus: Load 15 to 20 mg "phenytoin equivalents" (PE) per kg IM/IV no faster than 150 mg PE/min. Maintenance: 4 to 6 mg PE/kg/day in divided doses. Non-emergent use when oral phenytoin not possible: Load 10 to 20 mg PE IV (rate no faster than 150 mg PE/min) or IM. Initial maintenance dose 4 to 6 mg PE/kg/day in divided doses. When substituted for oral phenytoin an equivalent number of phenytoin equivalents may be used. ▸L ♀D ▸+ $

GABAPENTIN (*Neurontin, Horizant, Gralise*) Partial seizures, adjunctive therapy: Start 300 mg PO three times daily. Gradually increase to recommended dose of 300 to 600 mg PO three times per day. Doses of up to 2400 mg/day have been well tolerated. Max 3600 mg/day divided three times per day. Postherpetic neuralgia, immediate-release tabs: Start 300 mg PO on day 1; increase to 300 mg two times per day on day 2, and to 300 mg three times per day on day 3. Usual maintenance dose 1800 mg/day divided three times per day. Doses as high as 3600 mg/day have been used but are not more effective. Postherpetic neuralgia (Gralise): Start 300 mg PO once daily with evening meal. Increase to 600 mg on day 2, 900 mg on days 3 to 6, 1200 mg on days 7 to 10, 1500 mg on days 11 to 14, and 1800 mg on day 15. Max 1800 mg/day. Postherpetic neuralgia (Horizant): Start 600 mg PO q am for 3 days, then increase to 600 mg PO twice per day. Max 1200 mg/day. Restless legs syndrome (Horizant): 600 mg PO once daily around 5 pm taken with food. [Generic only: Tabs 100, 300, 400 mg. Generic/Trade: Caps 100, 300, 400 mg. Tabs 100, 300, 400, 600, 800 mg. Soln 50 mg/mL. Trade only: Tabs, extended-release 300, 600 mg (gabapentin enacarbil, Horizant). Trade only (Gralise): Tabs 300, 600 mg.] ▶K ♀C ▶? $$$$

LACOSAMIDE (*Vimpat*) Adjunctive therapy: Start 50 mg PO/IV two times per day. Increase weekly by 50 mg two times per day to recommended dose of 100 to 200 mg two times per day. Max recommended 400 mg/day (max 300 mg/day in mild/moderate hepatic or severe renal impairment). Alternative initiation: Load with 200 mg PO/IV followed 12 h later by 100 mg PO two times per day for 1 week. May then increase weekly as required by 50 mg two times per day to max recommended dose of 400 mg/day. Monotherapy: Start 100 mg PO/IV two times per day. May increase weekly by 50 mg two times per day to recommended range of 150 to 200 mg two times per day. Alternative initiation: Load with 200 mg PO/IV followed 12 h later by 100 mg twice daily for 1 week. May then increase weekly as required by 50

(cont.)

NEUROLOGY

mg two times per day to recommended range of 150 to 200 mg two times per day. Conversion to monotherapy: Initiate and titrate lacosamide to usual dose of 150 mg to 200 mg twice daily and maintain for at least 3 days before tapering off the concomitant drug. Loading and IV dosing should be monitored. Doses of 600 mg/day are not more effective than 400 mg/day. [Trade only: Tabs 50, 100, 150, 200 mg. Oral Sol 10 mg/mL.] ▶KL ♀C ▶? ⊙V $$$$$

LAMOTRIGINE—NEUROLOGY (*Lamictal, Lamictal CD, Lamictal ODT, Lamictal XR*) Partial seizures, Lennox-Gastaut syndrome, or generalized tonic–clonic seizures, adjunctive therapy with other anticonvulsants (not valproate or enzyme inducers):age older than 12 yo:Start 25 mg PO daily for 2 weeks, then 50 mg PO daily for 2 weeks. Increase by 50 mg/day every 1 to 2 weeks to usual maintenance dose of 225 to 375 mg/day divided twice per day. Extended-release (generalized tonic–clonic and partial seizures): Start 25 mg PO daily for weeks 1 to 2, then increase to 50 mg/day for weeks 3 to 4. Increase to 100 mg/day on week 5 then increase weekly by 50 mg/day to target dose of 300 to 400 mg/day. Partial seizures, Lennox-Gastaut syndrome, or generalized tonic–clonic seizures, adjunctive therapy (with an enzyme-inducing anticonvulsant) age older than 12 yo: Immediate-release: Start 50 mg PO daily for 2 weeks, then 50 mg PO twice per day for 2 weeks. Increase by 100 mg/day every 1 to 2 weeks to usual maintenance dose of 300 mg to 500 mg/day divided twice per day. Extended-release (generalized tonic–clonic and partial seizures):Start 50 mg PO daily for weeks 1 to 2, then increase to 100 mg PO daily for weeks 3 to 4. Then increase by 100 mg/day at weekly intervals to target dose of 400 to 600 mg/day. Partial seizures, Lennox-Gastaut syndrome, or generalized tonic–clonic seizures, adjunctive therapy (with valproate) age older than 12 yo: Start 25 mg PO every other day for 2 weeks, then 25 mg PO daily for 2 weeks. Increase by 25 to 50 mg/day every 1 to 2 weeks to usual maintenance dose of 100 to 400 mg/day (when used

(cont.)

with valproate + other inducers of glucuronidation) or 100 to 200 mg/day (when used with valproate alone) given once daily or divided twice per day. Extended-release (generalized tonic–clonic and partial seizures): Start 25 mg PO every other day for weeks 1 to 2, then increase to 25 mg/day for weeks 3 to 4. Then increase to 50 mg/day on week 5 and increase weekly by 50 mg/day to target dose of 200 to 250 mg/day. Partial seizures, conversion to monotherapy from adjunctive therapy (with a single enzyme-inducing anticonvulsant), immediate-release: (age 16 yo and older): Use preceding guidelines to gradually increase the dose to 250 mg PO twice per day; then taper the enzyme-inducing anticonvulsant by 20% per week over 4 weeks. Extended-release: Achieve dose of 500 mg/day then begin to reduce the enzyme-inducing AED by 20% decrements weekly over a 4-week period. Two weeks after the enzyme-inducing AED is discontinued Lamictal XR can be decreased no faster than 100 mg/day each week to the target dose of 250 to 300 mg/day. Partial seizures, conversion to monotherapy from adjunctive therapy (with valproate), immediate-release(ages 16 yo and older): Use preceding guidelines to achieve a dose of 200 mg/day and maintain it. Then begin to decrease valproate by decrements of no greater than 500 mg/day per week to a dose of 500 mg/day and maintain this for 1 week. Then increase lamotrigine to 300 mg/day and reduce valproate simultaneously to 250 mg/day and maintain for 1 week. Then stop the valproate and increase lamotrigine by 100 mg/day q week until a maintenance dose of 500 mg/day is achieved. Extended-release: Achieve a dose of 150 mg/day and maintain it. Then begin to decrease valproate by 500 mg/day per week to 500 mg/day and maintain for 1 week. Then simultaneously increase Lamictal XR to 200 mg/day and decrease valproate to 250 mg/day and maintain for 1 week. Then increase Lamictal XR to 250 mg to 300 mg per day and discontinue valproate. Partial seizures, conversion to monotherapy from other AEDs (not valproate or enzyme inducers) extended-release: Achieve

(cont.)

a dose of 250 to 300 mg/day of Lamictal XR then begin to withdraw the other AED by 20% decrements weekly over a 4-week period. No specific guidelines have been developed for conversion from other anticonvulsants (not inducers or valproate) to monotherapy with lamotrigine immediate-release. See psychiatry section for bipolar disorder dosing. Potentially life-threatening rashes reported in 0.3% of adults and 0.8% of children; discontinue at 1st sign of rash. [Generic/Trade: Tabs 25, 100, 150, 200 mg. Chewable dispersible tabs (Lamictal CD) 5, 25 mg. Extended-release tabs (Lamictal XR) 25, 50, 100, 200, 250, 300 mg. Orally disintegrating tabs (Lamictal ODT) 25, 50, 100, 200 mg.] ▶LK ♀C Possible risk of cleft palate or lip. ▶— $$$$ ■

LEVETIRACETAM (*Spritam, Keppra, Keppra XR*) Partial seizures, juvenile myoclonic epilepsy (JME), or primary generalized tonic-clonic seizures (GTC), adjunctive: Start 500 mg PO/IV twice per day (Keppra or Spritam) or 1000 mg PO once daily (Keppra XR, partial seizures only); increase by 1000 mg/day every 2 weeks prn to max 3000 mg/day (partial seizures) or to recommended dose of 3000 mg/day (JME or GTC, and doses less than 3000 mg/day have not been adequately studied). IV route not approved for GTC or if age younger than 16 yo. Doses above 3000 mg are not more effective. [Generic/Trade: Tabs 250, 500, 750, 1000 mg. Oral soln 100 mg/mL. Tabs, extended-release 500, 750 mg. Trade: orally disentegrating tablet (Spritam) 250, 500, 750, 1000 mg.] ▶K ♀C ▶? $$$

METHSUXIMIDE (*Celontin*) Start 300 mg PO daily for one week; increase weekly by 300 mg/day. Max 1200 mg/day. [Trade only: Caps 150, 300 mg.] ▶L ♀C ▶? $$$

OXCARBAZEPINE (*Trileptal, Oxtellar XR*) Immediate-release (adjunctive or conversion to monotherapy): Start 300 mg PO two times per day. If needed may titrate by no more than 600 mg/day to recommended dose of 1200 mg/day (adjunctive) or 2400 mg/day (monotherapy). Initiation of monotherapy: Start 300 mg PO twice daily. Increase every third day by 300

(cont.)

mg/day to recommended dose of 1200 mg/day. Extended-release (adjunctive): Start 600 mg PO daily. Increase by 600 mg/day weekly if needed, max 2400 mg/day. Peds 2 to 16 yo: Immediate-release: Start 8 to 10 mg/kg/day divided two times per day. Extended-release (adjunctive for 6 to 17 yo): Start 8 mg/kg to 10 mg/kg PO once daily not to exceed 600 mg/day. May increase weekly by 8 mg/kg to 10 mg/kg once daily if needed to max based on wt of 900 mg/day (20 to 29 kg), 1200 mg/day (29.1 to 39 kg), or 1800 mg/day (greater than 39 kg). Life-threatening rashes and hypersensitivity reactions. [Generic/Trade: Tabs (scored) 150, 300, 600 mg. Oral susp 300 mg/5 mL. Trade only: Extended-release tabs (Oxtellar XR) 150, 300, 600 mg.] ▶LK ♀C ▶– $$$$$

PERAMPANEL (*Fycompa*) Partial-onset seizures: Without other enzyme-inducing drugs: Start 2 mg PO once daily at bedtime. Increase by 2 mg/day weekly to usual range of 8 to 12 mg/day. Max 12 mg/day. With enzyme-inducing drugs: Start 4 mg PO once daily at bedtime. May increase weekly by 2 mg/day to max 12 mg/day. Mild to moderate hepatic impairment: Start 2 mg PO once daily at bedtime. May increase by 2 mg/day every 2 weeks to max 6 mg/day for mild disease and 4 mg/day for moderate. Avoid in severe hepatic impairment. Generalized tonic-clonic seizures, adjunctive: Without other enzyme-inducing drugs: Start 2 mg PO once daily at bedtime. Increase by 2 mg/day weekly to usual range of 8 to 12 mg/day. Max 12 mg/day. With enzyme-inducing drugs: Start 4 mg PO once daily at bedtime. May increase weekly by 2 mg/day to max 12 mg/day. Mild to moderate hepatic impairment: Start 2 mg PO once daily at bedtime. May increase by 2 mg/day every 2 weeks to max 6 mg/day for mild disease and 4 mg/day for moderate. Avoid in severe hepatic impairment. [Trade only:Tabs 2, 4, 6, 8, 10, 12 mg. Sus 0.5 mg/mL] ▶L ♀C ▶? ©III $$$$$ ■

PHENOBARBITAL (*Luminal*) Epilepsy: 50 mg to 100 mg PO twice to three times daily. Oral daytime sedation: 30 mg to 120 mg divided into two or three doses. Max 400 mg/24 hr. Hypnotic:

(cont.)

NEUROLOGY

100 mg to 320 mg PO at bedtime.   [Generic only: Tabs 15, 16.2, 30, 32.4, 60, 64.8, 97.2, 100 mg. Elixir 20 mg/5 mL.] ▶L ♀D Some manufacturers rate it as B ▶━ ⊚IV $

PHENYTOIN (*Dilantin, Phenytek*) Status epilepticus: Load 15 to 20 mg/kg IV no faster than 50 mg/min, then 100 mg IV/PO every 6 to 8 h. Epilepsy: Start 100 mg PO three times daily then titrate to a therapeutic serum concentration for maintenance. Once seizures are controlled may consider once-daily dosing for extended-release caps. Usual max 600 mg/day. Alternative oral loading: 400 mg PO initially, then 300 mg again in 2 h and 4 h. Then 24 hour later begin usual maintenance dosing. Limit dose increases to 10% or less due to saturable metabolism. [Generic/Trade: Extended-release caps 100 mg (Dilantin). Susp 125 mg/5 mL. Extended-release caps 200, 300 mg (Phenytek). Chewable tabs 50 mg (Dilantin Infatabs). Trade only: Extended-release caps 30 mg (Dilantin).] ▶L ♀D ▶━ $$

PREGABALIN (*Lyrica*) Painful diabetic peripheral neuropathy: Start 50 mg PO three times per day; may increase within 1 week to max 100 mg PO three times per day. Postherpetic neuralgia: Start 150 mg/day PO divided two to three times per day. May increase within 1 week to 300 mg/day divided two to three times per day. If needed and tolerated, may increase to 600 mg/day in two to three divided doses. Partial seizures (adjunctive): Start 75 mg PO twice daily or 50 mg PO three times daily. Increase as needed to max 600 mg/day. Fibromyalgia: Start 75 mg PO two times per day; may increase to 150 mg two times per day within 1 week; max 225 mg two times per day. Neuropathic pain associated with spinal cord injury: Start 75 mg PO two times per day; may increase to 150 mg two times per day within 1 week and then to 300 mg two times per day after 2 to 3 weeks if needed and tolerated.   [Trade only: Caps 25, 50, 75, 100, 150, 200, 225, 300 mg. Oral soln 20 mg/mL (480 mL).] ▶K ♀?/?/?R Evidence of teratogenicity in animals. Inadequate human data. Enroll in registry; refer to prescribing information ▶? ⊚V $$$$$

PRIMIDONE (*Mysoline*) Epilepsy: Start 100 to 125 mg PO at bedtime. Increase over 10 days to 250 mg three to four times per day. Max 2 g/day. Metabolized to phenobarbital. Essential tremor (unapproved): Up to 750 mg/day. [Generic/Trade: Tabs 50, 250 mg.] ▶LK ♀D ▶– $$

RUFINAMIDE (*Banzel*) Start 400 to 800 mg/day PO divided two times per day. Increase by 400 to 800 mg/day every 2 days to max/target 3200 mg/day. Give with food. Use lower initial doses of 10 mg/kg in children or 400 mg/d for adults if on valproate. [Trade only: Tabs 200, 400 mg. Susp 40 mg/mL.] ▶K ♀C ▶? $$$$$

TIAGABINE (*Gabitril*) Start 4 mg PO daily. Increase by 4 to 8 mg/day at weekly intervals prn to max 32 mg/day (age 12 to 18 yo) or max 56 mg/day (age older than 18 yo) divided two to four times per day. Use lower inital doses and slower titration for patients on non-inducing anticonvulsants. Avoid off-label use. Give with food. [Generic/Trade: Tabs 2, 4 mg. Trade only: Tabs 12, 16 mg.] ▶L ♀C ▶? $$$$$

TOPIRAMATE (*Qudexy XR, Topamax, Trokendi XR*) Partial seizures or primary generalized tonic-clonic seizures, monotherapy (immediate-release tabs): Start 25 mg PO two times per day (week 1), 50 mg two times per day (week 2), 75 mg two times per day (week 3), 100 mg two times per day (week 4), 150 mg two times per day (week 5), then 200 mg two times per day as tolerated. Extended-release (Trokendi XR and Qudexy XR): Start 50 mg PO daily. Increase weekly by 50 mg/day for 4 weeks then by 100 mg/day for weeks 5 and 6 to recommended dose of 400 mg once daily. Partial seizures, primary generalized tonic-clonic seizures or Lennox-Gastaut syndrome, adjunctive therapy: Start 25 to 50 mg PO at bedtime. Increase weekly by 25 to 50 mg per day to usual effective dose of 200 mg PO two times per day. Doses greater than 400 mg per day not shown to be more effective. Extended-release (Trokendi XR and Qudexy XR): Start 25 to 50 mg PO once daily. Increase weekly by 25 to 50 mg/day to effective dose. Recommended

(cont.)

NEUROLOGY

dose 200 to 400 mg/day for partial seizures or Lennox-Gastaut syndrome or 400 mg/day for generalized tonic–clonic seizures. Migraine prophylaxis: Start 25 mg PO at bedtime (week 1), then 25 mg two times per day (week 2), then 25 mg every am and 50 mg every pm (week 3), then 50 mg two times per day (week 4 and thereafter). Bipolar disorder (unapproved): Start 25 to 50 mg per day PO. Titrate prn to max 400 mg per day divided two times per day. [Generic/Trade: Tabs 25, 50, 100, 200 mg. Sprinkle caps 15, 25 mg. Extended-release caps (Qudexy XR) 25, 50, 100, 150, 200 mg. Trade only: Extended-release caps (Trokendi XR) 25, 50, 100, 200 mg.] ▸K ♀D ▸? \$\$\$\$\$

VALPROIC ACID—NEUROLOGY (*Depakene, Depakote, Depakote ER, Depacon, Stavzor, divalproex, sodium valproate, ✦Epival, Deproic*) Epilepsy (complex partial seizures), ages 10 yo and older: 10 to 15 mg/kg/day PO/IV in divided doses (immediate-release, delayed-release, or IV) or given once daily (Depakote ER). Titrate by 5 to 10 mg/kg/week to max 60 mg/kg/day. IV should be infused over 60 min (no faster than 20 mg/min). Simple and complex absence seizures, age 10 yo and older:Start 15 mg/kg/day and increase weekly as needed by 5 to 10 mg/kg/day to max dose 60 mg/kg/day. For both seizure types, give Depkaote ER once daily. Give delayed-release products (Depakote, Depakote Sprinkles) in divided doses for doses above 250 mg/day. Immediate-release products (Depakene, valproic acid) should be divided twice daily for 500 mg/day and above, and three times daily for doses of 750 mg/day and above. Migraine prophylaxis: Start 250 mg PO two times per day (Depakote or Stavzor) or 500 mg PO daily (Depakote ER) for 1 week, then increase to max 1000 mg/day PO divided two times per day (Depakote or Stavzor) or given once daily (Depakote ER). Hepatotoxicity, drug interactions, reduce dose in elderly. [Generic/Trade: Immediate-release caps 250 mg (Depakene), syrup (Depakene, valproic acid) 250 mg/5 mL. Delayed-release tabs (Depakote) 125, 250, 500 mg. Extended-release tabs (Depakote ER) 250, 500 mg.

(cont.)

Delayed-release sprinkle caps (Depakote) 125 mg. Trade only (Stavzor): Delayed-release caps 125, 250, 500 mg.] ▶L ♀D Category X when used for migraine prevention ▶+ $$$$ ■

ZONISAMIDE (*Zonegran*) Start 100 mg PO daily. Titrate every 2 weeks by 100 mg/day given once daily or divided two times per day. Max 600 mg/day but doses greater than 400 mg/day are not more effective. Drug interactions. Contraindicated in sulfa allergy. [Generic/Trade: Caps 25, 50, 100 mg.] ▶LK ♀?/?/?R ▶? $$$$

Migraine Therapy—Triptans (5-HT1 Receptor Agonists)

NOTE: *May cause vasospasm. Avoid in ischemic or vasospastic heart disease, cerebrovascular syndromes, peripheral arterial disease, uncontrolled HTN, and hemiplegic or basilar migraine. Do not use within 24 h of ergots or other triptans. Risk of serotonin syndrome if used with SSRIs or MAOIs. May be associated with medication overuse headaches if used 10 or more days per month.*

ALMOTRIPTAN (*Axert*) 6.25 to 12.5 mg PO. May repeat in 2 h prn. Max 25 mg/day. Avoid MAOIs. [Generic/Trade: Tabs 6.25, 12.5 mg.] ▶LK ♀C ▶? $$

ELETRIPTAN (*Relpax*) 20 to 40 mg PO. May repeat in 2 h prn. Max 40 mg/dose or 80 mg/day. Drug interactions. Avoid MAOIs. [Trade only: Tabs 20, 40 mg.] ▶LK ♀C ▶? $$$$

FROVATRIPTAN (*Frova*) 2.5 mg PO. May repeat in 2 h prn. Max 7.5 mg/24 h. [Generic/Trade: Tabs 2.5 mg.] ▶LK ♀C ▶? $$$$

NARATRIPTAN (*Amerge*) 1 to 2.5 mg PO. May repeat in 4 h prn. Max 5 mg/ 24 h. [Generic/Trade: Tabs 1, 2.5 mg.] ▶KL ♀C ▶? $$

RIZATRIPTAN (*Maxalt, Maxalt MLT*) 5 to 10 mg PO. May repeat in 2 h prn. Max 30 mg/24 h. MLT form dissolves on tongue without liquids. Avoid MAOIs. [Generic/Trade: Tabs 5, 10 mg. Orally disintegrating tabs 5, 10 mg.] ▶LK ♀C ▶? $$$

SUMATRIPTAN (*Zembrace SymTouch, Onzetra Xsail, Imitrex, Alsuma, Sumavel, Zecuity*) Migraine treatment: Imitrex: 1

(cont.)

to 6 mg (6 mg usual) SC. May repeat in 1 h prn if there was some response to first dose. Max 12 mg/24 h. If HA returns after initial SC injection, then single tabs may be used every 2 h prn, max 100 mg/24 h. Zembrace SymTouch: 3 mg SC. May repeat after 1 or more hours if needed up to three times or max of 12 mg/24 h. Tabs: 25 to 100 mg PO (50 mg most common). May repeat every 2 h prn with 25 to 100 mg doses. Max 200 mg/24 h. Initial oral dose of 50 mg appears to be more effective than 25 mg. Intranasal spray: 5 to 20 mg every 2 h. Max 40 mg/24 h. Intranasal powder: 22 mg (11 mg in each nostril). May repeat if needed at least 2 h after the first dose. Max 44 mg/24 h. Transdermal (Zecuity): 1 patch topically, max two patches/24 h with no less than 2 h before 2nd application. No evidence of increased benefit with 2nd patch. Zecuity manufacturing temporarily suspended June, 2016. Cluster headache treatment: 6 mg SC. May repeat after 1 h or longer prn if there was some response to first dose. Max 12 mg/24 h. Avoid MAOIs. [Generic/Trade: Tabs 25, 50, 100 mg. Injection (STATdose System) 4, 6 mg prefilled cartridges. Trade only: Nasal spray (Imitrex Nasal) 5, 20 mg (box of #6). Alsuma, Sumavel: Injection 6 mg prefilled cartridge. Injection (Zembrace SymTouch) 3 mg autoinjector. Zecuity Transdermal Patch (temporarily suspended June, 2016): 6.5 mg/4 h. Generic only: Nasal spray 5, 20 mg (box of #6). Intranasal powder: 11 mg/nosepiece.] ▶LK ♀C ▶+ $

TREXIMET (**sumatriptan + naproxen**) 1 tab (85/500) PO at onset of headache. Max 2 tabs/24 h separated by at least 2 h. [Trade only: Tabs 85 mg sumatriptan + 500 mg naproxen sodium and 10 mg sumatriptan + 60 mg of naproxen sodium.] ▶LK ♀C ▶– $$$$ ■

ZOLMITRIPTAN (**Zomig, Zomig ZMT**) 1.25 to 2.5 mg PO every 2 h. Max single dose 5 mg. Max 10 mg/24 h. Orally disintegrating tabs (ZMT) 2.5 mg PO. May repeat in 2 h prn. Max 10 mg/24 h. Nasal spray: 5 mg (1 spray) in 1 nostril. May repeat in 2 h. Max 10 mg/24 h. [Generic/Trade: Tabs 2.5, 5 mg. Orally

(cont.)

disintegrating tabs (ZMT) 2.5, 5 mg. Trade only: Nasal spray 5 mg/spray.] ▶L ♀C ▶? $$

Migraine Therapy—Other

CAFERGOT (ergotamine + caffeine, *Migergot*) Cafergot: 2 tabs PO at onset, then 1 tab every 30 min prn. Max 6 tabs/attack or 10/week. Migergot: Two supps PR is max dose for one headache. Total weekly dose should not exceed 5 supps. Drug interactions. Fibrotic complications. [Trade/generic: Tabs 1/100 mg ergotamine/caffeine.] ▶L ♀X ▶– $$$ ■

DIHYDROERGOTAMINE (*D.H.E. 45, Migranal*) Soln (D.H.E. 45) 1 mg IV/IM/SC. May repeat in 1 h prn. Max 2 mg (IV) or 3 mg (IM/SC) per day. Nasal spray (Migranal): 1 spray in each nostril. May repeat in 15 min prn. Max 6 sprays/24 h or 8 sprays/week. Drug interactions. Fibrotic complications. [Generic/Trade: Nasal spray 0.5 mg/spray (Migranal). Self-injecting soln (D.H.E. 45): 1 mg/mL.] ▶L ♀X ▶– $$$$$ ■

FLUNARIZINE Canada only. 10 mg PO at bedtime. [Generic/Trade: Caps 5 mg.] ▶L ♀C ▶– $$

Multiple Sclerosis

ALEMTUZUMAB (*Lemtrada*) First course: 12 mg/day by IV infusion over 4 h for 5 consecutive days (60 mg total dose). Second course (12 months after 1st course): 12 mg/day by IV infusion over 4 h for 3 consecutive days (36 mg total dose). Refer to package insert for infusion instructions and premedications required prior to infusions. See entry in Oncology for other uses. [Trade: Injection 12 mg/1.2 mL.] ▶proteolysis ♀C ▶? ■

DACLIZUMAB (*Zinbryta*) 150 mg SC monthly. Enroll in Zinbryta REMS. Monitor liver function and bilirubin. [Trade only: Inj 150 mg/mL] ▶proteolysis ♀?/?/? ▶? ■

DALFAMPRIDINE (*Ampyra*, *✦Fampyra*) 10 mg PO two times per day. Contraindicated in seizure disorders or moderate to severe renal impairment. [Trade: Extended-release tabs 10 mg.] ▶K – ♀C ▶? $$$$$

DIMETHYL FUMARATE (*Tecfidera*) Start 120 mg PO twice per day. Increase to maintenance dose after 7 days to 240 mg twice per day. [Trade only: delayed-release capsules 120, 240 mg.] ▶esterases – ♀C ▶? $$$$$

FINGOLIMOD (*Gilenya*) 0.5 mg PO once daily. Contraindicated in cerebral or cardiovascular disease. [Trade only: Caps 0.5 mg.] ▶L – ♀C ▶?

GLATIRAMER (*Copaxone, Glatopa*) Glatiramer acetate 20 mg/mL: 20 mg SC daily. Copaxone 40 mg/mL: 40 mg SC three times weekly with at least 48 hours between doses. [Trade and generic: Prefilled syringes 20 mg per mL for injection. Trade only (Copaxone): 40 mg/mL. The 20 mg/mL and 40 mg/mL are not interchangeable.] ▶tissues local hydrolysis ♀B ▶? $$$$$

INTERFERON BETA-1A (*Avonex, Rebif*) Avonex 30 mcg (6 million units) IM q week. May start with lower dose of 7.5 mcg and increase by 7.5 mcg each week until 30 mcg dose is achieved. Rebif: For 22 mcg maintenance dose, start 4.4 SC mcg three times weekly for 2 weeks, then increase to 11 mcg three times weekly for 2 weeks, then increase to 22 mcg three times weekly. For 44 mcg maintenance dose, start 8.8 mcg SC three times weekly for 2 weeks, then increase to 22 mcg three times weekly for 2 weeks, then increase to 44 mcg three times weekly. Give on the same days each week and at least 48 hours apart. Follow LFTs and CBC. [Trade only (Avonex): Injection 30 mcg single-dose vial with or without albumin. Prefilled syringe 30 mcg. Trade only (Rebif): Starter kit 20 mcg prefilled syringe. Prefilled syringe 22, 44 mcg.] ▶L ♀C ▶? $$$$$

INTERFERON BETA-1B (*Extavia, Betaseron*) Start 0.0625 mg SC every other day for weeks 1-2, then 0.125 mg weeks 3-4, then 0.1875 mg weeks 5-6, then increase to 0.25 mg (8 million units) SC every other day. Suicidality, hepatotoxicity, blood dyscrasias. Follow LFTs. [Trade only: Injection 0.3 mg (9.6 million units) single-dose vial.] ▶L ♀C ▶? $$$$$

NATALIZUMAB (*Tysabri*) Refractory, relapsing multiple sclerosis (monotherapy) and Crohn's disease: 300 mg IV infusion over 1 h every 4 weeks. ▶ Serum ♀C ▶? $$$$$ ■

PEGINTERFERON BETA-1A (*Plegridy*) Start 63 mcg SC on day 1, then 94 mcg on day 15, then 125 mcg on day 29 and every 14 days thereafter. [Trade only: Inj Starter pack (63 mcg and 94 mcg), pen 125 mcg] ▸K ♀C Enroll in registry ▸? $$$$$

Myasthenia Gravis

PYRIDOSTIGMINE (*Mestinon, Mestinon Timespan, Regonol*) 60 to 200 mg PO three times per day (immediate-release) or 180 mg PO daily or divided two times per day (extended-release). [Generic/Trade: Tabs 60 mg. Extended-release tabs 180 mg. Trade only: Syrup 60 mg/ 5 mL.] ▸Plasma, K ♀C ▸+ $$$$$

Parkinsonian Agents—Anticholinergics

BENZTROPINE MESYLATE (*Cogentin*) Parkinsonism: 0.5 to 2 mg IM/PO/IV given once daily or divided two times per day. Drug-induced extrapyramidal disorders (EPS): 1 to 4 mg PO/IM/IV given once daily or divided two times per day. [Generic only: Tabs 0.5, 1, 2 mg.] ▸LK ♀C ▸? $

TRIHEXYPHENIDYL (*Artane*) Start 1 mg PO daily. Gradually increase to 6 to 10 mg/day divided three times per day. Max 15 mg/day. [Generic only: Tabs 2, 5 mg. Elixir 2 mg/5 mL.] ▸LK ♀C ▸? $

Parkinsonian Agents—COMT Inhibitors

ENTACAPONE (*Comtan*) Start 200 mg PO with each dose of carbidopa-levodopa. Max 8 tabs (1600 mg)/day. [Generic/ Trade: Tabs 200 mg.] ▸L ♀C ▸? $$$$$

Parkinsonian Agents—Dopaminergic Agents and Combinations

APOMORPHINE (*Apokyn*) Start 0.2 mL SC prn. May increase in 0.1 mL increments every few days. Monitor for orthostatic

(cont.)

hypotension after initial dose and with dose escalation. Max 0.6 mL/dose or 2 mL/day. Potent emetic, pretreat with trimethobenzamide 300 mg PO three times per day starting 3 days prior to use and continue for at least 6 weeks. Do not use 5-HT3 antagonist antiemetics. Contains sulfites. [Trade only: Cartridges (for injector pen, 10 mg/mL) 3 mL. Ampules (10 mg/mL) 2 mL.] ▶L ♀C ▶? $$$$$

CARBIDOPA-LEVODOPA (*Rytary, DUOPA, Sinemet, Sinemet CR, Parcopa*) Start 1 tab (25/100 mg) PO three times per day. Increase every 1 to 4 days prn. Controlled-release: Start 1 tab (50/200 mg) PO two times per day; increase every 3 days prn. Extended-release caps (Rytary): Start 23.75/95 mg PO three times daily for 3 days. May then increase to 36.25/145 mg three times daily. Max daily dose 97.5/390 mg three times daily. Some patients may require shorter dosing intervals of up to 5 times per day with a max recommended dose of 612.5/2450 mg per day. Enteral susp (DUOPA): Dose is based on the amount of immediate-release carbidopa-levodopa the patient is taking and is administered via enteral feeding tube. Refer to the package insert for full dosing calculation information. [Generic/Trade: Tabs (carbidopa-levodopa) 10/100, 25/100, 25/250 mg. Tabs, sustained-release (Sinemet CR, carbidopa-levodopa ER) 25/100, 50/200 mg. Trade only: Orally disintegrating tabs (Parcopa) 10/100, 25/100, 25/250 mg. Enteral susp (DUOPA): 4.63 mg carbidopa/20 mg levodopa per mL. Caps, extended-release (Rytary): 23.75/95, 36.25/145, 48.75/195, 61.25/245 mg.] ▶L ♀C ▶− $$$$

PRAMIPEXOLE (*Mirapex, Mirapex ER*) Parkinson's disease: immediate-release, start 0.125 mg PO three times per day for one week. Then increase to 0.25 mg three times daily. Increase every 5 to 7 days by 0.25 mg/dose (0.75 mg/day) as needed and tolerated given three times per day. Usual effective range is 1.5 to 4.5 mg/day. When discontinuing reduce dose by 0.75 mg/day until the daily dose is 0.75 mg/day, then reduce the dose by 0.375 mg/day. Extended-release: Start 0.375 mg PO

(cont.)

daily. May increase after 5 to 7 days to 0.75 mg daily, then by 0.75 mg/day increments q 5 to 7 days to max 4.5 mg/day. When discontinuing, reduce dose by 0.75 mg/day until the daily dose is 0.75 mg/day, then reduce the dose by 0.375 mg/day. Restless legs syndrome: Start 0.125 mg PO 2 to 3 h before bedtime. May increase every 4 to 7 days to max 0.5 mg/day given 2 to 3 h before bedtime. [Generic/Trade: Tabs 0.125, 0.25, 0.5, 0.75, 1, 1.5 mg. Tabs, extended-release 0.375, 0.75, 1.5, 2.25, 3, 3.75, 4.5 mg.] ▶K ♀C ▶? $$$$$

ROPINIROLE (*Requip, Requip XL*) Parkinson's disease: Start 0.25 mg PO three times per day, then gradually increase over 4 weeks by 0.25 mg/dose to 1 mg PO three times per day. After this, if needed, the dose can be increased by 1.5 mg/day weekly to 9 mg/day. After this the dose can be increased weekly by 3 mg/day to max 24 mg/day (8 mg three times daily). Extended-release: Start 2 mg PO daily for 1 to 2 weeks, then gradually increase by 2 mg daily at weekly or longer intervals. Max 24 mg/day. Restless legs syndrome: Start 0.25 mg PO 1 to 3 h before bedtime for 2 days, then increase to 0.5 mg/day on days 3 to 7. Increase by 0.5 mg/day at weekly intervals prn to max 4 mg/day given 1 to 3 h before bedtime. [Generic/Trade: Tabs, immediate-release 0.25, 0.5, 1, 2, 3, 4, 5 mg. Tabs, extended-release 2, 4, 6, 8, 12 mg.] ▶L ♀C ▶? $$$

ROTIGOTINE (*Neupro*) Early-stage Parkinson's disease: Start 2 mg/24 h patch daily; may increase by 2 mg/24 h at weekly intervals to max 6 mg/24 h. Advanced-stage Parkinson's disease: Start 4 mg/24 h patch daily; may increase by 2 mg/24 h at weekly intervals to max 8 mg/24 h. Restless legs syndrome: Start 1 mg/24 h patch daily; may be increased by 1 mg/24 h at weekly intervals to max 3 mg/24 h. [Trade: Transdermal patch 1, 2, 3, 4, 6, 8 mg/24 h.] ▶L – ♀C ▶?

STALEVO (**carbidopa + levodopa + entacapone**) (Conversion from carbidopa-levodopa with or without entacapone): Start Stalevo tab that contains the same amount of carbidopa/levodopa as the patient was previously taking, then titrate

NEUROLOGY

(cont.)

to desired response. May need to reduce levodopa dose if not already taking entacapone. Max 8 tabs/24 h except for the Stalevo 200 tabs for which it is 6 tabs/24 h. [Trade/generic: Tabs (carbidopa/levodopa/entacapone): Stalevo 50 (12.5/50/200 mg), Stalevo 75 (18.75/75/200 mg), Stalevo 100 (25/100/200 mg), Stalevo 125 (31.25/125/200 mg), Stalevo 150 (37.5/150/200 mg), Stalevo 200 (50/200/200 mg).] ▶L ♀C ▶– $$$$$

Parkinsonian Agents—Monoamine Oxidase Inhibitors (MAOIs)

RASAGILINE (*Azilect*) Parkinson's disease, monotherapy or as adjunct but not taking levodopa: 1 mg PO q am. Parkinson's disease, adjunctive with levodopa: 0.5 mg PO q am. Max 1 mg/day. Requires an MAOI diet that avoids foods very high in tyramine content. [Trade only: Tabs 0.5, 1 mg.] ▶L ♀C ▶? $$$$$

SELEGILINE (*Eldepryl, Zelapar*) Parkinson's disease (adjunct to levodopa): 5 mg PO every am and at noon, max 10 mg/day. Zelapar ODT: 1.25 to 2.5 mg every am, max 2.5 mg/day. [Generic/Trade: Caps 5 mg. Tabs 5 mg. Trade only: Orally disintegrating tabs (Zelapar ODT) 1.25 mg.] ▶LK ♀C ▶? $$$$

Other Agents

ABOBOTULINUM TOXIN A (*Dysport*) Cervical dystonia: 500 units IM total dose divided among affected muscles. May repeat every 12 weeks or longer. Max dose 1000 units per treatment. Glabellar lines (age younger than 65 yo): 50 units IM total dose divided into 10 unit injections at 5 sites (see prescribing information). May repeat every 12 weeks or longer. Risk of distant spread with symptoms of systemic botulism. Botulinum toxin products are not interchangeable. [Trade: Vials 300, 500 units for reconstitution.] ▶ ♀C ▶? ∎

BOTULINUM TOXIN TYPE B (*Myobloc*) Start 2500 to 5000 units IM in affected muscles. Use lower initial dose if no prior history of botulinum toxin therapy. Benefits usually last for 12 to 16 weeks when a total dose of 5000 to 10,000 units has been administered. Titrate to effective dose. Give treatments at least 3 months apart to decrease the risk of producing neutralizing antibodies. ▶Not significantly absorbed ♀+ ▶? $$$$$

Dextromethorphan/Quinidine (**Nuedexta**) Start 1 cap PO daily for 7 days, then increase to maintenance dose of 1 cap PO every 12 h. [Trade only: Caps 10 mg dextromethorphan plus 20 mg quinidine.] ▶LK – ♀C ▶? $$$$$

INCOBOTULINUMTOXIN A (*Xeomin*) Cervical dystonia: Total 120 units IM divided among appropriate muscle groups. May repeat at intervals of at least 12 weeks. Blepharospasm in patients previously treated with Botox: Use same dose as Botox. If dose unknown, start 1.25 to 2.5 units per injection site. Do not exceed initial dose of 35 units/eye. May repeat at intervals of at least 12 weeks. Upper limb spasticity: Dose varies from 5 to 50 units depending on the problem and muscle group involved. Refer to package label for specific dosing. [Trade only: 50, 100 unit single-use vials.] ▶not absorbed ♀–C ▶? ■

MANNITOL (*Osmitrol, Resectisol*) Intracranial HTN: 0.25 to 2 g/kg IV over 30 to 60 min. ▶K ♀C ▶? $$

MILNACIPRAN (*Savella*) Day 1: 12.5 mg PO on day 1. Days 2 to 3: 12.5 mg two times per day. Days 4 to 7: 25 mg two times per day. After that: 50 mg two times per day. Max 200 mg/day. [Trade only: Tabs 12.5, 25, 50, 100 mg.] ▶KL ♀C ▶? $$$$ ■

NIMODIPINE (*Nimotop, Nymalize*) Subarachnoid hemorrhage: Start within 96 hours. 60 mg PO every 4 h for 21 days. [Generic only: Caps 30 mg. Trade only: 60 mg/20 mL oral solution (Nymalize)] ▶L ♀C ▶– $$$$$

ONABOTULINUM TOXIN TYPE A (*Botox, Botox Cosmetic*) Dose varies based on indication. Risk of distant spread with symptoms of systemic botulism. [Trade only: 100 unit single-use vials.] ▶Not absorbed ♀C ▶? $$$$$ ■

OXYBATE (*Xyrem, GHB, gamma hydroxybutyrate*) 2.25 g PO at bedtime. Repeat in 2.5 to 4 h. Increase by 1.5 g/day (0.75 g per dose) at 2-week intervals to effective range of 6 to 9 g/day. From a centralized pharmacy. [Trade only: Soln 180 mL (500 mg/mL) supplied with measuring device and child-proof dosing cups.] ▶L ♀C ▶? ©III $$$$$ ■

RILUZOLE (*Rilutek*) ALS: 50 mg PO q 12 h. Monitor LFTs. [Generic/Trade: Tabs 50 mg.] ▶LK ♀C ▶– $$$$$

TETRABENAZINE (*Xenazine, ✽Nitoman*) Start 12.5 mg PO every am. Increase after 1 week to 12.5 mg PO two times per day. May increase by 12.5 mg/day weekly. Doses greater than 37.5 to 50 mg/day should be divided and given three times per day. For doses greater than 50 mg/day, genotype for CYP2D6, titrate by 12.5 mg/day weekly and divide in doses three times per day to max 37.5 mg/dose and 100 mg/day (extensive/intermediate metabolizers) or 25 mg/dose and 50 mg/day (poor metabolizers). Risk of depression, suicidality, and orthostatic hypotension. [Generic/Trade: Tabs 12.5, 25 mg.] ▶L ♀C ▶? ? $$$$$ ■

OB/GYN

EMERGENCY CONTRACEPTION

Emergency contraception within 72 h of unprotected sex or contraception failure.

Progestin-only method (Causes less nausea and may be more effective. Some available OTC with no age restriction.): Dose is levonorgestrel 1.5 mg tab. Take 1 pill. Many brands and generics available; Aftera, Athentia Next, EContraEZ, Fallback Solo, Her Style, My Way, Next Choice One Dose, Opcicon One-Step, Plan B One-Step, Take Action.

Progestin and estrogen method: Dose goal of 0.5 mg levonorgestrel (or 1 mg norgestrel) plus 100 mcg ethinyl estradiol. Take 1st dose ASAP and repeat 12 hours later. If vomiting occurs within 1 h of taking dose, consider repeating that dose with an antiemetic 1 hr prior. Dose is defined as 2 pills of Ogestrel, 4 pills of Altavera, Amethia*, Camrese*, Chateal, Cryselle, Daysee*, Elifemme**, Elinest, Enpresse**, Introvale, Jolessa, Kurvelo, Levonest**, Levora, Low-Ogestrel, Marlissa, Myzilra**, Nordette, Portia, Quasense, Seasonale, Seasonique*, Trivora**, or 5 pills of Amathia Lo**, Amethyst, Ashlyna, Aviane, Camresse Lo**, Falmina, Lessina, LoSeasonique***, Lutera, Orsthia, Sronyx.

Anti-progestin: Emergency contraception within 120 h of unprotected sex. Ella (ulipristal 30 mg): Take 1 pill. More info at: www.not-2-late.com.

*Use 0.15 mg levonorgestres/30 mcg ethinyl estradiol tabs.
**Use 0.125 mg levonorgestrel/30 mcg ethinyl estradiol tabs.
***Use 0.1 mg levonorgestrel/20 mcg ethinyl estradiol tabs.

DRUGS GENERALLY ACCEPTED AS SAFE IN PREGNANCY (selected)

Analgesics	acetaminophen, codeine* , meperidine* , methadone* , oxycodone*
Antimicrobials	azithromycin, cephalosporins, clindamycin, clotrimazole, erythromycins (not estolate), metronidazole, penicillins, permethrin, nitrofurantoin*** , nystatin
Antivirals	acyclovir, famciclovir, oseltamivir, valacyclovir
CV	hydralazine* , labetalol, methyldopa, nifedipine
Derm	benzoyl peroxide, clindamycin, erythromycin
Endo	bromocriptine, cabergoline, glyburide, insulin, levothyroxine, liothyronine, metformin
ENT	certirizine, chlorpheniramine, diphenhydramine, dextromethorphan, guaifenesin, loratadine, nasal steroids, nasal cromolyn

(cont.)

GI	antacids*, bisacodyl, cimetidine, docusate, doxylamine, famotidine, lactulose, loperamide, meclizine, metoclopramide, nizatidine, ondansetron, psyllium, pyridoxine, ranitidine, simethicone, trimethobenzamide
Heme	Heparin, dalteparin, enoxaparin
Immunology	adalimumab, etanercept, infliximab
Psych	bupropion, buspirone, desipramine, doxepin
Pulmonary	beclomethasone, budesonide, cromolyn, montelukast, nedocromil, prednisone**, short-acting inhaled beta-2 agonists, theophylline
Vitamins	cholecalciferol, ergocalciferol, folic acid, folate, pyridoxine

*Except if used long-term or in high dose at term.

**Except 1st trimester.

***Contraindicated at term and during labor and delivery.

ORAL CONTRACEPTIVES* →L CX

	Estrogen (mcg)	Progestin (mg)
Monophasic		
Lo Loestrin Fe, Lo Minastrin Fe[c]	10 ethinyl estradiol	1 norethindrone
Beyaz, Gianvi, Loryna, Melamisa, Nikki, *Yaz*		3 drospirenone
Aubra, *Aviane*, Delyla, Falmina, Lessina, Lessina, Lutera, Orsythia, Sronyx, Vienva	20 ethinyl estradiol	0.1 levonorgestrel
Gildess Fe 1/20, Junel 1/20, Junel Fe 1/20, Larin 1/20, Larin Fe 1/20, *Loestrin-21 1/20*, Loestrin Fe 1/20, Loestrin-24 Fe, Lomedia 1/20, Lomedia 24 Fe, Microgestin 1/20, Microgestin Fe 1/20, Minastrin 24 Fe[c], Tarina Fe 1/20		1 norethindrone

(cont.)

(cont.)

Generess Fe[c], Layolis Fe[c]	25 ethinyl estradiol	0.8 norethindrone
Apri, Cyred, Desogen, Emoquette, *Enskyce*, Juleber, *Ortho-Cept*, Reclipsen, Solia		0.15 desogestrel
Ocella, Safyral, Syeda, Yaela, *Yasmin*, Zarah		3 drospirenone
Altavera, Chateal, Kurvelo, Levora, Jolessa, Marlissa, *Nordette*, Portia	30 ethinyl estradiol	0.15 levonorgestrel
Gildess Fe 1.5/30, Junel 1.5/30, Junel 1.5/30 Fe, Larin Fe 1.5/30, *Loestrin 1.5/30, Loestrin Fe 1.5/30*, Microgestin 1.5/30, Microgestin Fe 1.5/30		1.5 norethindrone
Cryselle, Elinest, Low-Ogestrel		0.3 norgestrel

ORAL CONTRACEPTIVES* →L CX (continued)

	Estrogen (mcg)	Progestin (mg)
Monophasic		
Kelnor 1/35, Zovia 1/35E		1 ethynodiol
Balziva, Briellyn, Femcon Fe, Gildagia, Ovcon 35, Philith, Vyfemla, Wymzya Fe[c], Zenchent Fe[c]	35 ethinyl estradiol	0.4 norethindrone
Brevicon, Modicon, Necon, Nortrel, Wera		0.5 norethindrone
Alyacen 1/35, Cyclafem 1/35, Dasetta 1/35, Necon 1/35, Norinyl 1+35, Nortrel 1/35, Norethin 1/35, Ortho-Novum 1/35, Pirmella 1/35		1 norethindrone
Estarylla, Mono-Linyah, MonoNessa, Ortho-Cyclen, Previfem, Sprintec		0.25 norgestimate

(cont.)

(cont.)

Zovia 1/50E	50 ethinyl estradiol	1 ethynodiol
Ogestrel		0.5 norgestrel
Necon 1/50, Norinyl 1+50	50 mestranol	1 norethindrone
Progestin only		
Camila, Debiltane, Errin, Heather, Jencycla, Jolivette, Lyza, Micronor, Nora-BE, Norlyrox, Nor-QD, Sharobel	None	0.35 norethindrone
Biphasic (estrogen and progestin contents vary)		
Azurette, Bekyree, Kariva, Kimidess, Mircette, Pimtrea, Viorele	20/10 ethinyl estradiol	0.15/0 desogestrel

ORAL CONTRACEPTIVES* → L CX (continued)

	Estrogen (mcg)	Progestin (mg)
Triphasic (estrogen and progestin contents vary)		
Estrostep Fe, Tilia-Fe, Tri-Legest, Tri-Legest Fe	20/30/35 ethinyl estradiol	1 norethindrone
Caziant, Cesia, *Cyclessa*, Velivet	25 ethinyl estradiol	0.1/0.125/0.150 desogestrel
Ortho Tri-Cyclen Lo, Tri-Lo-Marzia, Tri-Lo-Sprintec, TriNessa Lo		0.18/0.215/0.25 norgestimate
Enpresse, Levonest, Myzilra, *Trivora-28*	30/40/30 ethinyl estradiol	0.5/0.75/0.125 levonorgestrel

(cont.)

Alyacen 7/7/7, Cyclafem 7/7/7, Dasetta 7/7/7, Necon 7/7/7, Nortrel 7/7/7, Ortho-Novum 7/7/7, Primella 7/7/7	35 ethinyl estradiol	0.5/0.75/1 norethindrone
Aranelle, *Leena*, *Tri-Norinyl*		0.5/1/0.5 norethindrone
Ortho Tri-Cyclen, Tri-Estarylla, Tri-Linyah, Tri-Previfem, TriNessa, Tri-Sprintec		0.18/0.215/0.25 norgestimate
Quadphasic		
Natazia	3/2/2/1 mg estradiol valerate	0/2/3/0 dienogest

(cont.)

ORAL CONTRACEPTIVES* →L CX (continued)

Extended Cycle	Estrogen (mcg)	Progestin (mg)
Amethyst	20 ethinyl estradiol	0.09 levonorgestrel
Amethia Lo, Camrese Lo, LoSeasonique††	20/10 ethinyl estradiol	0.1 levonorgestrel
Quartette††	20/25/30/10 ethinyl estradiol	0.15 levonorgestrel
Introvale, Jolessa, Quasense, Seasonale, Setlakin	30 ethinyl estradiol	
Amethia, Ashlyna, Camrese, Daysee, Seasonique††	30/10 ethinyl estradiol	

(cont.)

Note: Brand names are in *italics*.

*****All:** Not recommended in smokers. Increases risk of thromboembolism, CVA, MI, hepatic neoplasia, and gallbladder disease. Nausea, breast tenderness, headache and breakthrough bleeding are common transient side effects. Effectiveness reduced by hepatic enzyme-inducing drugs such as certain anticonvulsants and barbiturates, rifampin, rifabutin, griseofulvin, and protease inhibitors. Coadministration with St. John's wort may decrease efficacy. Vomiting or diarrhea may also increase the risk of contraceptive failure. Consider an additional form of birth control in above circumstances. See product insert for absolute and relative contraindications and instructions on missing doses and initiation of use.

Progestin only: Must be taken at the same time every day. Because much of the literature regarding OC adverse effects pertains mainly to estrogen/progestin combinations, the extent to which progestin-only contraceptives cause these effects is unclear. No significant interaction has been found with broad-spectrum antibiotics. The effect of St. John's wort is unclear. No placebo days, start new pack immediately after finishing current one. Available in 28-day packs. Readers may find the following website useful: www.managingcontraception.com.

†Approved for continuous use without a "pill-free" period.

††84 active pills and 7 ethinyl estradiol only pills.

^cChewable

Contraceptives—Oral Monophasic

AVIANE (ethinyl estradiol + levonorgestrel, *Falmina, Lessina, Orsythia, ✦Alesse*) [Generic/Trade: Tabs 20 mcg ethinyl estradiol/0.1 mg levonorgestrel.] ▶L ♀X ▶– $$

LOESTRIN FE (ethinyl estradiol + norethindrone + ferrous fumarate, *Larin Fe 1/20, Gildess Fe 1/20, Junel Fe 1/20, Microgestin Fe 1/20*) [Generic/Trade: Tabs 1 mg norethindrone/20 mcg ethinyl estradiol with 7 days 75 mg ferrous fumarate (1/20); 1.5 mg norethindrone/30 mcg ethinyl estradiol with 7 days 75 mg ferrous fumarate (1.5/30).] ▶L ♀X ▶– $$$

LOSEASONIQUE (ethinyl estradiol + levonorgestrel, *Amethia Lo, Camrese Lo*) [Generic/Trade: Tabs 20 mcg ethinyl estradiol/0.1 mg levonorgestrel. 84 orange active pills followed by 7 yellow pills with 10 mcg ethinyl estradiol.] ▶L ♀X ▶– $$$

NORDETTE (ethinyl estradiol + levonorgestrel, *Altavera, Kurvelo, Levora, Marlissa, Portia, ✦Min-Ovral*) [Generic/Trade: Tabs 30 mcg ethinyl estradiol/0.15 mg levonorgestrel.] ▶L ♀X ▶– $$$

NORETHINDRONE (*Micronor, Camila, Errin, Heather, Jencycla, Jolivette, Nora BE, Nor-Q.D.*) 1 tab daily. [Generic/Trade: Tabs 0.35 mg.] ▶L ♀C ▶+

ORTHO CYCLEN (ethinyl estradiol + norgestimate, *Estarylla, Mono-Linyah, Previfem, Sprintec, ✦Cyclen*) [Generic/Trade: Tabs 35 mcg ethinyl estradiol/0.25 mg norgestimate.] ▶L ♀X ▶– $$

ORTHO-CEPT (ethinyl estradiol + desogestrel, *Apri, Desogen, Emoquette, Enskyce, Reclipsen, ✦Marvelon*) [Generic/Trade: Tabs 30 mcg ethinyl estradiol/0.15 mg desogestrel.] ▶L ♀X ▶– $$$

ORTHO-NOVUM 1/35 (ethinyl estradiol + norethindrone, *Alyacen 1/35, Cyclafem 1/35, Dasetta 1/35, Necon 1/35, Norinyl 1+35, Nortrel 1/35, Pirmella 1/35*) [Generic/Trade: Tabs 1 mg norethindrone/35 mcg ethinyl estradiol.] ▶L ♀X ▶– $$$

OVCON-35 (ethinyl estradiol + norethindrone, *Balziva, Briellyn, Gildagia, Philith, Vyfemla, Zenchent*) [Generic/Trade: Tabs 35 mcg ethinyl estradiol/0.4 mg norethindrone.] ▸L ♀X ▸– $$$

SEASONALE (ethinyl estradiol + levonorgestrel, *Introvale, Quasense*) [Generic/Trade: Tabs 30 mcg ethinyl estradiol/0.15 mg levonorgestrel. 84 pink active pills followed by 7 white placebo pills.] ▸L ♀X ▸– $$$

YASMIN (ethinyl estradiol + drospirenone, *Ocella, Syeda, Zarah*) [Generic/Trade: Tabs 30 mcg ethinyl estradiol/3 mg drospirenone.] ▸L ♀X ▸– $$$

YAZ (ethinyl estradiol + drospirenone, *Gianvi, Loryna, Nikki*) [Generic/Trade: Tabs 20 mcg ethinyl estradiol/3 mg drospirenone. 24 active pills are followed by 4 inert pills.] ▸L ♀X ▸– $$$

Contraceptives—Oral Biphasic

AZURETTE (ethinyl estradiol + desogestrel, *Bekyree, Kariva, Kimidess, Pimtrea, Viorele*) [Generic/branded generics only: Tabs 20 mcg ethinyl estradiol/0.15 mg desogestrel (21), 10 mcg ethinyl estradiol (5).] ▸L ♀X ▸– $$$

Contraceptives—Oral Triphasic

ESTROSTEP FE (ethinyl estradiol + norethindrone + ferrous fumarate, *Tilia Fe-28, Tri-Legest Fe*) [Generic/Trade: Tabs 20, 30, 35 mcg ethinyl estradiol/1 mg norethindrone + "placebo" tabs with 75 mg ferrous fumarate. Packs of 28 only.] ▸L ♀X ▸– $$$

ORTHO TRI-CYCLEN LO (ethinyl estradiol + norgestimate) [Generic/Trade: Tabs 25 mcg ethinyl estradiol/0.18 (7), 0.215 (7), 0.25 mg norgestimate (7).] ▸L ♀X ▸– $$$

ORTHO TRI-CYCLEN (ethinyl estradiol + norgestimate, *Tri-Estarylla, Tri-Linyah, Tri-Previfem, Tri-Sprintec, ✦Tri-Cyclen*) [Generic/Trade: Tabs 35 mcg ethinyl estradiol/0.18 (7), 0.215 (7), 0.25 mg norgestimate (7).] ▸L ♀X ▸– $$

ORTHO-NOVUM 7/7/7* (ethinyl estradiol + norethindrone,** ***Alyacen 7/7/7, Cyclafem 7/7/7, Dasetta 7/7/7, Necon 7/7/7, ***Nortrel 7/7/7, Pirmella 7/7/7)*** [Generic/Trade: Tabs 35 mcg ethinyl estradiol/0.5, 0.75, 1 mg norethindrone.] ▶L ♀X ▶– $$

TRIVORA-28* (ethinyl estradiol + levonorgestrel,** ***Enpresse, ***Levonest, Myzilra)*** [Generic/Trade: Tabs 30, 40, 30 mcg ethinyl estradiol/0.05, 0.075, 0.125 mg levonorgestrel.] ▶L ♀X ▶– $$

Contraceptives—Oral Four-Phasic

***NATAZIA* (estradiol valerate and estradiol valerate +** **dienogest)** Contraception: 1 tab PO daily, start on day 1 of menstrual cycle. Heavy menstrual bleeding: 1 tab PO daily. [Trade only: Tabs 3 mg estradiol valerate (2), 2 mg estradiol valerate/2 mg dienogest (5), 2 mg estradiol valerate/3 mg dienogest (17), 1 mg estradiol valerate (2), inert (2).] ▶L – stomach ♀X ▶– ■

Contraceptives—Other

LEVONORGESTREL—INTRAUTERINE (*Mirena*) Contraception: 1 intrauterine system q 5 years. [Trade only: Single intrauterine implant. 25 mg levonorgestrel.] ▶L – ♀X ▶+

LEVONORGESTREL—SINGLE DOSE (*Plan B One-Step, Next* ***Choice One-Step, Fallback Solo*)** Emergency contraception: 1 tab PO ASAP but within 72 h of intercourse. [OTC Trade only: Tabs 1.5 mg.] ▶L ♀X ▶– $$

***NUVARING* (ethinyl estradiol + etonogestrel vaginal ring)** Contraception: 1 ring intravaginally for 3 weeks each month. [Trade only: Flexible intravaginal ring, 15 mcg ethinyl estradiol/0.120 mg etonogestrel/day in 1, 3 rings/box.] ▶L ♀X ▶– $$$

ORTHO EVRA* (ethinyl estradiol + norelgestromin,** ***Xulane, **✦*Evra*)** Contraception: 1 patch q week for 3 weeks, then 1 week patch-free. [Trade only: Transdermal patch (Xulane) 150 mcg norelgestromin/20 mcg ethinyl estradiol/day in 1, 3 patches/ box.] ▶L ♀X ▶– $$$$ ■

Estrogens

NOTE: *See also Hormone Combinations.*

ESTERIFIED ESTROGENS (*Menest*) 0.3 to 1.25 mg PO daily. [Trade only: Tabs 0.3, 0.625, 1.25, 2.5 mg.] ▶L ♀X ▶– $$ ■

ESTRADIOL 1 to 2 mg PO daily. [Generic only: Tabs, micronized 0.5, 1, 2 mg, scored.] ▶L ♀X ▶– $ ■

ESTRADIOL ACETATE VAGINAL RING (*Femring*) Insert and replace after 90 days. [Trade only: 0.05 mg/day and 0.1 mg/day.] ▶L ♀X ▶– $$$ ■

ESTRADIOL CYPIONATE (*Depo-Estradiol*) 1 to 5 mg IM q 3 to 4 weeks. [Trade only: Injection 5 mg/mL in 5 mL vials.] ▶L ♀X ▶– $ ■

ESTRADIOL GEL (*Divigel, Estrogel, Elestrin*) Thinly apply contents of 1 complete pump depression to one entire arm (Estrogel) or upper arm (Elestrin) or contents of 1 foil packet (Divigel) to one upper thigh. [Trade only: Gel 0.06% in nonaerosol, metered-dose pump with #64 or #32 1.25 g doses (Estrogel), #100 0.87 g doses (Elestrin). Gel 0.1% in single-dose foil packets of 0.25, 0.5, 1.0 g, carton of 30 (Divigel).] ▶L ♀X ▶– $$$ ■

ESTRADIOL TRANSDERMAL PATCH (*Alora, Climara, Menostar, Vivelle Dot, Minivelle, ✦Estradot, Oesclim*) Apply 1 patch weekly (Climara, Estradiol, Menostar) or twice per week (Minivelle, Vivelle Dot, Alora). [Generic/Trade: Transdermal patches doses in mg/day: Climara (once a week) 0.025, 0.0375, 0.05, 0.06, 0.075, 0.1. Trade only: Vivelle Dot (twice per week) 0.025, 0.0375, 0.05, 0.075, 0.1. Alora (twice per week) 0.025, 0.05, 0.075, 0.1. Minivelle (twice per week) 0.0375, 0.05, 0.075, 0.1 mg/day. Menostar (once a week) 0.014 mg.] ▶L ♀X ▶– $$$ ■

ESTRADIOL TRANSDERMAL SPRAY (*Evamist*) 1 to 3 sprays daily to forearm. [Trade only: 1.53 mg estradiol per 90 mcL spray, 56 sprays per metered-dose pump.] ▶L ♀X ▶– $$$ ■

ESTRADIOL VAGINAL RING (*Estring*) Insert and replace after 90 days. [Trade only: 2 mg ring single pack.] ▶L ♀X ▶– $$$ ■

ESTRADIOL VAGINAL TAB (*Vagifem*) 1 tab vaginally daily for 2 weeks, then 1 tab vaginally two times per week. [Trade only: Vaginal tab 10 mcg in disposable single-use applicators, 8 or 18/pack.] ▶L ♀X ▶– $$$ ■

ESTROGEN VAGINAL CREAM (*Premarin, Estrace*) Menopausal atrophic vaginitis: Premarin: 0.5 to 2 g daily. Estrace: 2 to 4 g daily for 2 weeks, then reduce. Moderate to severe menopausal dyspareunia: Premarin: 0.5 g daily, then reduce to two times per week. [Trade only: Premarin: 0.625 mg conjugated estrogens/g in 30 g with calibrated applicator. Estrace: 0.1 mg estradiol/g in 42.5 g with calibrated applicator. Generic only: Cream 0.625 mg synthetic conjugated estrogens/g in 30 g with calibrated applicator.] ▶L ♀X ▶? $$$$ ■

ESTROGENS CONJUGATED (*Premarin, C.E.S., Congest*) 0.3 to 1.25 mg PO daily. Abnormal uterine bleeding: 25 mg IV/IM. Repeat in 6 to 12 h if needed. [Trade only: Tabs 0.3, 0.45, 0.625, 0.9, 1.25 mg.] ▶L ♀X ▶– $$$ ■

GnRH Agents

NOTE: *Anaphylaxis has occurred with synthetic GnRH agents.*

GANIRELIX (✷*Orgalutran*) Inhibition of premature LH surges in women undergoing controlled ovarian hyperstimulation. [Generic only: Injection 250 mcg/0.5 mL in prefilled, disposable syringe.] ▶Plasma ♀X ▶? $$$$$

LUPANETA PACK (leuprolide + norethindrone) Endometriosis: Leuprolide 3.75 mg IM injection q month. Norethindrone 5 mg PO daily. [Trade only: 3.75 mg leuprolide acetate IM injection + norethindrone acetate 5 mg PO tabs #30 (1 month kit). 11.25 mg leuprolide acetate IM injection and norethindrone acetate 5 mg PO tabs #90 (3-month kit).] ▶L ♀X ▶– $$$$$

Hormone Combinations

NOTE: *See also Estrogens.*

ACTIVELLA (estradiol + norethindrone, *Lopreeza*) 1 tab PO daily. [Trade only: Tabs 1/0.5 mg and 0.5/0.1 mg estradiol/norethindrone acetate in calendar dial pack dispenser.] ▶L ♀X ▶– $$$ ■

ANGELIQ (estradiol + drospirenone) 1 tab PO daily. [Trade only: Tabs 1 mg estradiol/0.5 mg drospirenone.] ▶L ♀X ▶– $$$ ■

CLIMARA PRO (estradiol + levonorgestrel) 1 patch weekly. [Trade only: Transdermal 0.045/0.015 estradiol/levonorgestrel in mg/day, 4 patches/box.] ▶L ♀X ▶– $$$ ■

COMBIPATCH (estradiol + norethindrone acetate, ✶*Estalis*) 1 patch twice per week. [Trade only: Transdermal patch 0.05 estradiol/0.14 norethindrone and 0.05 estradiol/0.25 norethindrone in mg/day, 8 patches/box.] ▶L ♀X ▶– $$$ ■

DUAVEE (conjugated estrogens/bazedoxifene) 1 tab daily. [Trade only: Conjugated estrogens 0.45 mg/bazedoxifene 20 mg tabs.] ▶glucuronidation ♀X ▶– ■

PREFEST (estradiol + norgestimate) 1 pink tab PO daily for 3 days followed by 1 white tab PO daily for 3 days, sequentially throughout the month. [Generic only: Tabs in 30-day blister packs 1 mg estradiol (15 pink), 1 mg estradiol/0.09 mg norgestimate (15 white).] ▶L ♀X ▶– $$$ ■

PREMPHASE (estrogens conjugated + medroxyprogesterone) 1 tab PO daily. [Trade only: Tabs in 28-day EZ-Dial dispensers: 0.625 mg conjugated estrogens (14), 0.625 mg/5 mg conjugated estrogens/medroxyprogesterone (14).] ▶L ♀X ▶– $$$ ■

PREMPRO (estrogens conjugated + medroxyprogesterone, ✶*PremPlus*) 1 tab PO daily. [Trade only: Tabs in 28-day EZ-Dial dispensers: 0.625 mg/5 mg, 0.625 mg/2.5 mg, 0.45 mg/1.5 mg (Prempro low dose), or 0.3 mg/1.5 mg conjugated estrogens/medroxyprogesterone.] ▶L ♀X ▶– $$$ ■

Labor Induction / Cervical Ripening

DINOPROSTONE (*PGE2, Prepidil, Cervidil, Prostin E2*) Cervical ripening: 1 syringe of gel placed directly into the cervical os for

(cont.)

cervical ripening or 1 insert in the posterior fornix of the vagina. [Trade only: Gel (Prepidil) 0.5 mg/3 g syringe. Vaginal insert (Cervidil) 10 mg. Vaginal supps (Prostin E2) 20 mg.] ▸Lung ♀C ▸? $$$$$

MISOPROSTOL—OB (*PGE1, Cytotec*) Cervical ripening: 25 mcg intravaginally q 3 to 6 h (or 50 mcg q 6 h). First trimester pregnancy failure: 800 mcg intravaginally, repeat on day 3 if expulsion incomplete. Postpartum hemorrhage: 800 mcg PR. [Generic/Trade: Oral tabs 100, 200 mcg.] ▸LK ♀X ▸– $$ ■

OXYTOCIN (*Pitocin*) Labor induction: 10 units in 1000 mL NS (10 milliunits/mL), start at 6 to 12 mL/h (1 to 2 milliunits/min). Postpartum bleeding: 10 units IM or 10 to 40 units in 1000 mL NS IV, infuse 20 to 40 milliunits/min. ▸LK ♀? ▸– $

Ovulation Stimulants

NOTE: *Potentially serious adverse effects include DVT/PE, ovarian hyperstimulation syndrome, adnexal torsion, ovarian enlargement and cysts, and febrile reactions.*

CHORIOGONADOTROPIN ALFA (*Ovidrel*) Specialized dosing for ovulation induction as part of ART. [Trade only: Prefilled syringe 250 mcg.] ▸L ♀X ▸? $$$

CLOMIPHENE CITRATE (*Clomid, Serophene*) Specialized dosing. [Generic/Trade: Tabs 50 mg, scored.] ▸L ♀D ▸? $$$$$

GONADOTROPINS (*menotropins, FSH and LH, Menopur, Pergonal, Repronex*) [Trade only: Powder for injection, 75 units FSH and 75 units LH activity.] ▸L ♀X ▸– $$$$$

Progestins

MEDROXYPROGESTERONE (*Provera*) 10 mg PO daily for last 10 to 12 days of month, or 2.5 to 5 mg PO daily. Secondary amenorrhea, abnormal uterine bleeding: 5 to 10 mg PO daily for 5 to 10 days. Endometrial hyperplasia: 10 to 30 mg PO daily for 12 to 14 days per month. [Generic/Trade: Tabs 2.5, 5, 10 mg, scored.] ▸L ♀X ▸– $

MEDROXYPROGESTERONE—INJECTABLE (*Depo-Provera, Depo-SubQ Provera 104*) Contraception/endometriosis: 150 mg IM in deltoid or gluteus maximus or 104 mg SC in anterior thigh or abdomen q 13 weeks. ▶L ♀X ▶+ $ ■

MEGESTROL (*Megace, Megace ES*) Endometrial hyperplasia: 40 to 160 mg PO daily for 3 to 4 months. AIDS anorexia, cachexia, or unexplained weight loss: 800 mg (20 mL) susp PO daily or 625 mg (5 mL) ES daily. [Generic/Trade: Tabs 20, 40 mg. Susp 40 mg/mL in 240 mL. Trade only: Megace ES susp 125 mg/mL (150 mL).] ▶L ♀D ▶? $$$$$

NORETHINDRONE ACETATE (*Aygestin, ✦Norlutate*) Amenorrhea, abnormal uterine bleeding: 2.5 to 10 mg PO daily for 5 to 10 days during the 2nd half of the menstrual cycle. Endometriosis: 5 mg PO daily for 2 weeks. Increase by 2.5 mg q 2 weeks to 15 mg. [Generic/Trade: Tabs 5 mg, scored.] ▶L ♀X ▶ $$

PROGESTERONE MICRONIZED (*Prometrium*) 200 mg PO at bedtime 10 to 12 days per month or 100 mg at bedtime daily. Secondary amenorrhea: 400 mg PO at bedtime for 10 days. Contraindicated in peanut allergy. [Generic/Trade: Caps 100, 200 mg.] ▶L ♀B ▶+ $$

Selective Estrogen Receptor Modulators

OSPEMIFENE (*Osphena*) Dyspareunia: 1 tab PO daily with food. [Trade only: Tabs 60 mg.] ▶L ♀X ▶– $$$$ ■

RALOXIFENE (*Evista*) Osteoporosis prevention/treatment, breast cancer prevention: 60 mg PO daily. [Generic/Trade: Tabs 60 mg.] ▶L ♀X ▶– $$$$ ■

TAMOXIFEN (*Soltamox, Tamone, ✦Tamofen*) Breast cancer prevention: 20 mg PO daily for 5 years. Breast cancer: 10 to 20 mg PO two times per day. [Generic/Trade: Tabs 10, 20 mg. Trade only (Soltamox): Sugar-free soln 10 mg/5 mL (150 mL).] ▶L ♀D ▶– $$ ■

Uterotonics

CARBOPROST (*Hemabate, 15-methyl-prostaglandin F2 alpha*)
Refractory postpartum uterine bleeding: 250 mcg deep IM. ▶LK
♀C ▶? $$$

METHYLERGONOVINE (*Methergine*) Refractory postpartum
uterine bleeding: 0.2 mg IM/PO three to four times per day prn.
[Trade only: Tabs 0.2 mg.] ▶LK ♀C ▶– $$

Vaginitis Preparations

NOTE: *See also STD/vaginitis table in antimicrobial section.*

BORIC ACID Resistant vulvovaginal candidiasis: 1 vaginal
suppository at bedtime for 2 weeks. [No commercial
preparation; must be compounded by pharmacist. Vaginal
supps 600 mg in gelatin caps.] ▶Not absorbed ♀? ▶– $

CLINDAMYCIN—VAGINAL (*Cleocin, Clindesse, ✦Dalacin*)
Bacterial vaginosis: Cleocin: 1 applicatorful cream at bedtime
for 7 days or 1 vaginal suppository at bedtime for 3 days.
Clindesse: 1 applicatorful once. [Generic/Trade: 2% vaginal
cream in 40 g tube with 7 disposable applicators (Cleocin).
Vaginal supp (Cleocin Ovules) 100 mg (3) with applicator.
2% vaginal cream in a single-dose prefilled applicator
(Clindesse).] ▶L ♀– ▶+ $$

CLOTRIMAZOLE—VAGINAL (*Mycelex 7, Gyne-Lotrimin,
✦Canesten, Clotrimaderm*) Vulvovaginal candidiasis: 1
applicatorful 1% cream at bedtime for 7 days. 1 applicatorful
2% cream at bedtime for 3 days. 1 vaginal suppository 100
mg at bedtime for 7 days. 200 mg suppository at bedtime for
3 days. [OTC Generic/Trade: 1% vaginal cream with applicator
(some prefilled). 2% vaginal cream with applicator and 1%
topical cream in some combination packs. OTC Trade only
(Gyne-Lotrimin): Vaginal supp 100 mg (7), 200 mg (3) with
applicators.] ▶LK ♀B ▶? $

METRONIDAZOLE—VAGINAL (*MetroGel-Vaginal*, *Nuvessa*, *Vandazole*, *★Nidagel*) Bacterial vaginosis: 1 applicatorful at bedtime or two times per day for 5 days. [Generic/Trade: 0.75% gel in 70 g tube with applicator (MetroGel, Vandazole). Trade only: 1.3% gel in single 5 g pre-filled applicator (Nuvessa).] ▶LK ♀B ▶? $$

MICONAZOLE (*Monistat*, *Femizol-M*, *M-Zole*, *Micozole*, *Monazole*) Vulvovaginal candidiasis: 1 applicatorful at bedtime for 3 (4%) or 7 (2%) days. 100 mg vaginal supp at bedtime for 7 days. 400 mg vaginal suppository at bedtime for 3 days. 1200 mg vaginal supp once. [OTC Generic/Trade: 2% vaginal cream in 45 g with 1 applicator or 7 disposable applicators. Vaginal supp 100 mg (7). OTC Trade only: 400 mg (3), 1200 mg (1) with applicator. Generic/Trade: 4% vaginal cream in 25 g tubes or 3 prefilled applicators. Some in combination packs with 2% miconazole cream for external use.] ▶LK ♀+ ▶? $

TERCONAZOLE (*Terazol*) Vulvovaginal candidiasis: 1 applicatorful of 0.4% cream at bedtime for 7 days, or 1 applicatorful of 0.8% cream at bedtime for 3 days, or 80 mg vaginal suppository at bedtime for 3 days. [All forms supplied with applicators: Generic/Trade: Vaginal cream 0.4% (Terazol 7) in 45 g tube, 0.8% (Terazol 3) in 20 g tube. Vaginal supp (Terazol 3) 80 mg (#3).] ▶LK ♀C ▶— $$

Other OB/GYN Agents

HYDROXYPROGESTERONE CAPROATE (*Makena*) Specialized dosing (1 mL IM weekly) to reduce risk of preterm birth. [Trade only: 5 mL MDV (250 mg/mL) hydroxyprogesterone caproate in castor oil soln.] ▶L + glucuronidation ♀B ▶? $$$$$

PREMESIS-RX (**pyridoxine + folic acid + cyanocobalamin + calcium carbonate**) Pregnancy-induced nausea: 1 tab PO daily. [Trade only: Tabs 75 mg vitamin B6 (pyridoxine), sustained-release, 12 mcg vitamin B12 (cyanocobalamin), 1 mg folic acid, and 200 mg calcium carbonate.] ▶L ♀A ▶+ $$

RHO IMMUNE GLOBULIN (*HyperRHO S/D, MICRhoGAM, RhoGAM, Rhophylac, WinRho SDF*) Prevention of hemolytic disease of the newborn if mother Rh− and baby is or might be Rh+: 300 mcg vial IM to mother at 28 weeks gestation followed by a 2nd dose within 72 h of delivery. Microdose (50 mcg, MICRhoGAM) is appropriate if spontaneous abortion less than 12 weeks gestation. ▶L ♀C ▶? $$$$$

ONCOLOGY

ONCOLOGY

ONCOLOGY

ALKYLATING AGENTS: altretamine (*Hexalen*), bendamustine (*Treanda*, Bendeka), busulfan (*Myleran, Busulfex*), carmustine (*BCNU, BiCNU, Gliadel*), chlorambucil (*Leukeran*), cyclophosphamide, dacarbazine (*DTIC-Dome*), ifosfamide (*Ifex*), lomustine (Gleostine, *CeeNu, CCNU*), mechlorethamine (*Mustargen*), melphalan (*Alkeran*), procarbazine (*Matulane*), streptozocin (*Zanosar*), temozolomide (*Temodar*, ✤*Temodal*), thiotepa (*Thioplex*).

ANTIBIOTICS: bleomycin (*Blenoxane-Canada only*), dactinomycin (*Cosmegen*), daunorubicin (*Cerubidine*), doxorubicin liposomal (*Doxil*, ✤ *Caelyx, Myocet*), doxorubicin, non-liposomal (*Adriamycin*), epirubicin (*Ellence*, ✤ *Pharmorubicin*), idarubicin (*Idamycin*), mitomycin (*Mutamycin, Mitomycin-C*), mitoxantrone (*Novantrone*), valrubicin (*Valstar*, ✤ *Valtaxin*).

ANTIMETABOLITES: azacitidine (*Vidaza*), capecitabine (*Xeloda*), cladribine (*Leustatin, chlorodeoxyadenosine*), clofarabine (*Clolar*), cytarabine (*Cytosar, AraC*), cytarabine liposomal (*Depo-Cyt*),decitabine (*Dacogen*) floxuridine (*FUDR*), fludarabine (*Fludara*), fluorouracil (*Adrucil, 5-FU*), gemcitabine (*Gemzar*), hydroxyurea (*Hydrea, Droxia*), mercaptopurine (*6-MP, Purinethol*), methotrexate (Otrexup, Rasuvo, Rheumatrex, Trexall), nelarabine (*Arranon*), pemetrexed (*Alimta*), pentostatin (*Nipent*), Pralatrexate (*Folotyn*), thioguanine (*Tabloid*, ✤ *Lanvis*).

(cont.)

ONCOLOGY (*continued*)

ONCOLOGY (*continued*)

CYTOPROTECTIVE AGENTS: amifostine (*Ethyol*), dexrazoxane (*Zinecard, Totect*), mesna (*Mesnex,* ✦ *Uromitexan*), palifermin (*Kepivance*). **HORMONES:** anastrozole (*Arimidex*), bicalutamide (*Casodex*), cyproterone, (✦*Androcur, Androcur Depot*), degarelix (*Firmagon*), estramustine (*Emcyt*), exemestane (*Aromasin*), flutamide (*Eulexin,* ✦ *Euflex*), fulvestrant (*Faslodex*), goserelin (*Zoladex*), histrelin (*Vantas, Supprelin LA*), letrozole (*Femara*), leuprolide (*Eligard, Lupron, Lupron Depot, Lupron Depot-Ped*), nilutamide (*Nilandron*), raloxifene (*Evista*) toremifene (*Fareston*), triptorelin (*Trelstar Depot*). **IMMUNOMODULATORS:** aldesleukin (*Proleukin, interleukin-2*),✦ BCG (*Bacillus of Calmette & Guerin, Pacis, TheraCys, Tice BCG,* ✦ *Oncotice,* ✦ *Immucyst*), everolimus (*Afinitor*), interferon alfa-2b (*Intron-A*), lenalidomide (*Revlimid*), temsirolimus (*Torisel*), thalidomide (*Thalomid*). **MITOTIC INHIBITORS:** cabazitaxel (*Jevtana*), docetaxel (*Taxotere*), ixabepilone (*Ixempra*), paclitaxel (*Taxol, Onxol*), vinblastine (*Velban, VLB*), vincristine (*Oncovin, Vincasar, VCR*), vinorelbine (*Navelbine*). **MONOCLONAL ANTIBODIES:** alemtuzumab (*Campath,* ✦ *MabCampath*), bevacizumab (*Avastin*), cetuximab (*Erbitux*), ibritumomab (*Zevalin*), ofatumumab (*Arzerra*), panitumumab (*Vecti bix*), rituximab (*Rituxan*), trastuzumab (*Herceptin*). **PLATINUM-CONTAINING AGENTS:** carboplatin (*Paraplatin*), cisplatin (*Platinol-AQ*),

(cont.)

ONCOLOGY (*continued*)

ONCOLOGY (*continued*)

oxaliplatin (*Eloxatin*). **RADIOPHARMACEUTICALS:** samarium 153 (*Quadramet*), strontium-89 (*Metastron*). **TOPOISOMERASE INHIBITORS:** etoposide (*VP-16, Etopophos, Toposar, VePesid*), irinotecan (*Camptosar*), teniposide (*Vumon, VM-26*), topotecan (*Hycamtin*) **TYROSINE KINASE INHIBITORS:** dasatinib (*Sprycel*), erlotinib (*Tarceva*) gefitinib (*Iressa*), imatinib (*Gleevec*), lapatinib (*Tykerb*), nilotinib (*Tasigna*), pazopanib (*Votrient*), sorafenib (*Nexavar*), sunitinib (*Sutent*). **MISCELLANEOUS:** arsenic trioxide (*Trisenox*), asparaginase (✿*Kidrolase*), bexarotene (*Targretin*), bortezomib (*Velcade*), leucovorin, *(folinic acid)*, levoleucovorin (*Fusilev*), mitotane (*Lysodren*), pegaspargase (*Oncaspar*), porfimer (*Photofrin*), rasburicase (*Elitek*), romidepsin (*Istodax*), tretinoin (*Vesanoid*), vorinostat (*Zolinza*).

(cont.)

OPHTHALMOLOGY

Antiallergy—Decongestants and Combinations

NOTE: *Most eye medications can be administered 1 gtt at a time despite common manufacturer recommendations of 1 to 2 gtts concurrently. Even a single gtt is typically more than the eye can hold, and thus a second gtt is wasteful and increases the possibility of systemic toxicity. If 2 gtts of the medication are desired, separate single gtt by at least 5 min.*

NAPHAZOLINE (*Albalon, All Clear, Naphcon, Clear Eyes*) 1 to 2 gtts in each affected eye four times per day for up to 3 days. [OTC Generic/Trade: Soln 0.012, 0.025% (15, 30 mL). Rx Generic/Trade: 0.1% (15 mL).] ▶? ♀C ▶? $

NAPHCON-A (naphazoline + pheniramine) 1 gtt in each affected eye four times per day prn for up to 3 days. [OTC Trade only: Soln 0.025% + 0.3% (15 mL).] ▶L ♀C ▶? $

VASOCON-A (naphazoline + antazoline) 1 gtt in each affected eye four times per day prn for up to 3 days. [OTC Trade only: Soln 0.05% + 0.5% (15 mL).] ▶L ♀C ▶? $

Antiallergy—Dual Antihistamine and Mast Cell Stabilizer

AZELASTINE—OPHTHALMIC (*Optivar*) 1 gtt in each affected eye two times per day. [Trade/Generic: Soln 0.05% (6 mL).] ▶L ♀C ▶? $$$

EPINASTINE (*Elestat*) 1 gtt in each affected eye two times per day. [Trade only: Soln 0.05% (5 mL).] ▶K ♀C ▶? $$$$

KETOTIFEN—OPHTHALMIC (*Alaway, Zaditor*) 1 gtt in each affected eye q 8 to 12 h. [OTC Generic/Trade: Soln 0.025% (5 mL, 10 mL).] ▶minimal absorption ♀C ▶? $

OLOPATADINE—OPHTHALMIC (*Pazeo, Pataday, Patanol*) 1 gtt of 0.1% soln in each affected eye two times per day (Patanol) or 1 gtt of 0.2% soln in each affected eye daily (Pataday) or 1 gtt of 0.7% soln in each affected eye daily (Pazeo). [Generic/Trade: Soln 0.1% (5 mL, Patanol). Trade **(cont.)**

only: Soln 0.2% (2.5 mL, Pataday), soln 0.7% (4 mL, Pazeo).]
▶K ♀C ▸? $$$$$

Antiallergy—Pure Antihistamines

ALCAFTADINE (*Lastacaft*) 1 gtt in each eye daily. [Trade: Soln 0.25%, 3 mL.] ▶not absorbed ♀B ▸? $$$

BEPOTASTINE (*Bepreve*) 1 gtt in each affected eye two times per day. [Trade only: Soln 1.5% (2.5, 5, 10 mL).] ▶L (but minimal absorption) – ♀C ▸? $$$

EMEDASTINE (*Emadine*) 1 gtt in each affected eye daily to four times per day. [Trade only: Soln 0.05% (5 mL).] ▶L ♀B ▸? $$$

Antiallergy—Pure Mast Cell Stabilizers

CROMOLYN—OPHTHALMIC (*Crolom, Opticrom*) 1 to 2 gtts in each affected eye 4 to 6 times per day. [Generic/Trade: Soln 4% (10 mL).] ▶LK ♀B ▸? $$

LODOXAMIDE (*Alomide*) 1 to 2 gtts in each affected eye four times per day. [Trade only: Soln 0.1% (10 mL).] ▶K ♀B ▸? $$$

NEDOCROMIL—OPHTHALMIC (*Alocril*) 1 to 2 gtts in each affected eye two times per day. [Trade only: Soln 2% (5 mL).] ▶L ♀B ▸? $$$

Antibacterials—Aminoglycosides

GENTAMICIN—OPHTHALMIC (*Garamycin, Genoptic, Gentak, ✦Diogent*) 1 to 2 gtts in each affected eye q 2 to 4 h; ½ inch ribbon of ointment two to three times per day. [Generic/Trade: Soln 0.3% (5, 15 mL). Oint 0.3% (3.5 g tube).] ▶K ♀C ▸? $

TOBRAMYCIN—OPHTHALMIC (*Tobrex*) 1 to 2 gtts in each affected eye q 1 to 4 h or ½ inch ribbon of ointment q 3 to 4 h or two or three times per day. [Generic/Trade: Soln 0.3% (5 mL). Trade only: Oint 0.3% (3.5 g tube).] ▶K ♀B ▸– $

Antibacterials—Fluoroquinolones

BESIFLOXACIN (*Besivance*) 1 gtt in each affected eye three times per day for 7 days. [Trade: Soln 0.6% (5 mL).] ▶LK ♀C ▸? $$$

CIPROFLOXACIN—OPHTHALMIC (*Ciloxan*) 1 to 2 gtts in each affected eye q 1 to 6 h or ½ inch ribbon ointment two to three times per day. [Generic/Trade: Soln 0.3% (2.5, 5, 10 mL). Trade only: Oint 0.3% (3.5 g tube).] ▶LK ♀C ▶? $$

LEVOFLOXACIN—OPHTHALMIC (*Iquix, Quixin*) Quixin: 1 to 2 gtts in each affected eye q 2 h while awake (up to 8 times per day) on days 1 and 2, then 1 to 2 gtts q 4 h (up to four times per day) on days 3 to 7. Iquix: 1 to 2 gtts q 30 min to 2 h while awake and q 4 to 6 h overnight on days 1 to 3, then 1 to 2 gtts q 1 to 4 h while awake on day 4 to completion of therapy. [Trade/Generic: Soln 0.5% (5 mL).] ▶KL ♀C ▶? $$$

MOXIFLOXACIN—OPHTHALMIC (*Vigamox, Moxeza*) 1 gtt in each affected eye three times per day for 7 days (Vigamox) or 1 gtt in each affected eye two times per day for 7 days (Moxeza). [Trade only: Soln 0.5% (3 mL, Vigamox and Moxeza).] ▶LK ♀C ▶? $$$

OFLOXACIN—OPHTHALMIC (*Ocuflox*) 1 to 2 gtts in each affected eye q 1 to 6 h for 7 to 10 days. [Generic/Trade: Soln 0.3% (5, 10 mL).] ▶LK ♀C ▶? $$

Antibacterials—Other

AZITHROMYCIN—OPHTHALMIC (*AzaSite*) 1 gtt in each affected eye two times per day for 2 days, then 1 gtt once daily for 5 more days. [Trade only: Soln 1% (2.5 mL).] ▶L ♀B ▶? $$$

BACITRACIN—OPHTHALMIC (*AK Tracin*) ¼ to ½ inch ribbon of ointment in each affected eye q 3 to 4 h or two to four times per day for 7 to 10 days. [Generic/Trade: Oint 500 units/g (3.5 g tube).] ▶minimal absorption ♀C ▶? $

ERYTHROMYCIN—OPHTHALMIC (*Ilotycin, AK-Mycin*) ½ inch ribbon of ointment in each affected eye q 3 to 4 h or two to six times per day. [Generic only: Oint 0.5% (1, 3.5 g tube).] ▶L ♀B ▶+ $

✦FUSIDIC ACID—OPHTHALMIC (*✦Fucithalmic*) Canada only. 1 gtt in both eyes twice daily for 7 days. [Canada trade only: gtts 1%. Multidose tubes of 3, 5 g. Single-dose, preservative-free tubes of 0.2 g in a box of 12.] ▶L ♀? ▶? $

NEOSPORIN OINTMENT—OPHTHALMIC (neomycin—ophthalmic + bacitracin—ophthalmic + polymyxin—ophthalmic) ½ inch ribbon of ointment in each affected eye q 3 to 4 h for 7 to 10 days or ½ inch ribbon two to three times per day for mild to moderate infection. [Generic only: Oint. (3.5 g tube).] ▶KL ♀C ▶? $

NEOSPORIN SOLUTION—OPHTHALMIC (neomycin—ophthalmic + polymyxin—ophthalmic + gramicidin) 1 to 2 gtts in each affected eye q 4 to 6 h for 7 to 10 days. [Generic/Trade: Soln (10 mL).] ▶KL ♀C ▶? $$

POLYSPORIN—OPHTHALMIC (polymyxin—ophthalmic + bacitracin—ophthalmic) ½ inch ribbon of ointment in each affected eye q 3 to 4 h for 7 to 10 days or ½ inch ribbon two to three times per day for mild to moderate infection. [Generic only: Oint (3.5 g tube).] ▶K ♀C ▶? $

POLYTRIM—OPHTHALMIC (polymyxin—ophthalmic + trimethoprim—ophthalmic) 1 to 2 gtts in each affected eye q 4 to 6 h (up to 6 gtts per day) for 7 to 10 days. [Generic/Trade: Soln (10 mL).] ▶KL ♀C ▶? $

SULFACETAMIDE—OPHTHALMIC (*Bleph-10, Sulf-10*) 1 to 2 gtts in each affected eye q 2 to 6 h for 7 to 10 days or ½ inch ribbon of ointment q 3 to 8 h for 7 to 10 days. [Generic/Trade: Soln 10% (15 mL), Oint 10% (3.5 g tube). Generic only: Soln 30% (15 mL).] ▶K ♀C ▶– $

Antiviral Agents

GANCICLOVIR—OPHTHALMIC (*Zirgan*) 1 gtt five times per day (approximately q 3 h) until ulcer heals, then 1 gtt 3 times per day for 7 days. [Trade only: Gel 0.15% (5g).] ▶minimal absorption ♀C ▶? $$$$

TRIFLURIDINE (*Viroptic*) 1 gtt q 2 to 4 h for 7 to 14 days, max 9 gtts per day and max of 21 days of therapy. [Generic/Trade: Soln 1% (7.5 mL).] ▶minimal absorption ♀C ▶– $$$

Corticosteroid & Antibacterial Combinations

NOTE: *Recommend that only ophthalmologists or optometrists prescribe due to infection, cataract, corneal/scleral perforation, and glaucoma risk from prolonged use. Monitor intraocular pressure.*

***BLEPHAMIDE* (prednisolone—ophthalmic + sulfacetamide—ophthalmic)** 2 gtts in each affected eye q 4 h and at bedtime or ½ inch ribbon to lower conjunctival sac 3 to 4 times per day and at bedtime. [Generic/Trade: Soln/Susp (5, 10 mL). Trade only: Oint (3.5 g tube).] ▶KL ♀C ▶? $

***CORTISPORIN—OPHTHALMIC* (neomycin—ophthalmic + polymyxin—ophthalmic + hydrocortisone—ophthalmic)** 1 to 2 gtts or ½ inch ribbon of ointment in each affected eye q 3 to 4 h or more frequently prn. [Generic only: Susp (7.5 mL). Oint (3.5 g tube).] ▶LK ♀C ▶? $

***FML-S liquifilm* (prednisolone—ophthalmic + sulfacetamide—ophthalmic)** 1 to 2 gtts in each affected eye q 1 to 8 h. [Trade only: Susp (10 mL).] ▶KL ♀C ▶? $$

***MAXITROL* (dexamethasone—ophthalmic + neomycin—ophthalmic + polymyxin—ophthalmic)** Small amount (about ½ inch) ointment in affected eye three to four times per day or at bedtime as an adjunct with gtts. 1 to 2 gtts susp into affected eye four to six times daily; in severe disease, gtts may be used hourly and tapered to discontinuation. [Generic/Trade: Susp (5 mL). Oint (3.5 g tube).] ▶KL ♀C ▶? $

***PRED G* (prednisolone—ophthalmic + gentamicin—ophthalmic)** 1 to 2 gtts in each affected eye two to four times per day or ½ inch ribbon of ointment one to three times per day. [Trade only: Susp (2, 5, 10 mL). Oint (3.5 g tube).] ▶KL ♀C ▶? $$

***TOBRADEX* (tobramycin—ophthalmic + dexamethasone—ophthalmic)** 1 to 2 gtts in each affected eye q 2 to 6 h or ½ inch ribbon of ointment three to four times per day. [Trade/Generic: Susp (tobramycin 0.3%/dexamethasone 0.1%, 2.5, 5, 10 mL). Trade: Oint (tobramycin 0.3%/dexamethasone 0.1%, 3.5 g tube).] ▶L ♀C ▶? $$$

TOBRADEX ST **(tobramycin—ophthalmic + dexamethasone—ophthalmic)** 1 gtt in each affected eye q 2 to 6 h. [Trade only: Tobramycin 0.3%/dexamethasone 0.05% susp (2.5, 5, 10 mL).] ▶L ♀C ▶? $$$

VASOCIDIN **(prednisolone—ophthalmic + sulfacetamide—ophthalmic)** 1 to 2 gtts in each affected eye q 1 to 8 h or ½ inch ribbon of ointment one to four times per day. [Generic only: Soln (5, 10 mL).] ▶KL ♀C ▶? $

ZYLET **(loteprednol + tobramycin—ophthalmic)** 1 to 2 gtts in each affected eye q 1 to 2 h for 1 to 2 days then 1 to 2 gtts q 4 to 6 h. [Trade only: Susp 0.5% loteprednol + 0.3% tobramycin (2.5, 5, 10 mL).] ▶LK ♀C ▶? $$$

Corticosteroids

NOTE: *Recommend that only ophthalmologists or optometrists prescribe due to infection, cataract, corneal/scleral perforation, and glaucoma risk from prolonged use. Monitor intraocular pressure.*

DIFLUPREDNATE (*Durezol*) Inflammation and pain associated with ocular surgery: 1 gtt in each affected eye four times per day, beginning 24 h after surgery for 2 weeks, then 1 gtt in each affected eye two times per day for 1 week, then taper based on response. Endogenous anterior uveitis: 1 gtt in each affected eye four times daily for 14 days followed by tapering as indicated. [Trade only: Ophthalmic emulsion 0.05% (2.5, 5 mL).] ▶not absorbed ♀C ▶? $$$$

FLUOROMETHOLONE (*FML, FML Forte, Flarex*) 1 to 2 gtts in each affected eye q 1 to 12 h or ½ inch ribbon of ointment q 4 to 24 h. [Trade only: Susp 0.1% (5, 10, 15 mL), 0.25% (2, 5, 10, 15 mL). Oint 0.1% (3.5 g tube).] ▶L ♀C ▶? $$

LOTEPREDNOL (*Alrex, Lotemax*) 1 to 2 gtts in each affected eye four times per day or ½ inch ointment four times daily beginning 24 h after surgery. [Trade only: Susp 0.2% (Alrex 5, 10 mL), 0.5% (Lotemax 2.5, 5, 10, 15 mL). Oint 0.5% 3.5 g, Gel drop 0.5% (Lotemax 10 mL).] ▶L ♀C ▶? $$$

PREDNISOLONE—OPHTHALMIC (*Pred Forte, Pred Mild, Inflamase Forte, Econopred Plus*) Soln: 1 to 2 gtts in each affected eye (up to q 1 h during day and q 2 h at night); when response observed, then 1 gtt in each affected eye q 4 h, then 1 gtt three to four times per day. Susp: 1 to 2 gtts in each affected eye two to four times per day. [Generic/Trade: Soln, Susp 1% (5, 10, 15 mL). Trade only (Pred Mild): Susp 0.12% (5, 10 mL), Susp (Pred Forte) 1% (1 mL).] ▶L ♀C ▶? $$

RIMEXOLONE (*Vexol*) 1 to 2 gtts in each affected eye q 1 to 6 h. [Trade only: Susp 1% (5, 10 mL).] ▶L ♀C ▶? $$

Glaucoma Agents—Beta-Blockers

NOTE: *Use caution in cardiac conditions and asthma.*

BETAXOLOL—OPHTHALMIC (*Betoptic, Betoptic S*) 1 to 2 gtts in each affected eye two times per day. [Trade only: Susp 0.25% (10, 15 mL). Generic only: Soln 0.5% (5, 10, 15 mL).] ▶LK ♀C ▶? $$

CARTEOLOL—OPHTHALMIC (*Ocupress*) 1 gtt in each affected eye two times per day. [Generic only: Soln 1% (5, 10, 15 mL).] ▶KL ♀C ▶? $

LEVOBUNOLOL (*Betagan*) 1 to 2 gtts in each affected eye one to two times per day. [Generic/Trade: Soln 0.25% (5, 10 mL), 0.5% (5, 10, 15 mL).] ▶? ♀C ▶– $$

METIPRANOLOL (*Optipranolol*) 1 gtt in each affected eye two times per day. [Generic/Trade: Soln 0.3% (5, 10 mL).] ▶? ♀C ▶? $

TIMOLOL—OPHTHALMIC (*Betimol, Timoptic, Timoptic XE, Istalol, Timoptic Ocudose*) 1 gtt in each affected eye two times per day. Timoptic XE, Istalol: 1 gtt in each affected eye daily. [Generic/Trade: Soln 0.25, 0.5% (5, 10, 15 mL). Preservative-free soln (Timoptic Ocudose) 0.25% (0.2 mL). Gel-forming soln (Timoptic XE) 0.25, 0.5% (5 mL).] ▶LK ♀C ▶+ $$

Glaucoma Agents—Carbonic Anhydrase Inhibitors

NOTE: *Sulfonamide derivatives; verify absence of sulfa allergy before prescribing.*

ACETAZOLAMIDE (*Diamox, Diamox Sequels*) Glaucoma: 250 mg PO up to four times per day (immediate-release) or 500 mg PO up to two times per day (sustained-release). Max 1 g/day. Acute glaucoma: 250 mg IV q 4 h or 500 mg IV initially with 125 to 250 mg q 4 h, followed by oral therapy. Mountain sickness prophylaxis: 125 to 250 mg PO two to three times per day, beginning 1 to 2 days prior to ascent and continuing at least 5 days at higher altitude. Edema: Rarely used, start 250 to 375 mg IV/PO q am given intermittently (every other day or 2 consecutive days followed by none for 1 to 2 days) to avoid loss of diuretic effect. Urinary alkalinization: 5 mg/kg IV, may repeat two or three times daily prn to maintain an alkaline diuresis. [Generic only: Tabs 125, 250 mg. Generic/Trade: Caps, extended-release 500 mg.] ▶LK ♀C ▶+ $$

BRINZOLAMIDE (*Azopt*) 1 gtt in each affected eye three times per day. [Trade only: Susp 1% (10, 15 mL).] ▶LK ♀C ▶? $$$

DORZOLAMIDE (*Trusopt*) 1 gtt in each affected eye three times per day. [Generic/Trade: Soln 2% (10 mL).] ▶KL ♀C ▶− $$$

METHAZOLAMIDE 25 to 50 mg PO daily (up to three times per day). [Generic only: Tabs 25, 50 mg.] ▶LK ♀C ▶? $$

Glaucoma Agents—Combinations and Other

COMBIGAN (brimonidine + timolol—ophthalmic) 1 gtt in each affected eye twice a day. Contraindicated in children younger than 2 yo. [Trade only: Soln brimonidine 0.2% + timolol 0.5% (5, 10 mL).] ▶LK ♀C ▶− $$$

COSOPT (dorzolamide + timolol—ophthalmic) 1 gtt in each affected eye two times per day. [Generic/Trade: Soln dorzolamide 2% + timolol 0.5% (5, 10 mL). Trade only: Soln, preservative-free dorzolamide 2% + timolol 0.5% (30 single-use containers).] ▶LK ♀D ▶− $$$

SIMBRINZA (brinzolamide + brimonidine) 1 gtt in each affected eye three times per day. [Trade: Brinzolamide 1% and brimonidine 0.2% 8 mL.] ▶LK − ♀C ▶? $$$$

OPHTHALMOLOGY

Glaucoma Agents—Miotics

CARBACHOL (*Isopto Carbachol, Miostat*) [Trade only: Soln (Isopto Carbachol) 1.5, 3% (15 mL). Intraocular soln (Miostat) 0.01%.] ▶? ♀C ▶? $$
PILOCARPINE—OPHTHALMIC (*Isopto Carpine, ✦Diocarpine, Akarpine*) 1 gtt in each affected eye up to four times per day. [Generic/Trade: Soln 0.5% (15 mL), 1% (2 mL, 15 mL), 2% (2 mL, 15 mL), 4% (2 mL, 15 mL), 6% (15 mL).] ▶plasma ♀C ▶? $

Glaucoma Agents—Prostaglandin Analogs

BIMATOPROST (*Lumigan, Latisse*) Glaucoma (Lumigan): 1 gtt in each affected eye at bedtime. Hypotrichosis of the eyelashes (Latisse): 1 gtt to eyelashes at bedtime. [Generic only: Soln 0.03% 2.5, 5, 7.5 mL. Trade only: Soln 0.01% (Lumigan), 2.5, 5, 7.5 mL. Soln 0.03% (Latisse) 3 mL with 70 disposable applicators, 5 mL with 140 disposable applicators.] ▶LK ♀C ▶? $$$$
LATANOPROST (*Xalatan*) 1 gtt in each affected eye at bedtime. [Generic/Trade: Soln 0.005% (2.5 mL).] ▶LK ♀C ▶? $
TAFLUPROST (*Zioptan*) 1 gtt in each affected eye q pm. [Trade: Soln 0.0015%] ▶L ♀C ▶? $$$
TRAVOPROST (*Travatan Z*) 1 gtt in each affected eye at bedtime. [Trade only: Benzalkonium chloride-free (Travatan Z) 0.004% (2.5, 5 mL). Generic only: Travoprost 0.004% (2.5, 5 mL).] ▶L ♀C ▶? $$$$

Glaucoma Agents—Sympathomimetics

NOTE: *Do not administer while wearing soft contact lenses. Wait 10 min after use before inserting contact lenses. On average, each mL of eye drop soln contains approximately 20 gtts. Reserve ointment formulations for bedtime use due to severe vision blurring. Most eye medications can be administered 1 gtt at a time despite common manufacturer recommendations of 1 to 2 gtts concurrently. Even a single gtt is*

(cont.)

typically more than the eye can hold and thus a second gtt is both wasteful and increases the possibility of systemic toxicity. If 2 gtts of the medication are desired, separate single gtts by at least 5 min.

BRIMONIDINE (*Alphagan P, ✦Alphagan*) 1 gtt in each affected eye three times per day. [Trade only: Soln 0.1% (5, 10, 15 mL). Generic/Trade: Soln 0.15% (5, 10, 15 mL). Generic only: Soln 0.2% (5, 10, 15 mL).] ▶L ♀B ▶? $$

Mydriatics and Cycloplegics

ATROPINE—OPHTHALMIC (*Isopto Atropine, Atropine Care*) 1 to 2 gtts in each affected eye before procedure or daily to four times per day or ⅛ to ¼ inch ointment before procedure or one to three times per day. Cycloplegia may last up to 5 to 10 days and mydriasis may last up to 7 to 14 days. [Generic/Trade: Soln 1% (2, 5, 15 mL). Generic only: Oint 1% (3.5 g tube).] ▶L ♀C ▶+ $

CYCLOPENTOLATE (*AK-Pentolate, Cyclogyl, Pentolair*) 1 to 2 gtts in each affected eye for 1 to 2 doses before procedure. Cycloplegia may last 6 to 24 h; mydriasis may last 1 day. [Generic/Trade: Soln 1% (2, 15 mL). Trade only (Cyclogyl): 0.5% (15 mL), 1% (5 mL), 2% (2, 5, 15 mL).] ▶? ♀C ▶? $

HOMATROPINE—OPHTHALMIC (*Isopto Homatropine*) 1 to 2 gtts in each affected eye before procedure or two to three times per day. Cycloplegia and mydriasis last 1 to 3 days. [Trade only: Soln 2% (5 mL), 5% (15 mL). Generic/Trade: Soln 5% (5 mL).] ▶? ♀C ▶? $

PHENYLEPHRINE—OPHTHALMIC 1 to 2 gtts in each affected eye before procedure or three to four times per day. No cycloplegia; mydriasis may last up to 5 h. [Rx Generic: Soln 2.5% (2, 3, 5, 15 mL), 10% (5 mL).] ▶plasma L ♀C ▶? $

TROPICAMIDE (*Mydriacyl, Tropicacyl*) 1 to 2 gtts in each affected eye before procedure. Mydriasis may last 6 h. [Generic/Trade: Soln 0.5% (15 mL), 1% (3, 15 mL). Generic only: Soln 1% (2 mL).] ▶? ♀C ▶? $

Non-Steroidal Anti-Inflammatories

BROMFENAC—OPHTHALMIC (*Bromday, Prolensa*) 1 gtt in each affected eye once daily beginning 1 day prior to surgery and continuing for 14 days after surgery (Bromday, Prolensa) or twice daily (generic). [Trade only: Soln 0.09% (Bromday) 1.7, 3.4 mL (two 1.7 mL twin packs). Soln 0.07% (Prolensa) 1.6, 3 mL. Generic only: Soln 0.09% (twice-daily soln 2.5, 5 mL).] ▶minimal absorption ♀C, D (3rd trimester) ▶? $$$$$

DICLOFENAC—OPHTHALMIC (*Voltaren, ✦Voltaren Ophtha*) 1 gtt in each affected eye one to four times per day. [Generic/Trade: Soln 0.1% (2.5, 5 mL).] ▶L ♀C ▶? $$$

FLURBIPROFEN—OPHTHALMIC (*Ocufen*) Inhibition of intraoperative miosis: 1 gtt q 30 min beginning 2 h prior to surgery (total of 4 gtts). [Generic/Trade: Soln 0.03% (2.5 mL).] ▶L ♀C ▶? $

KETOROLAC—OPHTHALMIC (*Acular, Acular LS, Acuvail*) 1 gtt in each affected eye four times per day (Acular, Acular LS). 1 gtt in each affected eye twice daily (Acuvail). [Generic/Trade: Soln (Acular LS) 0.4% (5 mL). Trade only: Acular 0.5% (3, 5, 10 mL), preservative-free Acuvail 0.45% unit dose (0.4 mL).] ▶L ♀C ▶? $$$$

NEPAFENAC (*Nevanac, Ilevro*) 1 gtt in each affected eye three times per day for 2 weeks. [Trade only: Susp 0.1% (Nevanac-3 mL). Susp 0.3% (Ilevro-1.7 mL).] ▶minimal absorption ♀C C, D in 3rd trimester ▶? $$$$

Other Ophthalmologic Agents

AFLIBERCEPT (*Eylea*) Wet macular degeneration, macular edema after central retinal vein occlusion, diabetic retinopathy with diabetic macular edema, macular edema following retinal vein occlusion: 2 mg (0.05 mL) intravitreal injection, frequency varies by indication. [Sterile powder for reconstitution.] ▶minimal absorption – ♀C ▶– $$$$$

ARTIFICIAL TEARS (*Tears Naturale, Hypotears, Refresh Tears, GenTeal, Systane*) 1 to 2 gtts prn. [OTC Generic/Trade: Soln (15, 30 mL, among others).] ▶minimal absorption ♀A▶+ $

CYCLOSPORINE—OPHTHALMIC (*Restasis*) 1 gtt in each eye q 12 h. [Trade only: Emulsion 0.05% (0.4 mL single-use vials).] ▶minimal absorption ♀C▶ $$$$

HYDROXYPROPYL CELLULOSE (*Lacrisert*) Moderate to severe dry eyes: 1 insert in each eye daily. Some patients may require twice-daily use. [Trade only: Ocular insert 5 mg.] ▶minimal absorption ♀+▶+ $$$

LIDOCAINE—OPHTHALMIC Do not prescribe for unsupervised or prolonged use. Corneal toxicity and ocular infections may occur with repeated use. 2 gtts before procedure, repeat prn. [Generic only: Gel 3.5% (5 mL).] ▶L ♀B▶? $

LIFITEGRAST (*Xiidra*) Dry eye disease: 1 gtt in each eye q12h. [Rx, Trade: Ophthalmic solution: single-use containers .] ▶minimal absorption ♀? ?/?/? ▶? $$$$

PETROLATUM (*Lacri-lube, Dry Eyes, Refresh PM, ✦DuoLube*) Apply ¼ to ½ inch ointment to inside of lower lid prn. [OTC Trade only: Oint (3.5, 7 g) tube.] ▶minimal absorption ♀A▶+ $

PROPARACAINE (*Ophthaine, Ophthetic, ✦Alcaine*) Do not prescribe for unsupervised or prolonged use. Corneal toxicity and ocular infections may occur with repeated use. 1 to 2 gtts into affected eye before procedure. [Generic/Trade: Soln 0.5% (15 mL).] ▶L ♀C▶? $

TETRACAINE—OPHTHALMIC (*Pontocaine*) Do not prescribe for unsupervised or prolonged use. Corneal toxicity and ocular infections may occur with repeated use. 1 to 2 gtts in each affected eye before procedure. [Generic only: Soln 0.5% (15 mL), unit-dose vials (0.7, 2 mL).] ▶plasma ♀C▶? $

PSYCHIATRY

BODY MASS INDEX

BMI	Class	4' 10"	5' 0"	5' 4"	5' 8"	6' 0"	6' 4"
<19	Underweight	<91	<97	<110	<125	<140	<156
19–24	Healthy weight	91–119	97–127	110–144	125–163	140–183	156–204
25–29	Overweight	120–143	128–152	145–173	164–196	184–220	205–245
30–40	Obese	144–191	153–204	174–233	197–262	221–293	246–328
>40	Very Obese	>191	>204	>174–233	>262	>293	>328

*BMI = kg/m^2 = (wt in pounds)(703)/(height in inches)^2. Anorectants appropriate if BMI ≥30 (with comorbidities ≥27); surgery an option if BMI > 40 (with comorbidities 35–40). www.nhlbi.nih.gov

Antidepressants—Heterocyclic Compounds

NOTE: *Gradually taper when discontinuing cyclic antidepressants to avoid withdrawal symptoms. Seizures, orthostatic hypotension, arrhythmias, and anticholinergic side effects may occur. Do not use with MAOIs. Antidepressants increase the risk of suicidal thinking and behavior in children, adolescents, and young adults; carefully weigh the risks and benefits before starting and monitor patients closely. Use of serotonergic drugs in late third trimester of pregnancy can lead to prolonged hospitalizations, need for respiratory support, and tube feeding. Antidepressants have been associated with acute narrow angle glaucoma.*

AMITRIPTYLINE Start 50 to 100 mg PO at bedtime; gradually increase by 25 to 50 mg/day to usual effective dose of 50 to 300 mg/day. Primarily inhibits serotonin reuptake. Demethylated to nortriptyline, which primarily inhibits norepinephrine reuptake. Suicidality. [Generic: Tabs 10, 25, 50, 75, 100, 150 mg. Elavil brand name no longer available.] ▶L ♀C ▶– $$ ■

CLOMIPRAMINE (*Anafranil*) Start 25 mg PO at bedtime; gradually increase to 100 mg/day over first 2 weeks in divided doses with meals. May increase to usual effective dose of 150 to 250 mg/day. May give one daily dose at bedtime after titration. Max 250 mg/day. Primarily inhibits serotonin reuptake. Suicidality. [Generic/Trade: Caps 25, 50, 75 mg.] ▶L ♀C ▶+ $$$ ■

DESIPRAMINE (*Norpramin*) Start 25 to 100 mg PO given once daily or in divided doses. Gradually increase to usual effective dose of 100 to 200 mg/day, max 300 mg/day. Primarily inhibits norepinephrine reuptake. Suicidality. [Generic/Trade: Tabs 10, 25, 50, 75, 100, 150 mg.] ▶L ♀?/?/? ▶+ $$ ■

DOXEPIN (*Silenor*) Depression: Start 75 mg PO at bedtime. Gradually increase to usual effective dose of 75 to 150 mg/day, max 300 mg/day. Doses above 150 mg/day should be divided. Primarily inhibits norepinephrine reuptake. Insomnia (Silenor): 6 mg PO 30 min before bedtime, 3 mg in age 65 yo or older.

(cont.)

Suicidality. [Generic only: Caps 10, 25, 50, 75, 100, 150 mg. Oral concentrate 10 mg/mL. Trade only: Tabs 3, 6 mg (Silenor).] ▶L ♀C ▶– $$ ■

IMIPRAMINE (*Tofranil, Tofranil PM*) Depression: Hospitalized patients, start 100 mg/day PO in divided doses. Gradually increase to 200 mg/day as required. May increase to 250 to 300 mg/day after two weeks. Outpatients, start 75 mg/day in divided doses and may increase to 150 mg/day. Usual maintenance 50 to 150 mg/day. Geriatric patients, start 30 to 40 mg/day and increase as needed and tolerated to max 100 mg/day. Enuresis: 25 to 75 mg PO at bedtime. Suicidality. [Generic/Trade: Tabs 10, 25, 50 mg. Caps 75, 100, 125, 150 mg (as pamoate salt).] ▶L ♀?/?/? ▶– $$$ ■

NORTRIPTYLINE (*Pamelor*) Usual dose 25 mg PO three to four times daily. Start at lower doses and increase as required. Max 150 mg/day. Elderly: 30 to 50 mg/day in one or divided doses. Once titrated total daily dose may be given once daily. Primarily inhibits norepinephrine reuptake. Suicidality. [Generic/Trade: Caps 10, 25, 50, 75 mg. Oral soln 10 mg/5 mL.] ▶L ♀?/?/? ▶+ $$$ ■

Antidepressants—Monoamine Oxidase Inhibitors (MAOIs)

NOTE: *Must be on tyramine-free diet throughout treatment and for 2 weeks after discontinuation. Numerous drug interactions; risk of hypertensive crisis and serotonin syndrome with many medications, including OTC. Allow at least 2 weeks wash-out when converting from an MAOI to an SSRI (6 weeks after fluoxetine), TCA, or other antidepressant. Antidepressants increase the risk of suicidal thoughts and behavior, especially early in therapy and with changes in dose. Antidepressants have been associated with acute narrow-angle glaucoma.*

ISOCARBOXAZID (*Marplan*) Start 10 mg PO two times per day; may increase by 10 mg every 2 to 4 days to a dose of 40 mg/day. Max 60 mg/day divided into two to four doses. MAOI diet. Suicidality. [Trade only: Tabs 10 mg.] ▶L ♀C ▶? $$$ ■

PHENELZINE (*Nardil*) Start 15 mg PO three times per day. Usual effective dose is 60 to 90 mg/day in divided doses. MAOI diet. Suicidality. [Trade only: Tabs 15 mg.] ▶L Primarily monomine oxidase ♀?/?/? ▶? $$$ ■

SELEGILINE—TRANSDERMAL (*Emsam*) Start 6 mg/24 h patch, change daily. Max 12 mg/24 h. MAOI diet for doses 9 mg/day or higher. Suicidality. [Trade only: Transdermal patch 6 mg/day, 9 mg/24 h, 12 mg/24 h.] ▶L ♀C ▶? $$$$$ ■

TRANYLCYPROMINE (*Parnate*) Start 10 mg PO every am; increase by 10 mg/day at 1- to 3-week intervals to usual effective dose of 30 mg/day divided two times per day. Max 60 mg/day. MAOI diet. Suicidality. [Generic/Trade: Tabs 10 mg.] ▶L ♀?/?/? ▶– $$ ■

Antidepressants—Selective Serotonin Reuptake Inhibitors (SSRIs)

NOTE: *Gradually taper when discontinuing SSRIs to avoid withdrawal symptoms. Observe patients for worsening depression or the emergence of suicidality, anxiety, agitation, panic attacks, insomnia, irritability, hostility, impulsivity, akathisia, mania, or hypomania, particularly early in therapy or after increases in dose. Antidepressants increase the risk of suicidal thinking and behavior in children, adolescents, and young adults; carefully weigh the risks and benefits before starting treatment and then monitor patients closely. Use of SSRIs during the 3rd trimester of pregnancy has been associated with neonatal complications including respiratory (including persistent pulmonary HTN), GI, and feeding problems, as well as seizures and withdrawal symptoms. Balance these risks against those of withdrawal and depression for the mother. Paroxetine should be avoided throughout pregnancy. Increased risk of abnormal bleeding; use caution when combined with NSAIDs or aspirin. SSRIs have been associated with serotonin syndrome and neuroleptic malignant syndrome. Use cautiously*

(cont.)

and observe closely for serotonin syndrome if SSRI is used with a triptan or other serotonergic drugs. SSRIs and SNRIs have been associated with hyponatremia, which is often associated with SIADH. The elderly and those taking diuretics may be at increased risk. Avoid use with MAOIs used for psychiatric conditions or during active treatment with linezolid or IV methylene blue. Antidepressants have been associated with acute narrow-angle glaucoma. Antidepressants including some SSRIs and depression itself have been associated with an increased risk of bone fractures. The mechanism is unclear. However, this is not a consistent finding among studies. Monitor bone health in susceptible populations.

CITALOPRAM (*Celexa*) Start 20 mg PO daily. May increase after 1 or more weeks to max 40 mg daily or 20 mg daily if older than 60 yo. Suicidality. [Generic/Trade: Tabs 10, 20, 40 mg. Generic only: Orally disintegrating tabs 10, 20, 40 mg, oral soln 10 mg/5 mL.] ▶LK ♀C Use in 3rd trimester associated with complications at birth. ▶– $$$ ■

ESCITALOPRAM (*Lexapro*, ✦*Cipralex*) Depression, generalized anxiety disorder, adults, and age 12 yo or older: Start 10 mg PO daily; max 20 mg/day. Suicidality. [Generic/Trade: Tabs 5, 10, 20 mg. Oral soln 1 mg/mL.] ▶LK ♀C Use in 3rd trimester associated with complications at birth. ▶– $$$$ ■

FLUOXETINE (*Prozac, Prozac Weekly, Sarafem, Selfemra*) Depression, OCD: Start 20 mg PO every am; usual effective dose is 20 to 40 mg/day (depression) or 20 to 60 mg/day (OCD), max 80 mg/day. Depression, maintenance: 20 to 40 mg/day (standard-release) or 90 mg PO once a week (Prozac Weekly) starting 7 days after last standard-release dose. Bulimia: 60 mg PO daily in the morning; may need to titrate slowly to this dose over several days for some patieints. Panic disorder: Start 10 mg PO every am; titrate to 20 mg/day after 1 week, max 60 mg/day. Premenstrual dysphoric disorder (Sarafem): 20 mg PO daily, given either throughout the menstrual cycle or for 14 days

(cont.)

prior to menses; max 80 mg/day. Doses greater than 20 mg/day can be divided two times per day (in morning and at noon). Bipolar I depression, olanzapine + fluoxetine given separately: Start 5 mg olanzapine + 20 mg fluoxetine daily in the evening. Increase to usual range of 5 to 12.5 mg olanzapine + 20 to 50 mg fluoxetine as tolerated. See also Symbyax combination product entry. Treatment-resistant depression, olanzapine + fluoxetine given separately: Start 5 mg olanzapine + 20 mg fluoxetine daily in the evening. Increase to usual range of 5 to 20 mg olanzapine + 20 to 50 mg fluoxetine as tolerated. See also Symbyax combination product entry. Suicidality, many drug interactions. [Generic: Tabs 10, 20, 60 mg. Generic/Trade: Caps 10, 20, 40 mg. Generic: Oral soln 20 mg/5 mL. Trade: Tabs (Sarafem and Selfemra) 10, 15, 20 mg. Generic/Trade: Caps, delayed-release (Prozac Weekly and generics) 90 mg.] ▶L ♀C ▶– $$$ ■

FLUVOXAMINE (*Luvox, Luvox CR*) Immediate-release: Start 50 mg PO at bedtime. May increase every 4-7 days by 50 mg/day to usual effective dose of 100 to 300 mg/day divided two times per day, max 300 mg/day. Controlled-release: Start 100 mg PO at bedtime and increase by 50 mg/day weekly as tolerated to max 300 mg/day. Children age 8 yo or older: Start 25 mg PO at bedtime; usual effective dose is 50 to 200 mg/day divided two times per day, max 200 mg/day. Do not use with thioridazine, pimozide, alosetron, tizanidine, tryptophan, or MAOIs; use caution with benzodiazepines, TCAs, theophylline, and warfarin. Suicidality. [Generic/Trade: Tabs 25, 50, 100 mg. Caps, extended-release 100, 150 mg.] ▶L ♀C Use in 3rd trimester associated with complications at birth. ▶– $$$$ ■

PAROXETINE (*Paxil, Paxil CR, Pexeva*) Depression: Start 20 mg PO every am; increase by 10 mg/day at intervals of 1 week or more to usual effective dose of 20 to 50 mg/day, max 50 mg/day. Depression, controlled-release tabs: Start 25 mg PO every am; may increase by 12.5 mg/day at intervals of 1 week or more to usual effective dose of 25 to 62.5 mg/day; max

(cont.)

62.5 mg/day. OCD: Start 20 mg PO every am; increase by 10 mg/day at intervals of 1 week or more to usual recommended dose of 40 mg/day; max 60 mg/day. Panic disorder: Start 10 mg PO every am; increase by 10 mg/day at intervals of 1 week or more to target dose of 40 mg/day; max 60 mg/day. Panic disorder, controlled-release tabs: Start 12.5 mg/day; increase by 12.5 mg/day at intervals of 1 week or more to usual effective dose of 12.5 to 75 mg/day; max 75 mg/day. Social anxiety disorder: Start 20 mg PO every am (which is the usual effective dose); max 60 mg/day. Social anxiety disorder, controlled-release tabs: Start 12.5 mg PO every am; may increase at intervals of 1 week or more by 12.5 mg/day to max 37.5 mg/day. Generalized anxiety disorder: Start 20 mg PO every am (which is the usual effective dose); doses higher than 20 mg/day have not been shown to be more effective. Max 50 mg/day in trials. Posttraumatic stress disorder: Start 20 mg PO every am; doses higher than 20 mg/day have not been shown to be more effective. Max 50 mg/day in clincal trials. Premenstrual dysphoric disorder (PMDD), continuous dosing: Start 12.5 mg PO every am (controlled-release tabs); may increase dose after 1 week to max 25 mg every am. PMDD, intermittent dosing (given for 2 weeks prior to menses): Start 12.5 mg PO every am (controlled-release tabs), max 25 mg/day. Suicidality, many drug interactions. [Generic/Trade: Tabs 10, 20, 30, 40 mg. Oral susp 10 mg/5 mL. Controlled-release tabs 12.5, 25 mg. Trade only: (Paxil CR) 37.5 mg.] ▶LK ♀D ▶? $$$

SERTRALINE (*Zoloft*) Depression, OCD: Start 50 mg PO daily; usual effective dose is 50 to 200 mg/day, max 200 mg/day. Panic disorder, post-traumatic stress disorder, social anxiety disorder: Start 25 mg PO daily, max 200 mg/day. PMDD, continuous dosing: Start 50 mg PO daily, max 150 mg/day. Intermittent dosing: (given for 14 days prior to menses): Start 50 mg PO daily for 3 days, then increase to 100 mg/day. Suicidality. [Generic/Trade: Tabs 25, 50, 100 mg. Oral concentrate 20 mg/mL (60 mL).] ▶LK ♀C Use in 3rd trimester associated with complications at birth. ▶+ $$$

VORTIOXETINE (*Trintellix*, ✦*Trintellix*) Start 10 mg PO daily. Max 20 mg/day. Reduce dose if given with strong CYP2D6 inhibitors. [Trade only: Tabs 5, 10, 15, 20 mg.] ▶L ♀C ▶? $$$$$ ■

Antidepressants—Serotonin-Norepinephrine Reuptake Inhibitors (SNRIs)

NOTE: *Monitor for the emergence of anxiety, agitation, panic attacks, insomnia, irritability, hostility, impulsivity, akathisia, mania, or hypomania, and for worsening depression or the emergence of suicidality, particularly early in therapy or after increases in dose. Antidepressants increase the risk of suicidal thinking and behavior in children, adolescents, and young adults; carefully weigh the risks and benefits before starting treatment, and then monitor closely. Antidepressants have been associated with acute narrow-angle glaucoma. SSRIs and SNRIs have been associated with hyponatremia, which is often associated with SIADH. The elderly and those taking diuretics may be at increased risk. Do not use with MAOIs. SNRIs have been associated with serotonin syndrome and neuroleptic malignant syndrome when used alone and especially in combination with other serotonergic drugs.*

DESVENLAFAXINE (*Pristiq, Khedezla*) 50 mg PO daily. No evidence that doses higher than 50 mg/day are more effective. [Trade/generic: extended-release tabs 25, 50, 100 mg] ▶LK ♀C ▶? $$$$ ■

DULOXETINE (*Cymbalta*) Depression: Start: 20 mg PO twice daily or 60 mg/day given once daily or divided twice daily. May start 30 mg PO once daily in some patients to improve tolerability. Increase as tolerated to 60 mg/day given once daily or divided twice daily. Max 120 mg/day. Doses of 120 mg/day have been used but have not been shown to be more effective than 60 mg/day. Generalized anxiety disorder: Start 30 to 60 mg PO daily, max 120 mg/day. Elderly: Start 30 mg PO daily for 2 weeks. Then increase to target dose of 60 mg/day, max

(cont.)

120 mg/day. Doses above 60 mg/day have not been shown to be more effective. Diabetic peripheral neuropathic pain: 60 mg PO daily. Fibromyalgia: Start 30 mg PO daily for one week then increase to 60 mg/day if needed and tolerated. Max 60 mg/day. Chronic musculoskeletal pain: Start 30 mg PO once daily for 1 week. Then increase to 60 mg once daily. Max 60 mg/day. Suicidality, hepatotoxicity, many drug interactions. [Generic/Trade: Caps 20, 30, 60 mg.] ▶L ♀C ▶? $$$$ ■

LEVOMILNACIPRAN (Fetzima) Start 20 mg PO once daily. Increase after 2 days to 40 mg/day. May increase by 40 mg/day at intervals of 2 or more days to max 120 mg/day. [Trade only: Caps 20, 40, 80, 120 mg.] ▶KL ♀C ▶? ■

VENLAFAXINE (Effexor XR) Depression/anxiety: Start 37.5 to 75 mg PO daily (Effexor XR) or 75 mg/day divided two to three times per day (immediate-release tabs). Usual effective dose is 150 to 225 mg/day, max 225 mg/day (Effexor XR) or 375 mg/day (Effexor). Generalized anxiety disorder: Start 37.5 to 75 mg PO daily (Effexor XR), max 225 mg/day. Social anxiety disorder: 75 mg PO daily (Effexor XR). Panic disorder: Start 37.5 mg PO daily (Effexor XR), may titrate by 75 mg/day at weekly intervals to max 225 mg/day. Suicidality, seizures, HTN. Give with food. [Generic/Trade: Caps, extended-release 37.5, 75, 150 mg. Tabs 25, 37.5, 50, 75, 100 mg. Generic only: Tabs, extended-release 37.5, 75, 150, 225 mg.] ▶LK ♀C ▶? $$$$

Antidepressants—Other

NOTE: Monitor for the emergence of anxiety, agitation, panic attacks, insomnia, irritability, hostility, impulsivity, akathisia, mania, or hypomania, and for worsening depression or the emergence of suicidality, particularly early in therapy or after increases in dose. Antidepressants increase the risk of suicidal thinking and behavior in children, adolescents, and young adults; carefully weigh the risks and benefits before starting treatment, and then monitor closely. Antidepressants have been associated with acute narrow-angle glaucoma. Avoid use with MAOIs.

TRAZODONE (*Oleptro*) Depression: Start 50 to 150 mg/day PO in divided doses; usual effective dose is 400 to 600 mg/day. Extended-release: Start 150 mg PO at bedtime. May increase by 75 mg/day every 3 days to max 375 mg/day. Insomnia (unapproved): 50 to 150 mg PO at bedtime. [Trade only: Extended-release tabs (Oleptro) 150, 300 mg. Generic only: Tabs 50, 100, 150, 300 mg.] ▶L ♀C ▶– $

BUPROPION (*Wellbutrin, Wellbutrin SR, Wellbutrin XL, Aplenzin, Zyban, Buproban, Forfivo XL*) Depression: Start 100 mg PO two times per day (immediate-release tabs); can increase to 100 mg three times per day after 4 to 7 days. May gradually increase to 450 mg/day if no response after several weeks. Usual effective dose is 300 to 450 mg/day, max 150 mg/dose and 450 mg/day. Sustained-release: Start 150 mg PO every am; may increase to 150 mg two times per day after 3 days, max 400 mg/day. Give last dose no later than 5 pm. Extended-release: Start 150 mg PO every am; may increase to 300 mg every am after 4 days, max 450 mg every am. Extended-release (Aplenzin): Start 174 mg PO every am; increase to target dose of 348 mg/day after 4 days or more. Extended-release (Forfivo XL): 450 mg PO once daily. Do not use to initiate therapy. If standard tabs tolerated and patient requires more than 300 mg/day, may use 450 mg PO daily, max 450 mg/day. Seasonal affective disorder: Start 150 mg of extended-release PO every am in autumn; can increase to 300 mg every am after 1 week, max 300 mg/day. In the spring, decrease to 150 mg/day for 2 weeks and then discontinue. Extended-release (Aplenzin): Start 174 mg PO every am. Increase to 348 mg/day after 7 days. Smoking cessation (Zyban, Buproban): Start 150 mg PO every am for 3 days, then increase to 150 mg PO two times per day for 7 to 12 weeks. Max 150 mg PO two times per day. Give last dose no later than 5 pm. Seizures, suicidality. [Generic/Trade (for depression, bupropion HCl): Tabs 75, 100 mg. Sustained-release tabs 100, 150, 200 mg. Extended-release tabs 150, 300 mg (Wellbutrin XL). Generic/Trade (Smoking cessation): Sustained-release tabs 150

(cont.)

mg (Zyban, Buproban). Trade only: Extended-release (Aplenzin, bupropion hydrobromide) tabs 174, 348, 522 mg. Extended-release (Forfivo XL) tab 450 mg.] ▶LK ♀C ▶– $$ ■

MIRTAZAPINE (*Remeron, Remeron SolTab*)   Start 15 mg PO at bedtime. Usual effective dose is 15 to 45 mg/day. Agranulocytosis in 0.1% of patients. Suicidality. [Generic/Trade: Tabs 15, 30, 45 mg. Tabs, orally disintegrating (SolTab) 15, 30, 45 mg. Generic only: Tabs 7.5 mg.] ▶LK ♀C ▶? $$ ■

VILAZODONE (*Viibryd*)   Start 10 mg once daily for 7 days, then increase to 20 mg once daily. May increase to max 40 mg/day if needed. [Trade only: Tabs 10, 20, 40 mg.] ▶L ♀C Rated C by ACOG ▶? ■

Antimanic (Bipolar) Agents

LAMOTRIGINE—PSYCHATRY (*Lamictal, Lamictal CD, Lamictal ODT, Lamictal XR*)   Bipolar disorder (maintenance): Start 25 mg PO daily for 2 weeks, 50 mg PO daily if on enzyme-inducing drugs, or 25 mg PO every other day if on valproate; titrate over next 5 weeks to 200 mg/day, up to 400 mg/day divided two times per day if on enzyme-inducing drugs, or 100 mg/day if on valproate. Potentially life-threatening rashes in 0.3% of adults and 0.8% of children; discontinue at 1st sign of rash. Drug interaction with valproic acid; see prescribing information for adjusted dosing guidelines. Discontinuing enzyme-inducing drugs or valproate will necessessistate changes in the lamotrigine dose. [Generic/Trade: Chewable dispersible tabs (Lamictal CD) 5, 25 mg. Tabs 25, 100, 150, 200 mg. Extended-release tabs (XR) 25, 50, 100, 200, 250, 300 mg. Orally disintegrating tabs (ODT) 25, 50, 100, 200 mg. Trade only: Chewable dispersible tabs 2 mg.] ▶LK ♀C Possible risk of cleft palate or lip. ▶– $$$$ ■

LITHIUM (*Lithobid, ✦Lithane*)   Acute mania: Start 300 to 600 mg PO two to three times per day. Starting at the lower dose may improve tolerability. Usual effective dose is 900 to 1800 mg/day. Steady state is achieved in 5 days. Bipolar maintenance:

(cont.)

Usually 900 to 1200 mg/day in divided doses titrated to therapeutic trough level of 0.6 to 1.2 mEq/L. [Generic/Trade: Caps 300 mg; Extended-release tabs 300, 450 mg. Generic only: Caps 150, 600 mg; Tabs 300 mg; Syrup 300 mg/5 mL.] ▶K ♀D ▶− $ ■

TOPIRAMATE (*Topamax*) Bipolar disorder (unapproved): Start 25 to 50 mg/day PO. Titrate prn to max 400 mg/day divided two times per day. [Generic/Trade: Tabs 25, 50, 100, 200 mg. Sprinkle caps 15, 25 mg.] ▶K ♀D ▶? $$$$$

VALPROIC ACID—PSYCHIATRY (***Depakote, Depakote ER, Stavzor, divalproex, ✦Epival***) Mania: 250 mg PO three times per day (Depakote) or 25 mg/kg once daily (Depakote ER); max 60 mg/kg/day. Hepatotoxicity, drug interactions, reduce dose in the elderly. [Generic only: Syrup (valproic acid) 250 mg/5 mL. Generic/Trade: Delayed-release tabs (Depakote) 125, 250, 500 mg. Extended-release tabs (Depakote ER) 250, 500 mg. Delayed-release sprinkle caps (Depakote) 125 mg. Trade only (Stavzor): Delayed-release caps 125, 250, 500 mg.] ▶L ♀D ▶+ $$$$

Antipsychotics—First Generation (Typical)

NOTE: *Antipsychotic potency is determined by affinity for D2 receptors. Extrapyramidal side effects (EPS) including tardive dyskinesia and dystonia may occur with antipsychotics. Use cautiously in patients with Parkinson's disease. High-potency agents are more likely to cause EPS and hyperprolactinemia. Can be given at bedtime, but may be divided initially to decrease side effects and daytime sedation. Antipsychotics have been associated with an increased risk of venous thromboembolism, especially early in therapy. Assess for other risk factors and monitor carefully. Off-label use for dementia-related psychosis in the elderly has been associated with increased mortality. Newborns exposed during the 3rd trimester are at increased risk for abnormal muscle movements (EPS) and withdrawal symptoms.*

ANTIPSYCHOTIC RELATIVE ADVERSE EFFECTS[a]

Gene-ration	Antipsychotic	Anticholi-nergic	Seda-tion	Hypot-ension	EPS	Weight Gain	Diabetes/ Hyper-glycemia	Dyslipid-emia
1st	chlorpromazine	+++	+++	++	++	+++	+++	+++
1st	fluphenazine	++	+	+	++++	+	+	+
1st	haloperidol	+	+	+	++++	+	+	+
1st	loxapine	++	++	+	++	++	++	?
1st	molindone	++	++	+	++	+	?	?
1st	perphenazine	++	+	+	++	++	++	?
1st	pimozide	+	+	+	+++	+	+	?
1st	thioridazine	++++	+++	+++	+	++	++	?
1st	thiothixene	+	++	++	+++	++	++	?
1st	trifluoperazine	++	+	+	+++	++	++	?

(cont.)

ANTIPSYCHOTIC RELATIVE ADVERSE EFFECTS[a] (continued)

Gene-ration	Antipsychotic	Anticholi-nergic	Seda-tion	Hypot-ension	EPS	Weight Gain	Diabetes/Hyper-glycemia	Dyslipid-emia
2nd	aripiprazole	++	+	0	0	0/+	0/+	0
2nd	asenapine	+	+	++	++	++	++	0
2nd	brexipiprazole	+	+	0/+	+	+	?	?
2nd	cariprazine	+	+	+	++	+	?	?
2nd	clozapine	++++	+++	+++	0	++++	++++	++++
2nd	lurasidone	+	+	+	+	+	+	0
2nd	iloperidone	++	+	+++	0[b]	++	++	++
2nd	olanzapine	+++	++	+	++	++++	++++	++++
2nd	paliperidone	+	+	++	++	+++	+++	+
2nd	risperidone	+	++	+	+[b]	+++	+++	+

(cont.)

PSYCHIATRY

| 2nd | quetiapine | + | +++ | ++ | 0 | +++ | +++ | +++ |
| 2nd | ziprasidone | + | + | 0 | 0 | 0/+ | 0 | 0 |

Crismon M, Argo T, Bickley P. Schizophrenia. In: DiPiro J, Talbert R, Yee G, et al. ed, *Pharmacotherapy. A pathophysiologic approach*, 9th ed. New York: McGraw Hill Education, 2014 and Jibson M. Second generation antipsychotic medications: pharmacology, administration, and comparative side effects. UpToDate, 2015 (www.uptodate.com); Muench J, Hamer A. Adverse effects of antipsychotic medications, *Am Fam Physician* 2010;81(5):617-622.

[a]Risk of specific adverse effects is graded from 0 (absent) to ++++ (high). ? = Limited or inconsistent comparative data.

[b]Extrapyramidal symptoms (EPS) are dose-related and are more likely for risperidone greater than 6 to 8 mg/day, olanzapine greater than 20 mg/day. Akathisia risk remains unclear and may not be reflected in these ratings. There are limited comparative data for aripiprazole iloperidone, paliperidone, and asenapine relative to other 2nd-generation antipsychotics.

CHLORPROMAZINE Start 10 to 25 mg PO/IM two to four times per day. May increase by 25 to 50 mg/day semi-weekly until effective dose achieved. Usual dose 300 to 800 mg/day. Severe acute psychosis may require 400 mg IM every 4 to 6 h up to max 2000 mg/day IM. [Generic only: Tabs 10, 25, 50, 100, 200 mg.] ▶LK ♀C Per ACOG Guidelines ▶– $$$ ■

FLUPHENAZINE (✦*Modecate*) 1.25 to 10 mg/day IM divided every 6 to 8 h. Start 0.5 to 10 mg/day PO divided every 6 to 8 h. Usual effective dose 1 to 20 mg/day. Depot (fluphenazine decanoate/enanthate): 12.5 to 25 mg IM/SC every 3 to 6 weeks is equivalent to 10 to 20 mg/day PO fluphenazine. [Generic/Trade: Tabs 1, 2.5, 5, 10 mg. Elixir 2.5 mg/5 mL. Oral concentrate 5 mg/mL.] ▶LK ♀C ▶? $$$ ■

HALOPERIDOL (*Haldol*) 2 to 5 mg IM to max 20 mg/day IM. Start 0.5 to 5 mg PO two to three times per day, usual effective dose 6 to 20 mg/day. Max PO dose 100 mg/day. Therapeutic range 2 to 15 ng/mL. Depot haloperidol (haloperidol decanoate): 100 to 200 mg IM every 4 weeks is equivalent to 10 mg/day oral haloperidol. [Generic only: Tabs 0.5, 1, 2, 5, 10, 20 mg. Oral concentrate 2 mg/mL.] ▶LK ♀C ▶– $$ ■

PERPHENAZINE Start 4 to 8 mg PO three times per day or 8 to 16 mg PO two to four times per day (hospitalized patients), max 64 mg/day PO. Can give 5 to 10 mg IM every 6 h, max 30 mg/day IM. [Generic only: Tabs 2, 4, 8, 16 mg.] ▶LK ♀C ▶? $$$

PIMOZIDE (*Orap*) Start 1 to 2 mg/day PO in divided doses, increase every 2 days to usual effective dose of 1 to 10 mg/day. Max dose 0.2 mg/kg/day or 10 mg/day whichever is lower. Obtain ECG at baseline. [Trade only: Tabs 1, 2 mg.] ▶L ♀C ▶– $$$ ■

THIORIDAZINE Start 50 to 100 mg PO three times per day, usual dose 200 to 800 mg/day. Not 1st-line therapy. Causes QTc prolongation, torsades de pointes, and sudden death. Contraindicated with SSRIs, propranolol, pindolol. Monitor baseline ECG and potassium. Pigmentary retinopathy with doses greater than 800 mg/day. [Generic only: Tabs 10, 15, 25, 50, 100 mg.] ▶LK ♀C ▶? $$ ■

THIOTHIXENE Start 2 mg PO three times per day. Usual effective dose is 20 to 30 mg/day, max 60 mg/day. [Generic/Trade: Caps 1, 2, 5, 10 mg.] ▶LK ♀C ▷? $$$ ■

TRIFLUOPERAZINE Start 2 to 5 mg PO two times per day. Usual effective dose is 15 to 20 mg/day. [Generic only: Tabs 1, 2, 5, 10 mg.] ▶LK ♀C ▷– $$$ ■

Antipsychotics—Second Generation (Atypical)

NOTE: *Tardive dyskinesia, neuroleptic malignant syndrome, drug-induced parkinsonism, dystonia, and other extrapyramidal side effects may occur with antipsychotic medications. Atypical antipsychotics have been associated with wt gain, dyslipidemia, hyperglycemia, and diabetes mellitus; monitor closely. Off-label use for dementia-related psychosis in the elderly has been associated with increased mortality. Antipsychotics have been associated with an increased risk of venous thromboembolism, particularly early in therapy; assess for other risk factors and monitor carefully. Antipsychotics when used for schizophrenia or bipolar disorder have been associated with an increased risk of suicidal thinking and behavior. Monitor closely. Antipsychotics may increase prolactin levels through dopamine receptor antagonism. Consider obtaining prolactin levels if symptoms of excess appear.*

ARIPIPRAZOLE (*Abilify, Abilify Maintena, Aristada*) Schizophrenia: Start 10 to 15 mg PO daily. Max 30 mg daily. Schizophrenia, maintenance (Maintena): 400 mg IM monthly. May reduce to 300 mg IM monthly if adverse reactions to higher dose. Schizophrenia, maintenance (Aristada): Establish tolerability with PO aripiprazole first. May start with 441 mg, 662 mg, or 882 mg IM monthly based on oral dose. The 882 mg dose may also be given every 6 weeks. The 441 mg dose can be substituted for the 10 mg/day oral dose, 662 mg for 15 mg/day, and 882 mg for 20 mg/day. In conjunction with the first IM Aristada dose, give oral aripiprazole for 21 consecutive days. See package insert for

(cont.)

PSYCHIATRY

missed doses. Bipolar disorder (acute manic or mixed episodes): Start 15 mg PO daily or 10 to 15 mg PO daily if used with lithium or valproate. Max 30 mg/day. Agitation associated with schizophrenia or bipolar disorder: 9.75 mg IM recommended. May consider 5.25 to 15 mg if indicated. May repeat in 2 h up to max 30 mg/day. Major depressive disorder, adjunctive therapy: Start 2 to 5 mg PO daily. Max 15 mg/day. [Generic/Trade: Tabs 2, 5, 10, 15, 20, 30 mg. Generic only: Orally disintegrating tabs 10, 15 mg. Trade only: Susp, extended-release for injection (Abilify Maintena) 300 mg and 400 mg/vial. Pre-filled susp, extended-release injection (Abilify Maintena) 300 mg and 400 mg/syringe. Generic only: oral solution 1 mg/mL.] ▶L ♀C ▷? $$$$$ ■

ASENAPINE (*Saphris*) Schizophrenia: Acute and maintenance: Start 5 mg SL twice per day. Max 10 mg twice per day; however may not be more effective than the lower dose. Bipolar disorder, acute manic or mixed episodes: Start 5 mg SL two times per day (adjunctive) or 10 mg SL two times per day (monotherapy). Max 20 mg/day. [Trade: SL tabs 5, 10 mg.] ▶L ♀C ?/?/?R withdrawal and EPS in neonates exposed in 3rd trimester. ▶− ■

BREXPIPRAZOLE (*Rexulti*) Major depressive disorder, adjunctive: Start 0.5 mg to 1 mg PO once daily. Increase weekly by 1 mg/day to max 3 mg/day. Schizophrenia: Start 1 mg PO daily for days 1-4. Then increase to 2 mg once daily for days 5-7. Then increase to max 4 mg/day as needed and tolerated. Reduce dose with hepatic or severe renal impairment. [Trade only: Tabs 0.25, 0.5, 1, 2, 3, 4 mg.] ▶L ♀? ?/?/?R withdrawal and extrapyramidal symptoms for neonate at birth ▶? ■

CARIPRAZINE (*Vraylar*) Schizophrenia: Start 1.5 mg PO once daily. The dose can be increased to 3 mg/day on day 2. May increase by 1.5 mg/day to 3 mg/day as needed and tolerated to max 6 mg/day. Bipolar I disorder, acute manic or mixed episodes: Start 1.5 mg PO once daily. May increase to 3 mg/day on day 2. May increase by 1.5 mg/day to 3 mg/day to recommended range of 3-6 mg/day, max 6 mg/day. [Trade only: Caps 1.5 , 3, 4.5, 6 mg.] ▶L ♀? ?/?/?R Neonates who have

(cont.)

been exposed in the third trimester are at increased risk for extrapyramidal or withdrawal reactions at delivery. ▶? ■

CLOZAPINE (*Clozaril, FazaClo ODT, Versacloz*) Start 12.5 mg PO one to two times per day. Titrate by 25 to 50 mg increments over two weeks to achieve a target dose of 300 to 450 mg/day divided two times per day. May then increase the dose every 1 to 2 weeks by up to 100 mg/day to max 900 mg/day. Must re-titrate if stopped for 2 days or more. Agranulocytosis 1 to 2%; check ANC weekly for 6 months, then every 2 weeks for 6 months and then monthly thereafter. Enroll patients in the national registry at www.clozapinerems.com. Agranulocytosis, infections, seizures, myocarditis, cardiopulmonary arrest. [Generic/Trade: Tabs 25, 100 mg. Orally disintegrating tabs 12.5, 25, 100, 150, 200 mg. Generic only: Tabs 50, 200 mg. Trade only: Susp (Versacloz): 50 mg/mL.] ▶L ♀B ▶– $$$$$ ■

ILOPERIDONE (*Fanapt*) Start 1 mg PO two times per day. Increase by no more than 2 mg twice daily to usual effective range of 6 to 12 mg PO two times per day. Max 24 mg/day. Retitrate if stopped for more than 3 days. [Trade: Tabs 1, 2, 4, 6, 8, 10, 12 mg.] ▶L ♀? ?/?/?R withdrawal reactions and EPS in neonates exposed during third trimester. ▶– ? ■

LURASIDONE (*Latuda*) Schizophrenia: Start 40 mg PO daily. Effective dose range 40 to 160 mg daily, max 160 mg/day. Take with food. Reduce starting dose to 20 mg PO daily if moderate to severe renal or hepatic insufficiency or use with moderate CYP3A4 inhibitors, max 80 mg/day unless severe hepatic insufficiency which is 40 mg/day. Depression associated with bipolar I disorder (monotherapy or adjunctive with lithium or valproate): Start 20 mg PO daily. Usual range 20 to 120 mg/day. Doses greater than 20 to 60 mg/day did not provide further efficacy as monotherapy in clinical trials. [Trade only: Tabs 20, 40, 60, 80, 120 mg.] ▶K – ♀B ▶? ■

OLANZAPINE (*Zyprexa, Zyprexa Zydis, Zyprexa Relprevv*) Agitation in acute bipolar mania or schizophrenia: Start 10 mg IM (may use 5 to 7.5 mg if warranted or 2.5 to 5 mg in elderly

(cont.)

or debilitated patients); may repeat in 2 h and again in 4 h if warranted. Max 30 mg/day. Schizophrenia, oral therapy: Start 5 to 10 mg PO daily. Target dose is 10 mg/day. Max 20mg/day; however, doses above 10 mg/day have not been shown to be more effective. Reduce to 5 mg in debilitated patients or those predisposed to hypotension. Schizophrenia, long-acting injection: dose based on prior oral dose and ranges from 150 mg to 300 mg deep IM (gluteal) every 2 weeks or 300 mg to 405 mg q 4 weeks. See prescribing information. Bipolar disorder, maintenance treatment, or monotherapy for acute manic or mixed episodes: Start 10 to 15 mg PO daily. Increase by 5 mg/day at intervals of 24 h or more if needed. Usual effective dose range 5 to 20 mg/day, max 20 mg/day. Bipolar disorder, adjunctive for acute manic or mixed episodes: Start 10 mg PO daily; usual effective dose is 5 to 20 mg/day, max 20 mg/day. Bipolar depression, olanzapine + fluoxetine given separately: Start 5 mg olanzapine + 20 mg fluoxetine daily in the evening. Increase to usual range of 5 to 12.5 mg olanzapine plus 20 to 50 mg fluoxetine as tolerated. Also see Symbyax combination product entry. Treatment-resistant depression, olanzapine + fluoxetine given separately: Start 5 mg olanzapine + 20 mg fluoxetine daily in the evening. Increase to usual range of 5 to 20 mg olanzapine plus 20 to 50 mg fluoxetine as tolerated. See also Symbyax combination product entry. [Generic/Trade: Tabs 2.5, 5, 7.5, 10, 15, 20 mg. Tabs, orally disintegrating (Zyprexa Zydis) 5, 10, 15, 20 mg. Trade only: Long-acting injection (Zyprexa Relprevv) 210, 300, 405 mg/vial.] ▶L ♀C ▶– $$$$$ ■

PALIPERIDONE (*Invega Trinza, Invega, Invega Sustenna*) Schizophrenia and schizoaffective disorder (adjunctive and monotherapy): Start 6 mg PO every am. 3 mg/day may be sufficient in some. Max 12 mg/day. Extended-release injection: Schizophrenia (Invega Sustenna): Start 234 mg IM (deltoid) and then 156 mg IM 1 week later. Recommended monthly dose 117 mg IM (deltoid or gluteal) or within range of 39 to 234 mg, based on response. Patient must be able to tolerate

(cont.)

oral paliperidone or risperidone prior to starting Sustenna. Schizophrenia (Invega Trinza): Use only after tolerability to Invega Sustenna has been established for at least 4 months. The dose of Trinza is given IM every 3 months based on the prior dose of Sustenna. For Sustenna 78 mg use Trinza 273 mg; Sustenna 117 mg, use Trinza 410 mg; Sustenna 156 mg, use Trinza 546 mg; and Sustenna 234 mg, use Trinza 819 mg. Adjust dose at intervals of 3 months. Schizoaffective disorder (Invega Sustenna): Start 234 mg IM (deltoid) and then 156 mg IM on day 8. Usual dose range 78 to 234 mg, max 234 mg. [Generic/Trade: Extended-release tabs 1.5, 3, 6, 9 mg. Trade only: Depot formulation (Sustenna): 39, 78, 117, 156, 234 mg. Depot formulation (Trinza) 273, 410, 546, 819 mg.] ▶KL ♀C ▶– $$$$$ ■

PIMAVANSERIN (*Nuplazid*) 34 mg PO once daily. [Trade only: tabs 17 mg] ▶L ♀?/?/? ▶? ■

QUETIAPINE (*Seroquel, Seroquel XR*) Schizophrenia: Start 25 mg PO two times per day (regular tabs); increase by 25 to 50 mg two to three times per day on days 2 and 3, and then to target dose of 300 to 400 mg/day divided two to three times per day on day 4. Usual effective dose is 150 to 750 mg/day, max 750 mg/day initial therapy or 800 mg/day maintenance. Schizophrenia, Extended-release tabs: Start 300 mg PO daily in evening, increase by up to 300 mg/day at intervals of more than 1 day to usual effective range of 400 to 800 mg/day. Max 800 mg/day. Acute bipolar mania, monotherapy, or adjunctive: Start 50 mg PO two times per day on day 1, then increase to no higher than 100 mg two times per day on day 2, 150 mg two times per day on day 3, and 200 mg two times per day on day 4. May increase prn to 300 mg two times per day on day 5 and 400 mg two times per day thereafter. Usual effective dose is 400 to 800 mg/day. Max 800 mg/day. Bipolar disorder, acute manic or mixed, monotherapy or adjunctive, extended-release: Start 300 mg PO evening of day 1, 600 mg day 2, and 400 to 800 mg/day thereafter. Max 800 mg/day. Bipolar depression,

(cont.)

regular and extended release: 50 mg, 100 mg, 200 mg and 300 mg once daily at bedtime for days 1 to 4 respectively, and 300mg/day thereafter. Max 300 mg/day. Bipolar maintenance: Continue dose required to maintain remission. Major depressive disorder, adjunctive to antidepressants, extended-release: Start 50 mg evening of days 1 and 2, may increase to 150 mg on day 3. Max 300 mg/day. Eye exam for cataracts recommended q 6 months. [Generic/Trade: Tabs 25, 50, 100, 200, 300, 400 mg. Trade only: Extended-release tabs 50, 150, 200, 300, 400 mg.] ▶LK ♀C ▶– $$$$

RISPERIDONE (*Risperdal, Risperdal Consta, Risperdal M-Tab*)
Schizophrenia: Start 2 mg/day PO given once daily or divided two times per day (0.5 mg two times per day in the elderly, debilitated, or with hypotension, severe renal or hepatic disease); increase by 1 to 2 mg/day (no more than 0.5 mg two times per day in elderly and debilitated) at intervals of 24 h or more to usual effective dose of 4 to 8 mg/day given once daily or divided two times per day, max 16 mg/day; however, doses above 6 mg/day have not been shown to be more effective. Schizophrenia, bipolar type 1 maintenance: Long-acting injection (Consta): Start 25 mg IM every 2 weeks while continuing oral dose for 3 weeks. May increase at 4-week intervals to max 50 mg q 2 weeks. Schizophrenia (13 to 17 yo): Start 0.5 mg PO daily; increase by 0.5 to 1 mg/day at intervals of 24 h or more to target dose of 3 mg/day. Max 6 mg/day. Bipolar mania or mixed episodes, monotherapy or adjunctive (adults): Start 2 to 3 mg PO daily; may increase by 1 mg/day at 24 h intervals to max 6 mg/day. Bipolar mania or mixed episodes, monotherapy (10 to 17 yo): Start 0.5 mg PO daily; increase by 0.5 to 1 mg/day at intervals of 24 h to recommended dose of 1 to 2.5 mg/day. Max 6 mg/day; however, doses greater than 2.5 mg/day have not been shown to be more effective. Autistic disorder irritability (age 5 to 16 yo): Start 0.25 mg (for wt less than 20 kg) or 0.5 mg (wt 20 kg or greater) PO daily. May

(cont.)

increase after 4 days to target dose of 0.5 mg/day (for wt less than 20 kg) or 1.0 mg/day (wt 20 kg or greater). Maintain at least 14 days. May then increase if needed at 14-day intervals or more by increments of 0.25 mg/day (for wt less than 20 kg) or 0.5 mg/day (wt 20 kg or greater). Usual effective range 0.5 to 3 mg/day. [Generic/Trade: Tabs 0.25, 0.5, 1, 2, 3, 4 mg. Oral soln 1 mg/mL (30 mL). Orally disintegrating tabs 0.5, 1, 2, 3, 4 mg. Generic only: Orally disintegrating tabs 0.25 mg. Trade only: IM injection (Risperdal Consta) 12.5, 25, 37.5, 50 mg.] ▶LK ♀C ▶– $$$$ ■

ZIPRASIDONE (*Geodon*, *✦Zeldox*) Schizophrenia: Start 20 mg PO two times per day with food; may adjust at more than 2-day intervals to max 80 mg PO two times per day. Acute agitation in schizophrenia: 10 to 20 mg IM. May repeat 10 mg every 2 h or 20 mg every 4 h up to max 40 mg/day. Bipolar I disorder, monotherapy for acute manic or mixed episodes and adjunctive for maintenance: Start 40 mg PO two times per day with food; may increase to 60 to 80 mg two times per day on day 2. Usual effective dose is 40 to 80 mg two times per day. Must be taken with a meal of at least 500 Cal for adequate absorption. [Trade/Generic: Caps 20, 40, 60, 80 mg. Trade only: 20 mg/mL injection.] ▶L ♀C ▶– $$$$$ ■

Anxiolytics/Hypnotics—Benzodiazepines—Short Half-Life (<12 h)

NOTE: *To avoid withdrawal, gradually taper when discontinuing after prolonged use. Sedative-hypnotics have been associated with severe allergic reactions and complex sleep behaviors including sleep driving. Use caution and discuss with patients.*

ALPRAZOLAM (*Xanax, Xanax XR, Niravam*) Anxiety: 0.25 to 0.5 mg PO two to three times per day. Max 4 mg/day. Panic disorder: Start 0.5 mg PO three times per day (or 0.5 to 1 mg PO

(cont.)

daily of Xanax XR), may increase by up to 1 mg/day every 3 to 4 days to usual effective dose of 5 to 6 mg/day (3 to 6 mg/day for Xanax XR), max dose is 10 mg/day. Half-life 12 h. Multiple drug interactions. [Generic/Trade: Tabs 0.25, 0.5, 1, 2 mg. Tabs, extended-release 0.5, 1, 2, 3 mg. Orally disintegrating tabs (Niravam) 0.25, 0.5, 1, 2 mg. Generic only: Oral concentrate (Intensol) 1 mg/mL.] ▶LK ♀D ▬ ©IV $

OXAZEPAM 10 to 30 mg PO three to four times per day. Half-life 8 h. [Generic/Trade: Caps 10, 15, 30 mg. Trade only: Tabs 15 mg.] ▶LK ♀D ▬ ©IV $$$

TRIAZOLAM (*Halcion*) 0.125 to 0.5 mg PO at bedtime. 0.125 mg/day in elderly. Half-life 2 to 3 h. [Generic/Trade: Tabs 0.25 mg. Generic only: Tabs 0.125 mg.] ▶LK ♀X ▬ ©IV $

Anxiolytics/Hypnotics—Benzodiazepines—Medium Half-Life (10 to 15 h)

NOTE: *To avoid withdrawal, gradually taper when discontinuing after prolonged use. Sedative-hypnotics have been associated with complex sleep behaviors including sleep driving. Use caution and discuss with patients.*

ESTAZOLAM (*ProSom*) 1 to 2 mg PO at bedtime. [Generic/Trade: Tabs 1, 2 mg.] ▶LK ♀X ▬ ©IV $$

LORAZEPAM (*Ativan*) Anxiety: Start 0.5 to 1 mg PO two to three times per day, usual effective dose is 2 to 6 mg/day. Max dose is 10 mg/day PO. Insomnia: 2 to 4 mg PO at bedtime. Status epilepticus: Adult: 4 mg IV over 2 min; may repeat in 10 to 15 min. Status epilepticus: Peds: 0.05 to 0.1 mg/kg (max 4 mg) IV over 2 to 5 min; may repeat 0.05 mg/kg once in 10 to 15 min. Half-life 10 to 20 h. [Generic/Trade: Tabs 0.5, 1, 2 mg. Generic only: Oral concentrate 2 mg/mL.] ▶LK ♀D Per ACOG guidelines ▬ ©IV $

TEMAZEPAM (*Restoril*) 7.5 to 30 mg PO at bedtime (usual dose 15 mg). Half-life 8 to 25 h. [Generic/Trade: Caps 7.5, 15, 22.5, 30 mg.] ▶LK ♀X ▬ ©IV $

Anxiolytics/Hypnotics—Benzodiazepines—Long Half-Life (25-100 h)

NOTE: *To avoid withdrawal, gradually taper when discontinuing after prolonged use. Use cautiously in the elderly; may accumulate and lead to side effects, psychomotor impairment. Sedative-hypnotics have been associated with complex sleep behaviors including sleep driving. Use caution and discuss with patients.*

BROMAZEPAM (✦*Lectopam*) Canada only. 6 to 18 mg/day PO in divided doses. [Generic/Trade: Tabs 1.5, 3, 6 mg.] ▶L ♀D ▶− $

CHLORDIAZEPOXIDE Anxiety: 5 to 25 mg PO three to four times per day. Acute alcohol withdrawal: 50 to 100 mg PO, repeat every 3 to 4 h prn up to 300 mg/day. Half-life 5 to 30 h. [Generic/Trade: Caps 5, 10, 25 mg.] ▶LK ♀D ▶−©IV $$

CLONAZEPAM (*Klonopin, Klonopin Wafer, ✦Rivotril, Clonapam*) Panic disorder: Start 0.25 mg PO two times per day, max 4 mg/day; however, doses greater than 1 mg/day have not been shown to be more effective for most patients. Akinetic, Lennox-Gastaut syndrome, or myoclonic seizures: Start 0.5 mg PO three times per day. Max 20 mg/day. Half-life 18 to 50 h. [Generic/Trade: Tabs 0.5, 1, 2 mg. Orally disintegrating tabs (approved for panic disorder only) 0.125, 0.25, 0.5, 1, 2 mg.] ▶LK ♀X/?/? Category D per ACOG guidelines ▶−©IV $

CLORAZEPATE (*Tranxene*) Anxiety: Start 7.5 to 15 mg PO at bedtime or two to three times per day, usual effective dose is 15 to 60 mg/day. Acute alcohol withdrawal: 60 to 90 mg/day on 1st day divided two to three times per day, reduce dose to 7.5 to 15 mg/day over 5 days. Partial seizures, adjunctive: 13 yo and older, start no higher than 7.5 mg PO three times daily. May increase by no more than 7.5 mg per week to max 90 mg/day. Age 9 to 12 yo: Start 7.5 mg PO twice daily. May increase by no more than 7.5 mg per week to max of 60 mg/day. [Generic/Trade: Tabs 3.75, 7.5, 15 mg.] ▶LK ♀D ▶− ©IV $$$$

DIAZEPAM (*Valium, Diastat, Diastat AcuDial, Diazemuls*)
Active seizures: 5 to 10 mg IV q 10 to 15 min to max 30 mg, or 0.2 to 0.5 mg/kg rectal gel PR. Skeletal muscle spasm, spasticity related to cerebral palsy, paraplegia, athetosis, "stiff man syndrome": 2 to 10 mg PO/PR three to four times per day. Anxiety: 2 to 10 mg PO two to four times per day. Half-life 20 to 80 h. Alcohol withdrawal: 10 mg PO three to four times per day for 24 h then 5 mg PO three to four times per day prn. [Generic/Trade: Tabs 2, 5, 10 mg. Rectal gel 2.5 mg ($$$$$). Generic only: Oral soln 5 mg/5 mL. Oral concentrate (Intensol) 5 mg/mL. Rectal gel 10, 20 mg ($$$$$). Trade only: Rectal gel (Diastat AcuDial-$$$$$) 10, 20 mg syringes. Available doses from 10 mg AcuDial syringe 5, 7.5, 10 mg. Available doses from 20 mg AcuDial syringe 12.5, 15, 17.5, 20 mg.] ▶LK ♀D ▶– ©IV $

FLURAZEPAM 15 to 30 mg PO at bedtime. Half-life 70 to 90 h. [Generic/Trade: Caps 15, 30 mg.] ▶LK ♀X ▶– ©IV $

Anxiolytics/Hypnotics—Other

NOTE: *Sedative-hypnotics have been associated with complex sleep behaviors including sleep driving. Use caution and discuss with patients.*

BUSPIRONE Start 15 mg "dividose" daily (7.5 mg PO two times per day), usual effective dose 30 mg/day. Max 60 mg/day. [Generic/Trade: Tabs 5, 10 mg. Dividose tabs 15, 30 mg (scored to be easily bisected or trisected). Generic only: Tabs 7.5 mg.] ▶K ♀B ▶– $$$

ESZOPICLONE (*Lunesta*) 2 mg PO at bedtime prn. Max 3 mg. Elderly: 1 mg PO at bedtime prn, max 2 mg. [Generic/Trade: Tabs 1, 2, 3 mg.] ▶L ♀C ▶? ©IV $$$$$

RAMELTEON (*Rozerem*) 8 mg PO at bedtime. [Trade only: Tabs 8 mg.] ▶L ♀C ▶? $$$$

SUVOREXANT (*Belsomra*) Start 10 mg PO once nightly 30 minutes before bedtime. May increase if needed to max 20 mg once nightly. [Trade: Tabs 5, 10, 15, 20 mg.] ▶L ♀C ▶? ©IV

TASIMELTEON (*Hetlioz*) Non 24-h sleep/wake disorder: 20 mg before bedtime. Take on empty stomach. [Trade only: Caps 20 mg.] ▶L ♀C ▶?

ZALEPLON (*Sonata*) 5 to 10 mg PO at bedtime prn, max 20 mg. Do not use for benzodiazepine or alcohol withdrawal. [Generic/Trade: Caps 5, 10 mg.] ▶L ♀C ▶− ⊚IV $$$$

ZOLPIDEM (*Ambien, Ambien CR, ZolpiMist, Intermezzo, Edluar, ✦Sublinox*) Insomnia: Standard tabs: women, 5 mg and men 5-10 mg PO at bedtime. The 5 mg dose may be increased to 10 mg if needed. For age older than 65 yo or debilitated: 5 mg PO at bedtime. Oral spray: women, 5 mg and men 5-10 mg PO at bedtime. May increase the 5 mg dose to 10 mg if needed. For age older than 65 yo or debilitated: 5 mg PO at bedtime. Control-release tabs: women, 6.25 mg and men 6.25-12.5 mg PO at bedtime. May increase the 6.25 mg dose to 12.5 mg if needed. For age older than 65 yo or debilitated: give 6.25 mg PO at bedtime. Sublingual tabs (Edluar): women, 5 mg and men 5-10 mg SL at bedtime. May increase the 5 mg dose to 10 mg if needed. Sublingual tabs (Intermezzo) for middle of the night awakening: women 1.75 mg SL and men 3.5 mg once nightly with at least 4 hours of sleep remaining. Do not use for benzodiazepine or alcohol withdrawal. [Generic/Trade: Tabs 5, 10 mg. Controlled-release tabs 6.25, 12.5 mg. SL tabs 1.75, 3.5 mg (Intermezzo). Trade only: Oral spray 5 mg/actuation (ZolpiMist); SL tabs 5, 10 mg (Edluar).] ▶L ♀C ▶+ ⊚IV $$$$

ZOPICLONE (✦*Imovane*) Canada only. 5 to 7.5 mg PO at bedtime. Reduce dose in elderly. [Generic/Trade: Tabs 5, 7.5 mg. Generic only: Tabs 3.75 mg.] ▶L ♀D ▶− $

Combination Drugs

SYMBYAX (olanzapine + fluoxetine) Bipolar type 1 with depression and treatment-resistant depression: Start 6 mg olanzapine/25 mg fluoxetine PO at bedtime. Max 18/75 mg/day. [Generic/Trade: Caps (olanzapine/fluoxetine) 3/25, 6/25, 6/50, 12/25, 12/50 mg.] ▶LK ♀C ▶− $$$$$ ∎

Drug Dependence Therapy

ACAMPROSATE (*Campral*)   Maintenance of abstinence from alcohol: 666 mg (2 tabs) PO three times per day. Start after alcohol withdrawal and when patient is abstinent. [Generic/Trade: Tabs, delayed-release 333 mg.] ▶K ♀C ▶? $$$$$

BUPRENORPHINE (*Subutex, Probuphine*)   Treatment of opioid dependence - Induction (Subutex): 8 mg SL on day 1, and 16 mg on day 2. Maintenance dose 16 mg daily, but may individualize in a range of 4 to 24 mg daily. Treatment of opioid maintenance (Probuphine): Use only if stable on 8 mg/day or less of a transmucosal form. Four implants in the inner aspect of one arm and left in place for 6 months and then removed. May repeat at 6 months in the other arm one time only. Must undergo special training and be registered to prescribe for this indication. [Trade and generic: SL tabs 2 and 8 mg. Trade only: Implants (Probuphine): 74.2 mg (= 80 mg buprenorphine HCl)] ▶L ♀C ▶− ©lll ■

DISULFIRAM (*Antabuse*)   Maintenance of abstinence from alcohol: 125 to 500 mg PO daily. Patient must abstain from any alcohol for at least 12 h before using. Metronidazole and alcohol in any form (cough syrups, tonics, etc.) contraindicated. [Generic/Trade: Tabs 250, 500 mg.] ▶L ♀C ▶? $$

NALTREXONE (*ReVia, Depade, Vivitrol*)   Alcohol/opioid dependence: 25 to 50 mg PO daily. Extended-release injectable susp: 380 mg IM every 4 weeks or monthly. Avoid if recent ingestion of opioids (past 7 to 10 days). Hepatotoxicity with higher than approved doses. [Generic/Trade: Tabs 50 mg. Trade only (Vivitrol): Extended-release injectable susp kits 380 mg.] ▶LK ♀C ▶? $$$$

NICOTINE GUM (*Nicorette, Nicorette DS*)   Smoking cessation: Gradually taper: 1 piece every 1 to 2 h for 6 weeks, 1 piece every 2 to 4 h for 3 weeks, then 1 piece every 4 to 8 h for 3 weeks, max 30 pieces/day of 2 mg or 24 pieces/day of 4 mg. Use Nicorette DS 4 mg/piece in high cigarette use (more than 24 cigarettes/day). [OTC/Generic/Trade: Gum 2, 4 mg.] ▶LK ♀C ▶− $$$$

NICOTINE INHALATION SYSTEM (*Nicotrol Inhaler*, ✱*Nicorette Inhaler*) Smoking cessation: 6 to 16 cartridges/day for 12 weeks. [Trade only: Oral inhaler 10 mg/cartridge (4 mg nicotine delivered), 42 cartridges/box.] ▶LK ♀D ▶– $$$$$

NICOTINE LOZENGE (*Commit, Nicorette*) Smoking cessation: In those who smoke within 30 min of waking, use 4 mg lozenge; others use 2 mg. Take 1 to 2 lozenges every 1 to 2 h for 6 weeks, then every 2 to 4 h in weeks 7 to 9, then every 4 to 8 h weeks 10 to 12. Length of therapy 12 weeks. [OTC Generic/Trade: Lozenge 2, 4 mg.] ▶LK ♀D ▶– $$$$$

NICOTINE NASAL SPRAY (*Nicotrol NS*) Smoking cessation: 1 to 2 doses q 1 h, each dose is 2 sprays, 1 in each nostril (1 spray contains 0.5 mg nicotine). Minimum recommended: 8 doses/day, max 40 doses/day. [Trade only: Nasal soln 10 mg/mL (0.5 mg/inhalation); 10 mL bottles.] ▶LK ♀D ▶– $$$$$

NICOTINE PATCHES (*Habitrol, NicoDerm CQ, Nicotrol*) Smoking cessation: Start 1 patch (14 to 22 mg) daily, taper after 6 weeks. Patients who slip up and smoke when using patches can still use them but suggest curbing use. [OTC/Rx/Generic/Trade: Patches 11, 22 mg/24 h. 7, 14, 21 mg/24 h (Habitrol and NicoDerm). OTC/Trade: 15 mg/16 h (Nicotrol).] ▶LK ♀D ▶– $$$$

SUBOXONE (buprenorphine + naloxone, *Bunavail, Zubsolv*) Treatment of opioid dependence: Induction (Suboxone SL film): Day 1 start with 2 mg/0.5 mg SL or 4 mg/1 mg SL and titrate upward in increments of 2 or 4 mg of buprenorphine at approximately 2 h intervals to 8 mg/2 mg total dose. Day 2 a dose of up to 16 mg/4 mg is recommended. Maintenance (SL tabs and film): Target dose 16 mg/4 mg SL daily. Can individualize to range of 4 to 24 mg of buprenorphine daily. Induction (Zubsolv): Day 1 start with 1.4 mg/0.36 mg and titrate upward in increments of 1 or 2 of these tablets every 1.5-2 hours to a dose of 5.7 mg/1.4 mg. Some patients may tolerate three of the tablets as the second dose depending upon recent narcotic exposure. Day 2 a dose of 11.4 mg/2.9 mg is recommended. Maintenance (Zubsolv): 11.4

(cont.)

mg/2.8 mg SL daily. Can individualize to range of 2.8/0.72 to 17.1/4.2 mg SL daily. Use sublingual buprenorphine monotherapy (without naloxone) for induction in patients dependent on methadone or other long-acting opioids. [Generic only: SL tabs 2/0.5 mg and 8/2 mg buprenorphine/ naloxone. Trade only: SL film 2/0.5, 4/1, 8/2, 12/3 mg buprenorphine/naloxone, SL tabs (Zubsolv) 1.4/0.36, 5.7/1.4 mg.] ▶L ♀C ▶— ⊝III $$$$$

VARENICLINE (*Chantix*, ✦*Champix*) Smoking cessation: Start 0.5 mg PO daily for days 1 to 3, then 0.5 mg two times per day days 4 to 7, then 1 mg two times per day thereafter. Take after meals with full glass of water. Start 1 week prior to cessation and continue for 12 weeks, or patient may start the drug and stop smoking between days 8 and 35 of treatment. May cause suicidal thinking and behavior. [Trade only: Tabs 0.5, 1 mg.] ▶K ♀C ▶? $$$$ ■

Stimulants/ADHD/Anorexiants

NOTE: *Sudden cardiac death has been reported with stimulants and atomoxetine at usual ADHD doses; carefully assess prior to treatment and avoid if cardiac conditions or structural abnormalities. Amphetamines are associated with high abuse potential and dependence with prolonged administration. Stimulants may also cause or worsen underlying psychosis or induce a manic or mixed episode in bipolar disorder. Problems with visual accommodation have also been reported with stimulants. Stimulants have been associated with rhabdomyolysis.*

ADDERALL XR (dextroamphetamine + amphetamine, *Adderall*)

ADHD, standard-release tabs: Start 2.5 mg (3 to 5 yo) or 5 mg (age 6 yo or older) PO one to two times per day, increase by 2.5 mg (3 to 5 yo) to 5 mg (6 yo and older) every week, max 40 mg/day. Extended-release caps (Adderall XR): Age 6 to 12

(cont.)

yo, start 5 to 10 mg PO daily to a max of 30 mg/day. Age 13 to 17 yo, start 10 mg PO daily to a max of 20 mg/day. Adults: Give 20 mg PO daily. Narcolepsy, immediate-release: Start 5 to 10 mg PO every morning, increase by 5 to 10 mg every week, max 60 mg/day. Avoid evening doses. Monitor growth and use drug holidays when appropriate. [Generic/Trade: Tabs 5, 7.5, 10, 12.5, 15, 20, 30 mg. Caps, extended-release (Adderall XR) 5, 10, 15, 20, 25, 30 mg.] ▶L ♀C▶– ⊝II $$$$

AMPHETAMINE (*Adzenys XR, Dyanavel XR*) Adults and children 6 yo and older, Dyanavel XR: Start 2.5 mg to 5 mg PO once daily in the morning. May increase by 2.5 mg to 10 mg per day every 4-7 days to max dose of 20 mg/day. Adzenys XR, adults: 12.5 mg dissolved on the tongue once daily in the morning. Children: Start 6.3 mg dissolved on the tongue once daily in the morning. Increase at weekly intervals by 3.1 mg to 6.3 mg to max of 18.8 mg daily for ages 6-12 yo and 12.5 mg daily for ages 13-17 yo. [Trade: Extended-release susp 2.5 mg/mL] ▶L ♀? Limited data in humans. Premature delivery and low birth weight have been observed. ▶– ⊝II ■

ARMODAFINIL (*Nuvigil*) Obstructive sleep apnea/hypopnea syndrome and narcolepsy: 150 to 250 mg PO every am. Inconsistent evidence for improved efficacy of 250 mg/day dose. Shift work sleep disorder: 150 mg PO 1 h prior to start of shift. [Trade only: Tabs 50, 150, 200, 250 mg.] ▶L ♀C ▶? ⊝IV $$$$$

ATOMOXETINE (*Strattera*) All ages wt greater than 70 kg: Start 40 mg PO daily, then increase after more than 3 days to target of 80 mg/day divided one to two times per day. May increase after another 2 to 4 weeks to max 100 mg/day. [Trade only: Caps 10, 18, 25, 40, 60, 80, 100 mg.] ▶K ♀C ▶? $$$$$ ■

CAFFEINE (*NoDoz, Vivarin, Caffedrine, Stay Awake, Quick-Pep, Cafcit*) 100 to 200 mg PO every 3 to 4 h prn. [OTC Generic/Trade: Tabs/Caps 200 mg. Oral soln caffeine citrate (Cafcit) 20 mg/mL. OTC Trade only: Tabs, extended-release 200 mg. Lozenges 75 mg.] ▶L ♀B/C ▶? $

CLONIDINE—PSYCHIATRY (*Kapvay, Catapres, Catapres TTS*)
ADHD (Kapvay):Start 0.1 mg PO at bedtime. May increase by 0.1 mg/day weekly to max 0.4 mg given twice daily. Taper when discontinuing. Tourette syndrome: (unapproved peds and adult): 3 to 5 mcg/kg/day PO divided two to four times per day. Opioid withdrawal, adjunct (unapproved adult): 0.1 to 0.3 mg PO three to four times per day or 0.1 to 0.2 mg PO q 4 h prn. Smoking cessation (uapproved adult): Start 0.1 mg PO two times per day, increase 0.1 mg/day at weekly intervals to 0.75 mg/day as tolerated; transdermal (Catapres TTS): 0.1 to 0.2 mg/24 h patch once a week for 2 to 3 weeks after cessation. [Generic/Trade: Extended-release tabs 0.1 mg. Tabs, immediate-release, 0.1, 0.2, 0.3 mg. Transdermal weekly patch 0.1 mg/day (TTS-1), 0.2 mg/day (TTS-2), 0.3 mg/day (TTS-3).] ▶LK ♀C ▶? Present in human milk $$$$$

DEXMETHYLPHENIDATE (*Focalin, Focalin XR*) Extended-release, not already on stimulants: Start 5 mg (children) or 10 mg (adults) PO every am. Max 30 mg/day (children) or 40 mg/day (Adults). Immediate-release, not already on stimulants: 2.5 mg PO two times per day. Max 20 mg/day. If taking racemic methylphenidate, use conversion of 2.5 mg for each 5 mg of methylphenidate. [Generic/Trade: Tabs, immediate-release 2.5, 5, 10 mg. Extended-release caps ($$$$$) 5, 10, 15, 20, 30, 40 mg. Trade only: Extended-release caps (Focalin XR-$$$$$) 25, 35 mg.] ▶LK ♀C ▶? ⊙II $$$

DEXTROAMPHETAMINE (*Dexedrine Spansules, ProCentra, Zenzedi*) Narcolepsy: Age 6 to 12 yo: Start 5 mg PO every am, increase by 5 mg/day each week. Age older than 12 yo: Start 10 mg PO every am, increase by 10 mg/day each week. Usual dose range 5 to 60 mg/day in divided doses (tabs) or daily (extended-release). ADHD: 2.5 to 5 mg PO every am, usual max 40 mg/day. Avoid evening doses. Monitor growth and use drug holidays when appropriate. [Generic/Trade: Caps, extended-release 5, 10, 15 mg. Tabs 5, 10 mg. Oral soln 5 mg/5 mL. Trade only: Tabs 2.5, 7.5 mg (Zenzedi).] ▶L ♀C ▶— ⊙II $$$$$

GUANFACINE—PSYCHIATRY (*Intuniv*) Start 1 mg PO once daily. Increase by 1 mg/week to max 7 mg/day based on weight. Refer to package insert for target dose ranges based on weight. [Generic/Trade: Tabs, extended-release 1, 2, 3, 4 mg.] ▶LK – ♀B ▶?

LISDEXAMFETAMINE (*Vyvanse*) ADHD: Adults, adolescents, and children ages 6 yo and older: Start 30 mg PO every morning. May increase weekly by 10 to 20 mg/day to max 70 mg/day. Avoid evening doses. Monitor growth and use drug holidays when appropriate. Binge eating disorder, mild to moderate: Start 30 mg PO once daily. May increase weekly by 20 mg/day to suggested range of 50 mg to 70 mg daily. Max 70 mg/day. [Trade: Caps 20, 30, 40, 50, 60, 70 mg.] ▶L ♀C▶ ⊚ll $$$$

METHYLPHENIDATE (*Quillichew ER, Aptensio XR, Ritalin, Ritalin LA, Methylin, Methylin ER, Metadate ER, Metadate CD, Concerta, Daytrana, Quillivant XR, ✦Biphentin*) ADHD: 5 to 10 mg PO two to three times per day (immediate-release) or 20 mg PO every am (extended-release), max 60 mg/day. Extended-release (Concerta) 18 to 36 mg PO every am, max 72 mg/day. Extended-release, chewable (Quillichew ER): Start 20 mg PO (chewed) once daily in the morning. May increase at weekly intervals by 10 mg, 15 mg, or 20 mg daily based on efficacy and tolerability. Max 60 mg/day. Extended-release (Aptensio XR): Start 10 mg PO once daily in the morning. May increase by 10 mg/day at weekly intervals to max 60 mg/day. Sustained-release suspension (Quillivant XR) 6 yo and older: Start 20 mg PO in the morning. May increase weekly by 10 to 20 mg daily to max 60 mg/day. Avoid evening doses. Monitor growth and use drug holidays when appropriate. Narcolepsy (Ritalin): 10 mg PO two to three times per day before meals. Usual effective dose is 20 to 30 mg/day, max 60 mg/day. [Trade only: Tabs, extended-release 10, 20 mg (Methylin ER, Metadate ER). Tabs, extended-release, chewable 20, 30 mg. Transdermal patch (Daytrana) 10 mg/9 h, 15 mg/9 h, 20 mg/9 h, 30 mg/9 h. Susp, extended-release 5 mg/mL (Quillivant XR). Generic/Trade: Tabs,

(cont.)

PSYCHIATRY

chewable 2.5, 5, 10 mg (Methylin). Tabs, 5, 10, 20 mg (Ritalin). Tabs, extended-release 18, 27, 36, 54 mg (Concerta). Caps, extended-release 10, 20, 30, 40, 50, 60 mg (Metadate CD), may be sprinkled on food. Caps, extended-release 10, 20, 30, 40 mg (Ritalin LA). Caps, extended-release (Aptensio XR) 10, 15, 20, 30, 40, 50, 60 mg. Oral soln 5 mg/5 mL, 10 mg/5 mL. Generic only: Tabs 5, 10, 20 mg. Tabs, extended-release 10, 20 mg.] ▶LK ♀C ▶? ⊚II $$

MODAFINIL (*Provigil, ✦Alertec*) Narcolepsy and sleep apnea/hypopnea: 200 mg PO q am. Shift work sleep disorder: 200 mg PO 1 h before shift. [Generic/Trade: Tabs 100, 200 mg.] ▶L ♀C ▶? ⊚IV $$$$$

PHENTERMINE (*Adipex-P, Suprenza*) 15 mg to 37.5 mg/day every am before or 1 to 2 h after breakfast. Alternatively 18.75 mg PO two times daily. Avoid late evening dosing. For short-term use. [Generic/Trade: Caps 15, 30, 37.5 mg. Tabs 37.5 mg. Trade only: Orally disintegrating tabs (Suprenza) 15, 30, 37.5 mg. Generic only: Caps, extended-release 15, 30 mg.] ▶KL ♀C ▶– ⊚IV $

PULMONARY

INHALER COLORS (Body then cap—Generics may differ)

Inhaler	Colors
Advair Diskus	purple
Advair HFA	purple/light purple
Aerobid-M	grey/green
Aerospan	purple/grey
Alvesco 80 mcg 160 mcg	 brown/red red/red
Anoro Ellipta	grey/red
Arcapta Neohaler	white/red
Arnuity Ellipta	grey/red
Asmanex HFA	blue/red
Asmanex Twisthaler 110 mcg 220 mcg	 white/grey white/pink
Atrovent HFA	clear/green

(cont.)

PULMONARY

INHALER COLORS (Body then cap—Generics may differ)
(*continued*)

Inhaler	Colors
Bevepsi Aerosphere	grey/orange
Breo Ellipta	grey/blue
Combivent Respimat	grey/orange
Dulera	blue
Flovent Diskus	orange
Flovent HFA	orange/peach
Foradil Aerolizer	blue
Incruse Ellipta	white/green
ProAir HFA	red/white
Proair Respiclick	red/white
Proventil HFA	yellow/orange
Pulmicort Flexhaler	white/brown
QVAR 40 mcg 80 mcg	beige/grey mauve/grey

(cont.)

INHALER COLORS (Body then cap—Generics may differ)
(*continued*)

Inhaler	Colors
Seebri Neohaler	white/amber
Serevent Diskus	green
Spiriva	grey
Spiriva Respimat 1.25 mcg 2.5 mcg	grey/blue grey/green
Stiolto Respimat	grey/green
Striverdi Respimat	grey/yellow
Symbicort	red/grey
Tudorza Pressair	white/green
Utibron Neohaler	white/yellow
Ventolin HFA	light blue/navy
Xopenex HFA	blue/red

INHALED STEROIDS: ESTIMATED COMPARATIVE DAILY DOSES*

Adults and Children older than 12 yo

Drug	Form	Low dose	Medium dose	High dose
beclomethasone HFA MDI	40 mcg/puff 80 mcg/puff	2–6 puffs/day 1–3 puffs/day	6–12 puffs/day 3–6 puffs/day	>12 puffs/day >6 puffs/day
budesonide DPI	90 mcg/dose 180 mcg/dose	2–6 inhalations/day 1–3 inhalations/day	6–13 inhalations/day 3–7 inhalations/day	>13 inhalations/day >7 inhalations/day
budesonide	soln for nebs	—	—	—
flunisolide HFA MDI	80 mcg/puff	4 puffs/day	5–8 puffs/day	>8 puffs/day

(cont.)

	Low dose	Medium dose	High dose
fluticasone HFA MDI 44 mcg/puff	2–6 puffs/day	6–10 puffs/day	> 10 puffs/day
110 mcg/puff	1–2 puffs/day	2–4 puffs/day	> 4 puffs/day
220 mcg/puff	1 puff/day	1–2 puffs/day	> 2 puffs/day
fluticasone DPI 50 mcg/dose	2–6 inhalations/day	6–10 inhalations/day	> 10 inhalations/day
100 mcg/dose	1–3 inhalations/day	3–5 inhalations/day	> 5 inhalations/day
250 mcg/dose	1 inhalation/day	2 inhalations/day	> 2 inhalations/day
mometasone DPI 220 mcg/dose	1 inhalation/day	2 inhalations/day	> 2 inhalations/day

CHILDREN (age 5 to 11 yo)

Drug	Form	Low dose	Medium dose	High dose
beclomethasone HFA MDI	40 mcg/puff	2–4 puffs/day	4–8 puffs/day	> 8 puffs/day
	80 mcg/puff	1–2 puffs/day	2–4 puffs/day	> 4 puffs/day

PULMONARY

(cont.)

INHALED STEROIDS: ESTIMATED COMPARATIVE DAILY DOSES* *(continued)*

CHILDREN (age 5 to 11 yo)

Drug	Form	Low dose	Medium dose	High dose
budesonide DPI	90 mcg/dose 180 mcg/dose	2–4 inhalations/day 1–2 inhalations/day	4–9 inhalations/day 2–4 inhalations/day	> 9 inhalations/day > 4 inhalations/day
budesonide	soln for nebs	0.5 mg 0.25–0.5 mg (0–4 yo)	1 mg > 0.5–1 mg (0–4 yo)	2 mg > 1 mg (0–4 yo)
flunisolide HFA MDI	80 mcg/puff	2 puffs/day	4 puffs/day	≥ 8 puffs/day

(cont.)

fluticasone HFA MDI (0–11 yo)	44 mcg/puff	2–4 puffs/day	4–8 puffs/day	> 8 puffs/day
	110 mcg/puff	1–2 puff/day	2–3 puffs/day	> 4 puffs/day
	220 mcg/puff	n/a	1–2 puffs/day	> 2 puffs/day
fluticasone DPI	50 mcg/dose	2–4 inhalations/day	4–8 inhalations/day	> 8 inhalations/day
	100 mcg/dose	1–2 inhalations/day	2–4 inhalations/day	> 4 inhalations/day
	250 mcg/dose	n/a	1 inhalation/day	> 1 inhalation/day
mometasone DPI	220 mcg/dose	n/a	n/a	n/a

http://www.nhlbi.nih.gov/guidelines/asthma/asthsumm.pdf

*HFA = Hydrofluoroalkane (propellant). MDI = metered dose inhaler. DPI = dry powder inhaler.

PULMONARY

PREDICTED PEAK EXPIRATORY FLOW (liters/min)

Age (yo)	Women (height in inches)					Men (height in inches)					Child (height in inches)
	55"	60"	65"	70"	75"	60"	65"	70"	75"	80"	
20	390	423	460	496	529	554	602	649	693	740	44–160"
30	380	413	448	483	516	532	577	622	664	710	46–187"
40	370	402	436	470	502	509	552	596	636	680	48–214"
50	360	391	424	457	488	486	527	569	607	649	50–240"
60	350	380	412	445	475	463	502	542	578	618	52–267"
70	340	369	400	432	461	440	477	515	550	587	54–293"

Am Rev Resp Dis 1963;88:644.

Beta Agonists—Short-Acting

ALBUTEROL (***ProAir RespiClick, AccuNeb, Ventolin HFA, Proventil HFA, ProAir HFA, VoSpire ER, ✦Airomir, salbutamol, Apo-Salvent***) MDI: 2 puffs q 4 to 6 h prn. Soln: 0.5 mL of 0.5% soln (2.5 mg) nebulized three to four times per day. One 3 mL unit dose (0.083%) nebulized three to four times per day. Tabs: 2 to 4 mg PO three to four times per day or extended-release 4 to 8 mg PO q 12 h up to 16 mg PO q 12 h. Peds: 0.1 to 0.2 mg/kg/dose PO three times per day up to 4 mg three times per day for age 2 to 5 yo, 2 to 4 mg or extended-release 4 mg PO q 12 h for age 6 to 12 yo. Prevention of exercise-induced bronchospasm: MDI: 2 puffs 10 to 30 min before exercise. [Trade only: MDI 90 mcg/actuation, 200 metered doses/canister. "HFA" inhalers use hydrofluoroalkane propellant instead of CFCs but are otherwise equivalent. "RespiClick" is a breath-actuated DPI. Generic/Trade: Soln for inhalation 0.021% (AccuNeb), 0.042% (AccuNeb), and 0.083% in 3 mL vials, 0.5% (5 mg/mL) in 20 mL with dropper. Tabs, extended-release 4, 8 mg (VoSpire ER). Generic only: Syrup 2 mg/5 mL. Tabs, immediate-release 2, 4 mg.] ▶L ♀C ▶? $$

LEVALBUTEROL (***Xopenex Concentrate, Xopenex, Xopenex HFA***) MDI 2 puffs q 4 to 6 h prn. Nebulizer 0.63 to 1.25 mg q 6 to 8 h. Peds: 0.31 mg nebulized three times per day for age 6 to 11 yo. [Generic/Trade: Soln for inhalation 0.31, 0.63, 1.25 mg in 3 mL and 1.25 mg in 0.5 mL unit-dose vials. Trade only: HFA MDI 45 mcg/actuation, 15 g 200/canister. "HFA" inhalers use hydrofluoroalkane propellant.] ▶L ♀C ▶? $$$

METAPROTERENOL (***✦Orciprenaline***) MDI: 2 to 3 puffs q 3 to 4 h. Soln: 0.2 to 0.3 mL 5% soln nebulized q 4 h. Peds: Tabs: 20 mg PO three to four times per day age older than 9 yo, 10 mg PO three to four times per day if age 6 to 9 yo, 1.3 to 2.6 mg/kg/day divided three to four times per day if age 2 to 5 yo. [Trade only: MDI 0.65 mg/actuation, 14 g 200/canister. Generic/Trade: Soln for inhalation 0.4%, 0.6% in 2.5 mL unit-dose vials. Generic only: Syrup 10 mg/5 mL. Tabs 10, 20 mg.] ▶L ♀C ▶? $$

Beta Agonists—Long-Acting

ARFORMOTEROL (*Brovana*) COPD: 15 mcg nebulized two times per day. [Trade only: Soln for inhalation 15 mcg in 2 mL vial.] ▶L ♀C ▶? $$$$$ ■

FORMOTEROL (*Foradil Aerolizer, Perforomist, ✦Oxeze Turbuhaler*) 1 puff two times per day. Nebulized: 20 mcg q 12 h. Not for acute bronchospasm. For asthma, use only in combination with corticosteroids. [Trade only: DPI 12 mcg, 12, 60 blisters/pack (Foradil). To be used only with Aerolizer device. Soln for inhalation: 20 mcg in 2 mL vial (Perforomist). Canada only (Oxeze): DPI 6, 12 mcg 60 blisters/pack.] ▶L ♀C ▶? $$$ ■

INDACATEROL (*Arcapta Neohaler, ✦Onbrez Breezhaler*) COPD: DPI: 75 mcg inhaled once daily. [Trade only: DPI: 75 mcg caps for inhalation, 30 blisters. To be used only with Neohaler device. Contains lactose.] ▶L − ♀C ▶? ■

OLODATEROL (*Striverdi Respimat*) COPD: 2 inhalations once daily. [Trade only: Carton with canister containing 28 or 60 metered actuations for use with provided Striverdi Respimat device. Each actuation delivers 2.5 mcg olodaterol.] ▶LK ♀C ▶? ■

SALMETEROL (*Serevent Diskus, ✦Serevent Diskhaler disk*) 1 inhalation two times per day. Not for acute bronchospasm. For asthma, use only in combination with corticosteroids. [Trade only: DPI (Diskus): 50 mcg, 60 blisters.] ▶L ♀C ▶? $$$$ ■

Combinations

ADVAIR HFA (fluticasone—inhaled + salmeterol, *Advair Diskus, ✦Advair, Advair Diskus*) Asthma: DPI: 1 inhalation two times per day (all strengths). MDI: 2 puffs two times per day (all strengths). COPD: DPI: 1 inhalation two times per day (250/50 only). [Trade only: DPI: 100/50, 250/50, 500/50 mcg fluticasone/salmeterol per actuation; 60 doses/DPI. Trade only (Advair HFA): MDI 45/21, 115/21, 230/21 mcg fluticasone/salmeterol per actuation; 120 doses/canister.] ▶L ♀C ▶? $$$$$ ■

BEVESPI AEROSPHERE (glycopyrrolate—inhaled + formoterol) COPD: Two inhalations twice daily. [Trade only: MDI: 9/4.8 mcg glycopyrrolate/formoterol per inhalation. 120 inhalations (10.7 g) per canister.] ▶KL ♀C ▶? ■

BREO ELLIPTA (fluticasone—inhaled + vilanterol, ✦***Breo Ellipta***) Chronic asthma, COPD: 1 inhalation once daily. 200/25 mcg fluticasone/vilanterol strength only approved for asthma. [Trade only: DPI: 100/25 mcg, 200/25 mcg fluticasone/vilanterol per actuation.] ▶L – ♀C ▶? $$$$$ ■

COMBIVENT RESPIMAT (albuterol—inhaled + ipratropium—inhaled, ✦***Combivent Respimat***) Respimat: 1 inhalation four times per day, max 6 inhalations/day. [Trade only: Respimat: 100 mcg albuterol/20 mcg ipratropium per inhalation, 120/canister.] ▶L ♀C ▶? $$$$

DULERA (mometasone—inhaled + formoterol, ✦***Zenhale***) Chronic asthma: 2 puffs two times per day (all strengths). [Trade only: MDI 100/5, 200/5 mcg mometasone/formoterol per actuation; 120 doses/canister.] ▶L – ♀C ▶? $$$$$ ■

DUONEB (albuterol—inhaled + ipratropium—inhaled, ✦***Combivent inhalation soln***) 1 unit dose four times per day. [Generic/Trade: Unit dose: 2.5 mg albuterol/0.5 mg ipratropium per 3 mL vial, premixed; 30, 60 vials/carton.] ▶L ♀C ▶? $$$$$

STIOLTO RESPIMAT (tiotropium + olodaterol) COPD: 2 inhalations once per day using Respimat device. [Trade only: Inhalation spray: equivalent of 2.5/2.5 mcg tiotropium/olodaterol per inhalation. Canisters contain 60 inhalations each. For use with Respimat device only.] ▶KL ♀C ▶? ■

SYMBICORT (budesonide—inhaled + formoterol, ✦***Symbicort Turbuhaler***) Asthma: 2 puffs two times per day (both strengths). COPD: 2 puffs two times per day (160/4.5). [Trade only: MDI: 80/4.5, 160/4.5 mcg budesonide/formoterol per actuation; 120 doses/canister.] ▶L ♀C ▶? $$$$ ■

UTIBRON NEOHALER (indacaterol + glycopyrrolate—inhaled) COPD: Inhale powder contents of one capsule twice daily using Neohaler device. [Trade only: caps: 27.6 mcg/15.6 mcg

(cont.)

indacaterol/glycopyrrolate in blister packs in boxes of 6 or 60 caps for use with Neohaler device.] ▶L ♀C ▶? ■

Inhaled Steroids

NOTE: *See Endocrine-Corticosteroids when oral steroids necessary.*

BECLOMETHASONE—INHALED (*QVAR, ✦QVAR*) 1 to 4 puffs two times per day (40 mcg). 1 to 2 puffs two times per day (80 mcg). [Trade only: HFA MDI: 40, 80 mcg/actuation, 7.3 g 100 actuations/canister.] ▶L ♀C ▶? $$$

BUDESONIDE—INHALED (*Pulmicort Respules, Pulmicort Flexhaler, ✦Pulmicort Turbuhaler*) 1 to 2 puffs daily up to 4 puffs two times per day. Respules: 0.5 to 1 mg daily or divided two times per day. [Trade only: DPI (Flexhaler) 90, 180 mcg powder/actuation 60, 120 doses/canister, respectively. Generic/Trade: Respules 0.25, 0.5, 1 mg/2 mL unit dose.] ▶L ♀B ▶? $$$$

CICLESONIDE—INHALED (*Alvesco*) 80 mcg/puff: 1 to 4 puffs two times per day. 160 mcg/puff: 1 to 2 puffs two times per day. [Trade only: 80 mcg/actuation, 60 per canister. 160 mcg/actuation, 60, 120 per canister.] ▶L ♀C ▶? $$$$

FLUNISOLIDE—INHALED (*Aerospan*) 2 to 4 puffs two times per day. [Trade only: MDI: 250 mcg/actuation, 100 metered doses/canister. AeroBid-M (AeroBid + menthol flavor). Aerospan HFA MDI: 80 mcg/actuation, 60, 120 metered doses/canister.] ▶L ♀C ▶? $$$

FLUTICASONE FUROATE (*Flovent Diskus, Flovent HFA, Arnuity Ellipta, ✦Flovent Diskus, Flovent HFA, Arnuity Ellipta*) Chronic asthma: 1 inhalation once daily. [Trade only: Foil strip with 30 blisters each containing 100 or 200 mcg fluticasone furoate for use with Ellipta DPI device.] ▶L ♀C ▶?

FLUTICASONE—INHALED (*Arnuity Ellipta, Flovent HFA, Flovent Diskus, ✦Arnuity Ellipta, Flovent HFA, Flovent Diskus*) 2 to 4

(cont.)

puffs two times per day. [Trade only: HFA MDI: 44, 110, 220 mcg/actuation 120/canister. DPI (Diskus): 50, 100, 250 mcg/actuation delivering 44, 88, 220 mcg respectively.] ▶L ♀C ▶? $$$$

MOMETASONE—INHALED (*Asmanex HFA, Asmanex Twisthaler, ✦Asmanex Twisthaler*) 1 to 2 puffs in the evening or 1 puff two times per day. If prior oral corticosteroid therapy: 2 puffs two times per day. [Trade only: DPI: 110 mcg/actuation with #30 dosage units, 220 mcg/actuation with #30, 60, 120 dosage units.] ▶L ♀C ▶? $$$$

Leukotriene Inhibitors

MONTELUKAST (*Singulair*) Adults: 10 mg PO daily in the evening. Chronic asthma, allergic rhinitis: Give 4 mg (chew tab or oral granules) PO daily for age 2 to 5 yo, give 5 mg PO daily for age 6 to 14 yo. Asthma: Age 12 to 23 mo: 4 mg (oral granules) PO daily. Allergic rhinitis: Age 6 to 23 mo: 4 mg (oral granules) PO daily. Prevention of exercise-induced bronchoconstriction: 10 mg PO 2 h before exercise. [Generic/Trade only: Tabs 10 mg. Oral granules 4 mg packet, 30/box. Chewable tabs (cherry flavored) 4, 5 mg.] ▶L ♀B ▶? $$$$

ZAFIRLUKAST (*Accolate, ✦Accolate*) 20 mg PO two times per day. Peds age 5 to 11 yo, 10 mg PO two times per day. Take at least 1 h before or 2 h after meals. Potentiates warfarin and theophylline. [Trade only: Tabs 10, 20 mg.] ▶L ♀B ▶— $$$$

ZILEUTON (*Zyflo, Zyflo CR*) 1200 mg PO two times per day. Take within 1 h after morning and evening meals. Hepatotoxicity, potentiates warfarin, theophylline, and propranolol. [Trade only: Tabs, extended-release 600 mg.] ▶L ♀C ▶? $$$$$

Other Pulmonary Medications

ACETYLCYSTEINE—INHALED (*Mucomyst*) Mucolytic: 3 to 5 mL of 20% or 6 to 10 mL of 10% soln nebulized three to four times per day. [Generic/Trade: Soln for inhalation 10, 20% in 4, 10, 30 mL vials.] ▶L ♀B ▶? $

PULMONARY

ACLIDINIUM (*Tudorza Pressair*, ♦*Tudorza Genuair*) COPD: Pressair: 400 mcg two times per day. [Trade only: Sealed aluminum pouches 400 mcg per actuation. To be used with Pressair device only. Packages of 60 with Pressair device.] ▶L – ♀C ▶? $$$$$

CROMOLYN—INHALED (♦*Nu-Cromolyn*, *PMS-Sodium Cromoglycate*) Asthma: 2 to 4 puffs four times per day or 20 mg nebs four times per day. Prevention of exercise-induced bronchospasm: 2 puffs 10 to 15 min prior to exercise. Mastocytosis: Oral concentrate 100 mg four times per day in children 2 to 12 yo, 200 mg PO four times per day for adults. [Generic only: Soln for nebs: 20 mg/2 mL. Generic/Trade: Oral concentrate 100 mg/5 mL in individual amps.] ▶LK ♀B ▶? $

DORNASE ALFA (*Pulmozyme*, ♦*Pulmozyme*) Cystic fibrosis: 2.5 mg nebulized one to two times per day. [Trade only: Soln for inhalation: 1 mg/mL in 2.5 mL vials.] ▶L ♀B ▶? $$$$$

EPINEPHRINE RACEMIC (*S-2*, ♦*Vaponefrin*) Severe croup: 0.05 mL/kg/dose diluted to 3 mL w/NS. Max dose 0.5 mL. [Trade only: Soln for inhalation: 2.25% epinephrine in 15, 30 mL.] ▶Plasma ♀C ▶– $

GLYCOPYRROLATE—INHALED (*Seebri Neohaler*) COPD: Inhale powder contents of one cap twice daily using Neohaler device. [Trade only: caps: 15.6 mcg glycopyrrolate in blister packs in boxes of 60 caps for use with Neohaler device.] ▶KL ♀C ▶?

IPRATROPIUM—INHALED (*Atrovent HFA*, ♦*Atrovent HFA*, *Gen-Ipratropium*) 2 puffs four times per day, or one 500 mcg vial neb three to four times per day. Contraindicated with soy or peanut allergy (Atrovent MDI only). [Trade only: Atrovent HFA MDI: 17 mcg/actuation, 200/canister. Generic/Trade: Soln for nebulization: 0.02% (500 mcg/vial) in unit dose vials.] ▶Lung ♀B ▶? $$$$

KETOTIFEN (♦*Zaditen*) Canada only. For age 6 mo to 3 yo: Give 0.05 mg/kg PO two times per day. Age older than 3 yo: Give 1 mg PO two times per day. [Generic/Trade: Tabs 1 mg. Syrup 1 mg/5 mL.] ▶L ♀C ▶– $$

NINTEDANIB (*Ofev, ✦Ofev*) Idiopathic pulmonary fibrosis: 150 mg twice daily 12 h apart with food. [Trade only: Caps: 100, 150 mg.] ▶L ♀D ▶?

PIRFENIDONE (*Esbriet, ✦Esbriet*) Idiopathic pulmonary fibrosis: 267 mg three times a day for 7 days, then 534 mg three times a day for 7 days, then 801 mg three times a day thereafter. Should be taken with meals. [Trade only: Caps 267 mg.] ▶LK ♀C ▶?

ROFLUMILAST (*Daliresp, ✦Daxas*) Severe COPD due to chronic bronchitis: 500 mcg PO daily with or without food. [Trade only: Tabs 500 mcg.] ▶L – ♀C ▶– $$$$$

THEOPHYLLINE (*Elixophyllin, Uniphyl, Theo-24, T-Phyl, ✦Theo-Dur, Theolair*) 5 to 13 mg/kg/day PO in divided doses. Max dose 900 mg/day. Peds dosing variable. [Generic/Trade: Elixir 80 mg/15 mL. Trade only: Caps Theo-24: 100, 200, 300, 400 mg. T-Phyl: 12 h SR tabs 200 mg. Theolair: Tabs 125, 250 mg. Generic only: 12 h tabs 100, 200, 300, 450 mg, 12 h caps 125, 200, 300 mg.] ▶L ♀C ▶+ $

TIOTROPIUM (*Spiriva HandiHaler, Spiriva Respimat, ✦Spiriva, Spiriva Respimat*) COPD: HandiHaler: 18 mcg inhaled daily. Respimat: 2 inhalations of 2.5 mcg or 5 mcg/inhalation once daily. Asthma: Respimat: age 12 yo old or older: 2 inhalations of 2.5 mcg or 5 mcg/inhalation once daily. [Trade only: HandiHaler: caps for oral inhalation 18 mcg to be used with HandiHaler device only. Packages of 5, 30, 90 caps with HandiHaler device. Respimat: canister containing 1.25 or 2.5 mcg tiotropium/inhalation to be used with Respimat device only, 60 actuations/canister.] ▶K ♀C ▶– $$$$

UMECLIDINIUM (*Incruse Ellipta, ✦Incruse Ellipta*) COPD: 1 inhalation once daily. [Trade only: Foil blister strip with 30 blisters each containing 62.5 mcg for use with Ellipta device.] ▶L ♀C ▶?

RHEUMATOLOGY

INITIAL TREATMENT OF RHEUMATOID ARTHRITIS (RA): AMERICAN COLLEGE OF RHEUMATOLOGY RECOMMENDATIONS

Disease Activity Treatment-experience	Treatment Options
Early disease (duration <6 months)	
Low and DMARD-naive	Single DMARD (MTX 1st-line)[1]
Moderate or high and DMARD-naive	Consider single DMARD[1,4]
Moderate or high on single DMARD	Combination DMARD[2,4] *or* TNF-blocker ± MTX[4] *or* Non-TNF biologic[3] ± MTX[4]
Established disease (duration ≥6 months)	
Low and DMARD-naive	Single DMARD (MTX 1st-line) preferred over TNF-blocker
Moderate to high and DMARD-naive	Consider single DMARD (MTX 1st-line); see guideline for more options[4]
Moderate or high on single DMARD	Combination DMARD[4] *or* Add TNF-blocker ± MTX[4] *or* Non-TNF biologic[3] ± MTX[4] *or* Tofacinitib ± MTX[4]

RHEUMATOLOGY

(cont.)

INITIAL TREATMENT OF RHEUMATOID ARTHRITIS (RA): AMERICAN COLLEGE OF RHEUMATOLOGY RECOMMENDATIONS (*continued*)

Disease Activity Treatment-experience	Treatment Options
Established disease (duration ≥6 months)	
Moderate or high on TNF-blocker without DMARD	Add one or two DMARDs[4] see guideline for more options
Moderate or high on DMARD, TNF-blocker, or non-TNF biologic[3]	Consider ≤10 mg/day prednisone equivalent for <3 months; see guideline for more options

Adapted from: *Arthritis Rheumatol.* 2016 Jan;68(1): 1–26. Available online at: http://www.rheumatology.org.

DMARD = disease-modifying anti-rheumatic drug;

HCQ = hydroxychloroquine; LEF = leflunomide; MTX = methotrexate; SSZ = sulfasalazine; TNF = tumor necrosis factor.

Treatment target is low disease activity or remission, giving each regimen for at least 3 months before therapy escalation.

[1]Single DMARD: HCQ, LEF, MTX, or SSZ.

[2]DMARD combination: MTX + SSZ; MTX + HCQ; SSZ+ HCQ; MTX + SSZ + HCQ; combinations + LEF.

[3]Non-TNF biologics: abatacept, rituximab, tocilizumab.

[4]Consider adding ≤10 mg/day prednisone for patients with moderate or high disease activity when starting a DMARD or in patients with DMARD or biologic failure. Also consider corticosteroid to manage disease flares, using the lowest possible dose for the shortest possible duration (<3 months).

Biologic Response Modifiers—TNF-Blockers

NOTE: *TNF-blockers increase the risk of serious infections (e.g., TB, sepsis, invasive fungal and opportunistic infections); discontinue if serious infection. Screen for HBV and latent TB (treat if present) before using a TNF-blocker; monitor for active TB during treatment. Hold TNF-blockers for at least 1 week before and after surgery. Other adverse events include lymphoma and other malignancies in children and adolescents; new onset/exacerbation of demyelinating disorders and heart failure (avoid if NYHA Class III/IV heart failure), a lupus-like syndrome, and serious hypersensitivity reactions including anaphylaxis. Increased risk of HBV reactivation; refer to AGA guideline (www.gastro.org) for prevention and treatment. Avoid live vaccines. Do not coadminister other biologic response modifiers (e.g., abatacept, anakinra, tofacitinib). Refer to ACR RA guidelines (www.rheumatology.org) for advice on TB screening, vaccines, and other safety issues.*

ADALIMUMAB (*Humira*) RA, psoriatic arthritis, ankylosing spondylitis: 40 mg SC q 2 weeks, alone or in combination with methotrexate or other non-biologic DMARD. May increase frequency to q week if not on methotrexate. Plaque psoriasis, non-infectious uveitis: 80 mg SC on day 1, 40 mg SC on day 8, then 40 mg SC q 2 weeks. Crohn's disease, ulcerative colitis: 160 mg SC on day 1, 80 mg on day 15, then 40 mg q 2 weeks starting on day 29. Hidradenitis suppurativa: 160 mg SC on day 1, 80 mg on day 15, then 40 mg q week starting on day 29. Peds. Polyarticular JIA, age 2 yo or older: Give SC q 2 weeks at a dose of 10 mg for wt 10 to less than 15 kg; 20 mg for wt 15 to less than 30 kg; 40 mg for wt 30 kg or greater. Crohn's disease, age 6 yo or older. For wt 17 kg to less than 40 kg: 80 mg SC (two 40 mg injections) on day 1, then 40 mg SC 2 weeks later. Maintain with 20 mg SC q 2 weeks. For wt 40 kg and greater: 160 mg

(cont.)

RHEUMATOLOGY

SC on day 1, then 80 mg SC (two 40 mg injections) 2 weeks later. Maintain with 40 mg SC q 2 weeks. Can give initial 160 mg dose as four 40 mg injections on day 1 or two 40 mg injections per day for 2 days. Inject SC into thigh or abdomen, rotating injection sites. [Trade only: Single-use injection pen or syringe (2 per pack): 40 mg/0.8 mL. Crohn's disease/ulcerative colitis/hidradenitis suppurativa starter pack: Six 40 mg pens. Psoriasis/uveitis starter pack: Four 40 mg pens. Pediatric single-use syringe (2 per pack): 10 mg/0.2 mL, 20 mg/0.4 mL. Pediatric Crohn's disease starter pack: Three or six 40 mg/0.8 mL syringes.] ▶proteolysis ♀O/?/?/R Increased fetal exposure after 20th week. ▶? Caution advised, but no known risks. $$$$$ ■

CERTOLIZUMAB (*Cimzia*) Crohn's disease: 400 mg SC at 0, 2, and 4 weeks. If response occurs, then 400 mg SC q 4 weeks. RA, psoriatic arthritis: 400 mg SC at 0, 2, and 4 weeks. Then maintain with 200 mg SC q 2 weeks; can consider 400 mg SC q 4 weeks. Ankylosing spondylitis: 400 mg at 0, 2, and 4 weeks, then 200 mg q 2 weeks or 400 mg q 4 weeks. Give 400 mg dose as 2 separate 200 mg injections at different sites on thigh or abdomen. Rotate injection sites. Not indicated in children. [Trade only: Packs of 2 vials for reconstitution or 2 prefilled syringes, 200 mg/1 mL each. Starter pack of 6 syringes.] ▶K proteolysis ♀B Increased fetal exposure after 20th week. R ▶? $$$$$ ■

ETANERCEPT, ETANERCEPT-SZZS (*Enbrel, Erelzi*) RA, psoriatic arthritis, ankylosing spondylitis: 50 mg SC q week. Plaque psoriasis: 50 mg SC 2 times per week for 3 months, then 50 mg SC q week. JIA, age 2 yo or older: 0.8 mg/kg SC q week for wt less than 63 kg; 50 mg SC for wt of 63 kg or greater. Inject into thigh, abdomen, or outer upper arm. Rotate injection sites. [Trade only (Enbrel): Single-use prefilled syringe or autoinjector 50 mg/1 mL. Single-use prefilled syringe 25 mg/0.5 mL. Multidose vial 25 mg. Etanercept-szzs (Erelzi) is not available yet.] ▶proteolysis ♀B Increased fetal exposure after 20th week. R ▶? $$$$$ ■

GOLIMUMAB (*Simponi, Simponi Aria*) RA, psoriatic arthritis, ankylosing spondylitis: 50 mg SC q month. IV regimen (Simponi Aria) for RA: 2 mg/kg IV infused over 30 min at weeks 0 and 4, then q 8 weeks. Use IV/SC golimumab with methotrexate to treat RA. Ulcerative colitis: 200 mg SC at week 0, 100 mg SC at week 2, then 100 mg SC q 4 weeks. Give SC injection in thigh, abdomen, or upper outer arm. Rotate injection sites. Give at separate sites if a dose requires more than 1 injection. Not indicated in children. [Trade only: Single-dose autoinjector or prefilled syringe: 50 mg/0.5 mL, 100 mg/1 mL.] ▶? ♀B Increased fetal exposure after 20th week. ▶ $$$$$ ■

INFLIXIMAB, INFLIXIMAB-DYYB (*Remicade, Inflectra*) RA, with methotrexate: 3 mg/kg IV at weeks 0, 2, and 6, then q 8 weeks. Ankylosing spondylitis: 5 mg/kg IV at weeks 0, 2, and 6, then q 6 weeks. Plaque psoriasis, psoriatic arthritis, Crohn's disease, ulcerative colitis: 5 mg/kg IV at weeks 0, 2, and 6, then q 8 weeks. Peds, ulcerative colitis, Crohn's disease, age 6 yo or older: 5 mg/kg IV at weeks 0, 2, and 6, then q 8 weeks. Infuse over 2 h or more. [Infliximab-dyyb (Inflectra) is not available yet.] ▶proteolysis ♀B Increased fetal exposure after 20th week. ▶? $$$$$ ■

Biologic Response Modifiers—Other

ABATACEPT (*Orencia, ✽Orencia*) RA: IV regimen: Infuse IV over 30 minutes at wt-based dose of 500 mg for wt less than 60 kg, 750 mg for 60 to 100 kg, 1000 mg for greater than 100 kg. Give additional IV doses at weeks 2 and 4, then q 4 weeks. SC regimen: 125 mg SC q week after optional initial IV dose. Give 1st SC dose within 1 day of IV dose. Give SC in thigh, abdomen, or upper outer arm. Rotate injection sites. Peds, JIA, age 6 yo or older: 10 mg/kg IV infused over 30 min. Give additional IV doses at weeks 2 and 4, then q 4 weeks. Use adult dose if weight 75 kg or greater (max 1000 mg per IV dose). [Trade only: Prefilled single-dose syringe or autoinjector 125 mg/1 mL.] ▶serum ♀?/?/? R▶ $$$$$

ANAKINRA (_Kineret_) RA: 100 mg SC daily, alone or with non-biologic DMARDs. JIA: Initial dose of 1 to 2 mg/kg (max 100 mg) SC once daily. Inject SC into thigh, abdomen, outer area of upper arm, or upper outer area of buttocks. Rotate injection sites. [Trade only: Prefilled graduated syringe 100 mg/0.67 mL.] ▸K ♀B ▸? $$$$$

CANAKINUMAB (_Ilaris_) Systemic JIA, age 2 yo or older and wt 7.5 kg or greater: 4 mg/kg (max dose of 300 mg) SC q 4 weeks. Cryopyrin-associated periodic syndromes. Adults and children with wt greater than 40 kg: 150 mg SC q 8 weeks. Children age 4 yo or older and wt 15 to 40 kg: 2 mg/kg SC q 8 weeks, increasing to 3 mg/kg q 8 weeks if inadequate response. ▸? ♀?/?/? Increased fetal exposure expected after 20th week. ▸? $$$$$

RITUXIMAB (_Rituxan_) RA, with methotrexate: 1000 mg IV infusion weekly for 2 doses q 24 weeks. Give methylprednisolone 100 mg IV 30 min before infusion. Granulomatosis with polyangiitis (Wegener's), microscopic polyangiitis, with corticosteroids: 375 mg/m^2 q week for 4 weeks. Non-Hodgkin's lymphoma, chronic lymphocytic leukemia: Doses vary by indication. Can cause life-threatening infusion reactions. Premedicate with acetaminophen and antihistamine. ▸? ♀C ▸– $$$$$ ■

SECUKINUMAB (_Cosentyx_) Plaque psoriasis: 300 mg SC weekly for 5 weeks, then 300 mg SC q 4 weeks. Each 300 mg dose is two SC 150 mg injections at different sites. A dose of 150 mg may be adequate for some patients. Psoriatic arthritis (± methotrexate), ankylosing spondylitis: 150 mg SC weekly for 5 weeks, then 150 mg q 4 weeks; can also give 150 mg SC q 4 weeks with no loading regimen. Consider 300 mg dose for continued active psoriatic arthritis. [Trade only: 150 mg/mL prefilled syringe or pen. 150 mg vial for reconstitution by healthcare provider.] ▸proteolysis ♀B ▸? $$$$$

TOCILIZUMAB (_Actemra_) RA, moderate to severe: 162 mg SC q 2 weeks titrated to q week based on clinical response for wt less than 100 kg; 162 mg SC q week for wt 100 kg or

(cont.)

greater. RA, IV regimen: 4 mg/kg IV q 4 weeks, increasing to 8 mg/kg (max 800 mg) IV q 4 weeks based on clinical response. Polyarticular JIA, age 2 yo or older: 10 mg/kg IV q 4 weeks for wt less than 30 kg; 8 mg/kg q 4 weeks for wt 30 kg or greater. Systemic JIA, age 2 yo or older: 12 mg/kg q 2 weeks for wt less than 30 kg; 8 mg/kg q 2 weeks for 30 kg or greater. IV infused over 1 h. [Trade only: 162 mg/0.9 mL prefilled single-use syringe.] ▶? ♀C ▶– $$$$$ ■

TOFACITINIB (*Xeljanz, Xeljanz XR*) RA: 5 mg PO two times per day or Xeljanz XR 11 mg PO once daily. Reduce to 5 mg PO once daily if given with fluconazole, strong CYP3A4 inhibitor, or combination of moderate CYP3A4 inhibitor and strong CYP2C19 inhibitor (see P450 isozyme table). Do not crush, split, or chew Xeljanz XR. Dosage adjustments for lymphopenia, neutropenia, and anemia in product labeling. Indicated for moderate to severe RA with inadequate response or intolerance to methotrexate. For use as monotherapy or in combination with methotrexate or another nonbiologic DMARD. [Trade only: Tabs 5 mg. Extended-release tabs 11 mg.] ▶LK ♀C ▶– $$$$$ ■

Disease-Modifying Antirheumatic Drugs (DMARDs)

AZATHIOPRINE (*Azasan, Imuran, AZA*) RA: Initial dose 1 mg/kg (50 to 100 mg) PO daily or divided two times per day. Increase after 6 to 8 weeks. Prevention of rejection after renal transplant: Individualized dosing. Reduce azathioprine dose by 66% to 75% if allopurinol coadministered. Monitor CBC for myelosuppression. [Generic/Trade (Imuran-$$$$$): Tabs 50 mg, scored. Trade only (Azasan-$$$$$): 75, 100 mg, scored.] ▶LK ♀D ▶– $$$ ■

HYDROXYCHLOROQUINE (*Plaquenil, HCQ*) RA: Start 400 to 600 mg PO daily, then taper to 200 to 400 mg daily. SLE: 400 PO one to two times per day to start, then taper to 200 to 400 mg daily. Take with food or milk to improve GI

(cont.)

RHEUMATOLOGY

tolerability. Per American Academy of Opthalmology, avoid doses greater than 5 mg/kg/day (real weight) to reduce risk of irreversible retinopathy. See www.aao.org for retinopathy screening recommendations. [Generic/Trade: Tabs 200 mg hydroxychloroquine sulfate (200 mg sulfate equivalent to 155 mg base), scored.] ▶K ♀C ▶+ $ ■

LEFLUNOMIDE (*Arava, LEF*) RA: Optional loading dose for patients not receiving methotrexate or immunosuppressant: 100 mg PO daily for 3 days. Not for patients at risk of hepatotoxicity (eg, taking methotrexate) or myelosuppression (eg, taking an immunosuppressant). Maintenance dose: 10 to 20 mg PO daily. [Generic/Trade: Tabs 10, 20 mg. Trade only: Tabs 100 mg.] ▶LK ♀X/X/X. R ▶– $$$$$ ■

METHOTREXATE—RHEUMATOLOGY (*Otrexup, Rasuvo, Rheu-matrex, Trexall, MTX*) Severe RA: Initial dose of 7.5 mg PO/SC once weekly. Alternative regimen: 2.5 mg PO q 12 h for 3 doses given as a course once weekly. May increase dose gradually to max of 20 mg/week. After clinical response, reduce to lowest effective dose. Severe psoriasis: 10 to 25 mg PO/SC/IV/IM once weekly until response, then decrease to lowest effective dose. Max usual dose is 30 mg/week. Supplement with 1 mg/day of folic acid. Severe JIA: 10 mg/m² PO/SC q week. When converting between PO and SC administration, consider that SC administration has higher bioavailability. Give SC injection in abdomen or thigh. [Trade only (Trexall): Tabs 5, 7.5, 10, 15 mg. Dose Pak (Rheumatrex) 2.5 mg (# 8, 12, 16, 20, 24). Generic/Trade: Tabs 2.5 mg, scored. Trade only: Single-dose SC auto-injectors. Otrexup: 7.5, 10, 12.5, 15, 17.5, 20, 22.5, 25 mg/0.4 mL. Rasuvo: 7.5, 10, 12.5, 15, 17.5, 20, 22.5, 25, 27.5, 30 mg (volume ranges from 0.15 to 0.6 mL).] ▶LK ♀X ▶– $$ ■

SULFASALAZINE—RHEUMATOLOGY (*Azulfidine, Azulfidine EN-tabs, ✦Salazopyrin EN-tabs*) RA: 500 mg PO two times per day after meals up to 1 g PO two times per day. May turn body fluids, contact lenses, or skin orange-yellow. [Generic/Trade: Tabs 500 mg, scored. Enteric-coated, delayed-release (EN-tabs) 500 mg.] ▶L ♀B ▶? $$

Gout-Related—Xanthine Oxidase Inhibitors

ALLOPURINOL (*Aloprim, Zyloprim*) Prevention of recurrent gout: 100 mg PO daily initially, titrating upward q 1 to 5 weeks to achieve target serum urate level (usually less than 6 mg/dL, but may be less than 5 mg/dL). Maximum dose is 800 mg/day. Initial dose is 50 mg/day for CrCl less than 30 mL/min. Divide doses greater than 300 mg/day. To improve tolerability, take PO allopurinol after meals. Reduce azathioprine or mercaptopurine dose by 66% to 75% and monitor CBC. [Generic/Trade (Zyloprim-$$$$): Tabs 100, 300 mg.] ▶K ♀C ▶+ $

FEBUXOSTAT (*Uloric*) Hyperuricemia with gout: Start 40 mg PO daily, max 80 mg daily. [Trade only: Tabs 40, 80 mg.] ▶LK ♀C ▶? $$$$$

Gout-Related—Other

COLCHICINE (*Colcrys, Mitigare*) Treatment of gout flares: 1.2 mg PO at signs of attack then 0.6 mg 1 h later. Do not repeat this regimen for 3 days. Prevention of gout flares: 0.6 mg PO one or two times per day. Max dose of 1.2 mg/day. Familial Mediterranean fever: 1.2 to 2.4 mg PO daily or divided two times per day. See table for dosage reductions when given with strong/moderate CYP3A4 inhibitors or P-glycoprotein inhibitors. [Generic/Trade: Tabs 0.6 mg (Colcrys). Caps 0.6 mg (Mitigare).] ▶L ♀C ▶? $$$$$

COLCHICINE + PROBENECID Gout: 1 tab PO daily for 1 week, then 1 tab two times per day. [Generic only: Tabs 0.5 mg colchicine + 500 mg probenecid.] ▶KL ♀C ▶? $

LESINURAD (*Zurampic*) Gout, added to allopurinol or febuxostat: 200 mg PO each morning with food and water, at the same time as xanthine oxidase inhibitor. Tell patients to drink at least 2 L of fluid daily. Not for monotherapy due to increased risk of acute renal failure. Not for use with allopurinol doses <300 mg/day (<200 mg/day if CrCl <60 mL/min). Provide gout flare prophylaxis when starting lesinurad. [Trade only: Tab 200 mg.] ▶L ♀?/?/? ▶? $$$$$ ■

RHEUMATOLOGY

COLCHICINE: DOSAGE REDUCTIONS FOR COADMINISTRATION WITH INHIBITORS OF COLCHICINE METABOLISM

Usual colchicine dose	Colchicine dosage reduction for...		
	Strong CYP3A4 inhibitors[a]	Moderate CYP3A4 inhibitors[b]	P-glycoprotein inhibitors[c]
Prevention of gout flares: 0.6 mg PO two times per day	0.3 mg PO once daily	0.3 mg PO two times per day or 0.6 mg PO once daily	0.3 mg PO once daily
Prevention of gout flares: 0.6 mg PO once daily	0.3 mg PO once every other day	0.3 mg PO once daily	0.3 mg PO once every other day

(cont.)

Treatment of gout flares: 1.2 mg PO followed by 0.6 mg 1 hour later^d	0.6 mg PO followed by 0.3 mg 1 hour later^d	1.2 mg PO in a single dose^d	0.6 mg PO in a single dose^d
Familial Mediterranean Fever: Up to 1.2 to 2.4 mg/day PO	Up to 0.6 mg/day PO (can give as 0.3 mg two times per day)	Up to 1.2 mg/day PO (can give as 0.6 mg two times per day)	Up to 0.6 mg/day PO (can give as 0.3 mg two times per day)

Notes: Do not give colchicine to patients with renal or hepatic impairment who are taking a strong CYP3A4 or P-glycoprotein inhibitor. Do not treat gout flares with colchicine in patients already receiving it for prevention of gout flares and also receiving a CYP3A4 inhibitor. Dosage reductions of colchicine are recommended for patients who are currently taking or discontinued a CYP3A4 or P-glycoprotein inhibitor within the past 14 days. This table may not list all possible CYP3A4 and P-glycoprotein inhibitors that increase the risk of colchicine toxicity.

(cont.)

RHEUMATOLOGY

COLCHICINE: DOSAGE REDUCTIONS FOR COADMINISTRATION WITH INHIBITORS OF COLCHICINE METABOLISM (*continued*)

[a]**Strong CYP3A4 inhibitors:** atazanavir, clarithromycin, cobicistat (alone or in combination products), conivaptan, darunavir-ritonavir, fosamprenavir-ritonavir, indinavir, itraconazole, ketoconazole, lopinavir-ritonavir, nefazodone, nelfinavir, posaconazole, ritonavir, saquinavir-ritonavir, telithromycin, tipranavir-ritonavir, voriconazole.

[b]**Moderate CYP3A4 inhibitors:** aprepitant, ciprofloxacin, crizotinib, diltiazem, dronedarone, erythromycin, fluconazole, fosamprenavir (unboosted), grapefruit juice, imatinib, isavuconazole, netupitant (in Akynzeo) verapamil.

[c]**P-glycoprotein inhibitors:** cyclosporine, ranolazine.

[d]For colchicine treatment of gout flares, do not repeat earlier than 3 days.

PEGLOTICASE (*Krystexxa*) Chronic gout (refractory): 8 mg IV infusion q 2 weeks. ▶? ♀C ▶? $$$$$ ■

PROBENECID Gout: 250 mg PO two times per day for 7 days, then 500 mg PO two times per day. Adjunct to penicillin/cephalosporin: 1 g PO single dose to 500 mg PO four times per day. [Generic only: Tabs 500 mg.] ▶KL ♀B ▶? $

Other

APREMILAST (*Otezla*) Psoriatic arthritis, moderate to severe plaque psoriasis: Give PO 10 mg in am on day 1, 10 mg two times per day on day 2, 10 mg in am and 20 mg in pm on day 3, 20 mg two times per day on day 4, 20 mg in am and 30 mg in pm on day 5, 30 mg two times per day on day 6 and thereafter. Do not crush, split, or chew tabs. [Trade only: Tabs 30 mg. Two-week starter pack of 10, 20, and 30 mg tabs.] ▶L ♀C ▶? $$$$$

TOXICOLOGY

ANTIDOTES

Toxin	Antidote/Treatment
acetaminophen	N-acetylcysteine
TCAs	sodium bicarbonate
arsenic, mercury	dimercaprol (BAL)
benzodiazepine	flumazenil
beta-blockers	glucagon
calcium channel blockers	calcium chloride, glucagon
cyanide	Cyanokit (hydroxocobalamin)
dabigatran	idarucizumab
digoxin	dig immune Fab
ethylene glycol	fomepizole
heparin	protamine
iron	deferoxamine
lead	BAL, EDTA, succimer
local anesthetics	intralipid
methanol	fomepizole
methemoglobin	methylene blue
opioids/opiates	naloxone
organophosphates	atropine + pralidoxime
warfarin	vitamin K, FFP

ACETYLCYSTEINE (*N-acetylcysteine, Mucomyst, Acetadote, ✦Parvolex*) Acetaminophen toxicity: Mucomyst (Oral): Loading dose 140 mg/kg PO or NG, then 70 mg/kg q 4 h for 17 doses. May be mixed in water or soft drink diluted to a 5% soln. Acetadote (IV): Loading dose 150 mg/kg in 200 mL of D5W infused over 60 min; maintenance dose 50 mg/kg in 500 mL of D5W infused over 4 h followed by 100 mg/kg in 1000 mL of D5W infused over 16 h. Contrast nephropathy prophylaxis: 600 mg PO two times per day on the day before and on the day of contrast. [Generic/Trade: Soln 10, 20%. IV (Acetadote).] ▶L ♀B ▶? $$$$

CHARCOAL (*activated charcoal, Actidose-Aqua, CharcoAid, EZ-Char, ✦Charcodate*) 25 to 100 g (1 to 2 g/kg) PO or NG as soon as possible. May repeat q 1 to 4 h prn at doses equivalent to 12.5 g/h. When sorbitol is coadministered, use only with the 1st dose if repeated doses are to be given. [OTC/Generic/Trade: Powder 15, 30, 40, 120, 240 g. Soln 12.5 g/60 mL, 15 g/75 mL, 15 g/120 mL, 25 g/120 mL, 30 g/120 mL, 50 g/240 mL. Susp 15 g/120 mL, 25 g/120 mL, 30 g/150 mL, 50 g/240 mL. Granules 15 g/120 mL.] ▶Not absorbed ♀+ ▶+ $

DEFEROXAMINE (*Desferal*) Chronic iron overload: 500 to 1000 mg IM daily and 2 g IV infusion (no faster than 15 mg/kg/h) with each unit of blood or 1 to 2 g SC daily (20 to 40 mg/kg/day) over 8 to 24 h via continuous infusion pump. Acute iron toxicity: IV infusion up to 15 mg/kg/h. ▶K ♀C ▶? $$$$$

FAT EMULSION (*Intralipid, Nutrilipid*) Local anesthetic toxicity: Bolus of 1.5 mL/kg of 20% intralipid over 1 minute, may repeat once in 5 min PRN, followed by infusion at a rate of 0.25 mL/kg/min for 20 to 60 min until hemodynamics improve. Max of 10 mL/kg over first 30 min. ▶L ♀C ▶? $$$$$

FLUMAZENIL Benzodiazepine sedation reversal: 0.2 mg IV over 15 sec, then 0.2 mg q 1 min prn up to 1 mg total dose. Overdose reversal: 0.2 mg IV over 30 sec, then 0.3 to 0.5 mg q 30 sec prn up to 3 mg total dose. Contraindicated in mixed drug overdose or chronic benzodiazepine use due to seizure risk. ▶LK ♀C ▶? $$$$ ■

FOMEPIZOLE (*Antizol*) Ethylene glycol or methanol toxicity: 15 mg/kg IV (load), then 10 mg/kg IV q 12 h for 4 doses, then 15 mg/kg IV q 12 h until ethylene glycol or methanol level is below 20 mg/dL. Administer doses as slow IV infusions over 30 min. Increase frequency to q 4 h during hemodialysis. ▶L ♀C ▶? $$$$$

HYDROXOCOBALAMIN (*Cyanokit*) Cyanide poisoning: 5 g IV over 15 min; may repeat prn. ▶K ♀C ▶? $$$$$

METHYLENE BLUE (*Urolene blue*) Methemoglobinemia: 1 to 2 mg/kg IV over 5 min. Dysuria: 65 to 130 mg PO three times per day after meals with liberal water. May turn urine/contact lenses blue. [Trade only: Tabs 65 mg.] ▶K ♀C ▶? $

PHYSOSTIGMINE (*Antilirium*) Life-threatening anticholinergic toxicity: 2 mg IV/IM, administer IV no faster than 1 mg/min. May repeat q 10 to 30 min for severe toxicity. Peds: 0.02 mg/kg IM/IV injection, administer IV no faster than 0.5 mg/min. [Generic/Trade: 1 mg/mL in 2 mL ampules.] ▶LK ♀D ▶? $

PRALIDOXIME (*Protopam, 2-PAM*) Organophosphate poisoning: 1 to 2 g IV infusion over 15 to 30 min or slow IV injection over 5 min or longer (max rate 200 mg/min). May repeat dose after 1 h if muscle weakness persists. High-dose regimen (unapproved): 2 g over 30 min, followed by 1 g/h for 48 h, then 1 g/h q 4 h until improved. Peds: 20 to 50 mg/kg/dose IV over 15 to 30 min. ▶K ♀C ▶? $$$$

SUCCIMER (*Chemet*) Lead toxicity in children 1 yo or older: Start 10 mg/kg PO or 350 mg/m2 q 8 h for 5 days, then reduce the frequency to q 12 h for 2 weeks. [Trade only: Caps 100 mg.] ▶K ♀C ▶? $$$$$

UROLOGY

Benign Prostatic Hyperplasia

ALFUZOSIN (*UroXatral*, ✦*Xatral*) 10 mg PO daily after the same meal each day. [Generic/Trade: Tabs, extended-release 10 mg.] ▶KL ♀B ▶– $

COMBODART (dutasteride + tamsulosin, *Duodart*, *Jalyn*) 0.5 mg dutasteride + 0.4 mg tamsulosin daily 30 minutes after the same meal each day. [Trade only: Caps 0.5 mg dutasteride + 0.4 mg tamsulosin.] ▶LK - ♀X ▶– $$$$

DUTASTERIDE (*Avodart*) BPH: 0.5 mg PO daily. [Generic/Trade: Caps 0.5 mg.] ▶L ♀X Capsules should not be touched by a woman who is pregnant or may become pregnant due to transdermal absorption resulting in fetal exposure. ▶– $$

FINASTERIDE (*Proscar*, *Propecia*) To reduce the risk of symptomatic progression of BPH: Proscar: 5 mg PO daily alone or in combination with doxazosin. Androgenetic alopecia in men: Propecia: 1 mg PO daily. [Generic/Trade: Tabs 1 mg (Propecia), 5 mg (Proscar).] ▶L ♀X ▶– $

SILODOSIN (*RAPAFLO*) 8 mg PO daily with a meal. [Trade: Caps 8 mg.] ▶LK ♀–B ▶– $$$$$

TAMSULOSIN (*Flomax*) 0.4 mg PO daily, 30 min after a meal. Max 0.8 mg/day. [Generic/Trade: Caps 0.4 mg.] ▶LK ♀B ▶– $$$$

Bladder Agents—Anticholinergics and Combinations

DARIFENACIN (*Enablex*) Overactive bladder with symptoms of urinary urgency, frequency, and urge incontinence: 7.5 mg PO daily. May increase to max dose 15 mg PO daily in 2 weeks. Max dose 7.5 mg PO daily with moderate liver impairment or when coadministered with potent CYP3A4 inhibitors (ketoconazole, itraconazole, ritonavir, nelfinavir, clarithromycin, and nefazodone). [Trade only: Tabs, extended-release 7.5, 15 mg.] ▶LK ♀C ▶– $$$$

FESOTERODINE (*Toviaz*) Overactive bladder: 4 to 8 mg PO daily. [Trade only: Tabs, extended-release 4, 8 mg.] ▶Plasma ♀C ▶ – $$$$

OXYBUTYNIN (*Ditropan, Ditropan XL, Gelnique, Oxytrol, ★Oxybutyn, Uromax*) Bladder instability: 2.5 to 5 mg PO two to three times per day, max 5 mg PO four times per day. Extended-release tabs: 5 to 10 mg PO daily, increase 5 mg/day q week to 30 mg/day. Oxytrol: 1 patch twice a week on abdomen, hips, or buttocks. Gelnique: Apply gel once daily to abdomen, upper arms/shoulders, or thighs. [Generic/Trade: Tabs, 5 mg. Syrup 5 mg/5 mL. Tabs, extended-release 5, 10, 15 mg. Trade only: OTC Transdermal patch (Oxytrol) 3.9 mg/day. Gelnique 3, 10% gel, 1 g unit dose.] ▶LK ♀B ▶? $$

PROSED/DS **(methenamine + phenyl salicylate + methylene blue + benzoic acid + hyoscyamine)** Bladder spasm: 1 tab PO four times per day with liberal fluids. May turn urine/contact lenses blue. [Trade only: Tabs (methenamine 81.6 mg/phenyl salicylate 36.2 mg/methylene blue 10.8 mg/benzoic acid 9.0 mg/hyoscyamine sulfate 0.12 mg).] ▶KL ♀C ▶? $$

SOLIFENACIN (*VESIcare*) Overactive bladder with symptoms of urinary urgency, frequency, or urge incontinence: 5 mg PO daily. Max dose: 10 mg daily (5 mg daily if CrCl less than 30 mL/min, moderate hepatic impairment, or concurrent ketoconazole or other potent CYP3A4 inhibitors). [Trade only: Tabs 5, 10 mg.] ▶LK ♀C ▶ – $$$$

TOLTERODINE (*Detrol, Detrol LA*) Overactive bladder: 1 to 2 mg PO two times per day (Detrol) or 4 mg PO daily; may be reduced to 2 mg PO daily based on response and tolerability (Detrol LA). [Generic/Trade: Tabs 1, 2 mg. Caps, extended-release 2, 4 mg.] ▶L ♀C ▶ – $$$$$

TROSPIUM (*Sanctura, Sanctura XR, ★Trosec*) Overactive bladder with urge incontinence: 20 mg PO two times per day; give 20 mg at bedtime if CrCl less than 30 mL/min. If age 75 yo or older may taper down to 20 mg daily. Extended-release: 60 mg PO q am, 1 h before food. [Generic only: Tabs 20 mg. Caps, extended-release 60 mg.] ▶LK ♀C ▶? $$$$

URISED (*methenamine* + *phenyl salicylate* + *atropine* + *hyoscyamine* + *benzoic acid* + *methylene blue*) Dysuria: 2 tabs PO four times per day. May turn urine/contact lenses blue. Do not use with sulfa. [Trade only: Tabs (methenamine 40.8 mg/phenyl salicylate 18.1 mg/atropine 0.03 mg/hyoscyamine 0.03 mg/4.5 mg benzoic acid/5.4 mg methylene blue).] ▶K ♀C ▶? $

UTA (*methenamine* + *sodium phosphate* + *phenyl salicylate* + *methylene blue* + *hyoscyamine*) Bladder spasm: 1 cap PO four times per day with liberal fluids. [Trade only: Caps (methenamine 120 mg/sodium phosphate 40.8 mg/phenyl salicylate 36 mg/methylene blue 10 mg/hyoscyamine 0.12 mg).] ▶KL ♀C ▶? $

UTIRA-C (*methenamine* + *sodium phosphate* + *phenyl salicylate* + *methylene blue* + *hyoscyamine*) Bladder spasm: 1 cap PO four times per day with liberal fluids. [Trade only: Tabs (methenamine 81.6 mg/sodium phosphate 40.8 mg/phenyl salicylate 36.2 mg/methylene blue 10.8 mg/hyoscyamine 0.12 mg).] ▶KL ♀C ▶? $$

Bladder Agents—Other

BETHANECHOL (*Urecholine, Duvoid, ✦Myotonachol*) Urinary retention: 10 to 50 mg PO three to four times per day. [Generic/Trade: Tabs 5, 10, 25, 50 mg.] ▶L ♀C ▶? $$$$

MIRABEGRON (*Myrbetriq*) Overactive bladder with symptoms of urge urinary incontinence, urgency, and urinary frequency: 25 mg PO daily. May increase to 50 mg unless severe renal impairment or moderate hepatic impairment. [Trade only: Extended-release tabs 25, 50 mg.] ▶LK – ♀C ▶?

PHENAZOPYRIDINE (*Pyridium, Azo-Standard, Urogesic, Prodium, Pyridiate, Urodol, Baridium, UTI Relief, Azourinary Pain Relief, Uristat, Azo-Gesic, Azo-Septic, Phenazo, Re-Azo, Uricalm*) Dysuria: 200 mg PO three times per day for 2 days. May turn urine/contact lenses orange. [OTC Generic/Trade: Tabs 95, 97.2 mg. Rx Generic/Trade: Tabs 100, 200 mg.] ▶K ♀B ▶? $

Erectile Dysfunction

ALPROSTADIL (*Muse, Caverject, Caverject Impulse, Edex, Prostin VR Pediatric, prostaglandin E1, ✳Prostin VR*) 1 intraurethral pellet (Muse) or intracavernosal injection (Caverject, Edex) at lowest dose that will produce erection. Onset of effect is 5 to 20 min. [Trade only: Syringe system (Edex) 10, 20, 40 mcg; (Caverject) 5, 10, 20, 40 mcg; (Caverject Impulse) 10, 20 mcg. Pellet (Muse) 125, 250, 500, 1000 mcg. Intracorporeal injection of locally compounded combination agents (many variations): "Bi-mix" can be 30 mg/mL papaverine + 0.5 to 1 mg/mL phentolamine, or 30 mg/mL papaverine + 20 mcg/mL alprostadil in 10 mL vials. "Tri-mix" can be 30 mg/mL papaverine + 1 mg/mL phentolamine + 10 mcg/mL alprostadil in 5, 10, or 20 mL vials.] ▶L ♀— ▶— $$$$

AVANAFIL (*Stendra*) Start 100 mg PO as early as 15 min prior to sexual activity. Max 1 dose/day. May increase to 200 mg or decrease to 50 mg prn. Contraindicated with nitrates and strong CYP3A4 inhibitors. Start at 50 mg if concurrent alpha blocker or moderate CYP3A4 inhibitor. Contraindicated in severe renal or hepatic impairment. [Trade only (Stendra): Tabs 50, 100, 200 mg.] ▶L — ♀C ▶? $$$$

SILDENAFIL—UROLOGY (*Viagra*) Start 50 mg PO 0.5 to 4 h prior to intercourse. Max 1 dose/day. Usual effective range 25 to 100 mg. Start at 25 mg if for age 65 yo or older or liver/renal impairment. Contraindicated with nitrates. [Trade only (Viagra): Tabs 25, 50, 100 mg. Unscored tab but can be cut in half.] ▶LK ♀B ▶— $$$$

TADALAFIL (*Cialis*) ED: 2.5 to 5 mg PO daily without regard to timing of sexual activity. Daily dosing should not exceed 2.5 mg if on concomitant CYP3A4 inhibitor. As-needed dosing: Start 10 mg PO at least 30 to 45 min prn prior to sexual activity. May increase to 20 mg or decrease to 5 mg prn. Max 1 dose/day. Start 5 mg (max 1 dose/day) if CrCl is 31 to 50 mL/min. Max 5 mg/day if CrCl < 30 mL/min including patients on dialysis.

(cont.)

Max 10 mg/day if mild to moderate hepatic impairment; avoid in severe hepatic impairment. Max 10 mg once in 72 h if concurrent potent CYP3A4 inhibitors. BPH with or without erectile dysfunction: 5 mg PO daily. Contraindicated with nitrates and alpha-blockers (except tamsulosin 0.4 mg daily). Not FDA approved for women. [Trade only (Cialis): Tabs 2.5, 5, 10, 20 mg.] ▶L ♀B ▶– $$$$

VARDENAFIL (*Levitra, Staxyn*) Start 10 mg PO 1 h before sexual activity. Usual effective dose range 5 to 20 mg. Max 1 dose/day. Use lower dose (5 mg) if age 65 yo or older or moderate hepatic impairment (max 10 mg). Contraindicated with nitrates and alpha-blockers. Not FDA approved for women. [Trade only: Tabs 2.5, 5, 10, 20 mg. Orally disintegrating tabs, 10 mg (Staxyn).] ▶LK ♀B ▶– $$$$$

Nephrolithiasis

CITRATE (*Polycitra-K, Urocit-K, Bicitra, Oracit, Polycitra, Polycitra-LC*) Urinary alkalinization: 1 packet in water/juice PO three to four times per day. [Generic/Trade: Polycitra-K packet 3300 mg potassium citrate/ea, Polycitra-K oral soln (1100 mg potassium citrate/5 mL, 480 mL). Oracit oral soln (490 mg sodium citrate/5 mL, 15, 30, 480 mL). Bicitra oral soln (500 mg sodium citrate/5 mL, 480 mL). Urocit-K wax (potassium citrate): Tabs 5, 10 mEq. Polycitra-LC oral soln (550 mg potassium citrate/500 mg sodium citrate per 5 mL, 480 mL). Polycitra oral syrup (550 mg potassium citrate/500 mg sodium citrate per 5 mL, 480 mL).] ▶K ♀C ▶? $$$

NOTE: Information in tables is denoted with a "*t*" after the page number. Entries in bold indicate page number of main drug monograph.

T

APPENDIX
ADULT EMERGENCY DRUGS (selected)

ALLERGY	diphenhydramine (*Benadryl*): 25 to 50 mg IV/IM/PO. epinephrine: 0.1 to 0.5 mg IM/SC (1:1000 solution), may repeat after 20 minutes. methylprednisolone (*Solu-Medrol*): 125 mg IV/IM.
HYPERTENSION	esmolol (*Brevibloc*): 500 mcg/kg IV over 1 minute, then titrate 50 to 200 mcg/kg/min. fenoldopam (*Corlopam.*): Start 0.1 mcg/kg/min, titrate up to 1.6 mcg/kg/min. labetalol: Start 20 mg slow IV, then 40 to 80 mg IV q10 min prn up to 300 mg total cumulative dose. nitroglycerin: Start 10 to 20 mcg/min IV infusion, then titrate prn up to 100 mcg/min. nitroprusside (*Nitropress*): Start 0.3 mcg/kg/min IV infusion, then titrate prn up to 10 mcg/kg/min.
DYSRHYTHMIAS / ARREST	adenosine (*Adenocard*): PSVT (not A-fib): 6 mg rapid IV and flush, preferably through a central line or proximal IV. If no response after 1-2 minutes, then 12 mg. A third dose of 12mg may be given prn. amiodarone: V-fib or pulseless V-tach: 300 mg IV/IO; may repeat 150 mg just once. Life-threatening ventricular arrhythmia: Load 150 mg IV over 10 min, then 1 mg/min × 6 h, then 0.5 mg/min × 18 h. atropine: 0.5 to 1 mg IV, repeat q 3-5 minutes prn to maximum of 3 mg. diltiazem (*Cardizem*): Rapid A-fib: bolus 0.25 mg/kg or 20 mg IV over 2 min. May repeat 0.35 mg/kg or 25 mg 15 min after 1st dose. Infusion 5-15 mg/h. epinephrine: 1 mg IV/IO q 3-5 minutes for cardiac arrest [1:10,000 solution]. lidocaine (*Xylocaine*): Load 1 mg/kg IV, then 0.5 mg/kg q 8-10 min prn to max 3 mg/kg. Maintenance 2 g in 250 mL D5W (8 mg/mL) at 1 to 4 mg/min drip (7-30 mL/h).

(cont.)

ADULT EMERGENCY DRUGS (selected) (*continued*)

PRESSORS	dobutamine: 2 to 20 mcg/kg/min. 70 kg: 5 mcg/kg/min with 1 mg/mL concentration (e.g. 250 mg in 250 mL D5W) = 21 mL/h. dopamine: Start at 5 mcg/kg/min, increase prn by 5 to 10 mcg/kg/min increments at 10 min intervals, max 50 mcg/kg/min. 70 kg: 5 mcg/kg/min with 1600 mcg/mL concentration (e.g. 400 mg in 250 mL D5W) = 13 mL/h. Doses in mcg/kg/min: 2–4 = (traditional renal dose, apparently ineffective) dopaminergic receptors; 5–10= (cardiac dose) dopaminergic and beta1 receptors; >10 = dopaminergic, beta1, and alpha1 receptors. norepinephrine (*Levophed*): 4 mg in 500 mL D5W (8 mcg/mL), start 8 to 12 mcg/min (1 to 1.5 mL/h), usual dose once BP is stabilized 2 to 4 mcg/min. 22.5 mL/h = 3 mcg/min. phenylephrine: 20 mg in 250 mL D5W (80 mcg/mL), start 100 to 180 mcg/min (75 to 135 mL/h), usual dose once BP is stabilized 40 to 60 mcg/min (30 to 45 mL/h).
INTUBATION	etomidate (*Amidate*): 0.3 mg/kg IV. methohexital (*Brevital*): 1 to 1.5 mg/kg IV. propofol (*Diprivan*): 2.0 to 2.5 mg/kg IV. rocuronium (*Zemuron*): 0.6 to 1.2 mg/kg IV. succinylcholine (*Anectine, Quelicin*): 0.6 to 1.1 mg/kg IV. Peds (<5 yo): 2 mg/kg IV. thiopental: 3 to 5 mg/kg IV.
SEIZURES	diazepam (*Valium*): 5 to 10 mg IV, or 0.2 to 0.5 mg/kg rectal gel up to 20 mg PR. fosphenytoin (*Cerebyx*): Load 15 to 20 mg "phenytoin equivalents" (PE)/ kg IV, no faster than 100 to 150 mg PE/min. lorazepam (Ativan): Status epilepticus: 4 mg IV over 2 min, may repeat in 10-15 min. Anxiolytic/sedation: 0.04 to 0.05 mg/kg IV/IM; usual dose 2 mg, max 4 mg. phenobarbital: Status epilepticus: 15 to 20 mg/kg IV load; may give additional 5 mg/kg doses q 15-30 mins to max total dose of 30 mg/kg. phenytoin (*Dilantin*): 15 to 20 mg/kg up to 1000mg IV no faster than 50 mg/min.

CARDIAC DYSRHYTHMIA PROTOCOLS (for adults and adolescents)

Chest compressions ~100/min. Ventilations 8–10/min if intubated; otherwise 30:2 compression/ventilation ratio. Drugs that can be administered down ET tube (use 2–2.5 × usual dose): epinephrine, atropine, lidocaine, naloxone, vasopressin*.

V-Fib, Pulseless V-Tach

Airway, oxygen, CPR until defibrillator ready
Defibrillate 360 J (old monophasic), 120–200 J (biphasic), or with AED
Resume CPR × 2 min (5 cycles)
Repeat defibrillation if no response
Vasopressor during CPR:
- Epinephrine 1 mg IV/IO q 3–5 minutes, or
- Vasopressin* 40 units IV to replace 1st or 2nd dose of epinephrine
Rhythm/pulse check every ~2 minutes
Consider antiarrhythmic during CPR:

Bradycardia, <60 bpm and Inadequate Perfusion

Airway, oxygen, IV
Prepare for transcutaneous pacing; don't delay if advanced heart block
Consider atropine 0.5 mg IV; may repeat q 3–5 min to max 3 mg
Consider epinephrine (2–10 mcg/min) or dopamine(2–10 mcg/kg/min)
Prepare for transvenous pacing

Tachycardia with Pulses

Airway, oxygen, IV
If unstable and heart rate >150 bpm, then synchronized cardioversion

CARDIAC DYSRHYTHMIA PROTOCOLS (for adults and adolescents) *(continued)*

- Amiodarone 300 mg IV/IO; may repeat 150 mg just once
- Lidocaine 1.0–1.5 mg/kg IV/IO, then repeat 0.5–0.75 mg/kg to max 3 doses or 3 mg/kg
- Magnesium sulfate 1–2 g IV/IO if suspect torsades de pointes

Asystole or Pulseless Electrical Activity (PEA)

Airway, oxygen, CPR
Vasopressor (when IV/IO access):
- Epinephrine 1 mg IV/IO q 3–5 min, or
- Vasopressin* 40 units IV/IO to replace 1st or 2nd dose of epinephrine

If stable narrow-QRS (<120 ms):
- Regular: Attempt vagal maneuvers, If no success, adenosine 6 mg IV, then 12 mg prn (may repeat x 1),
- Irregular: Control rate with diltiazem or beta blocker (caution in CHF or severe obstructive disease).

If stable wide-QRS (>120 ms):
- Regular and suspect V-tach: Amiodarone 150 mg IV over 10 min; repeat prn to max 2.2 g/24 h. Prepare for elective synchronized cardioversion.
- Regular and suspect SVT with aberrancy: adenosine as per narrow-QRS above.

(cont.)

Consider atropine 1 mg IV/IO for asystole or slow PEA. Repeat q 3–5 min up to 3 doses.

Rhythm/pulse check every ~2 minutes

Consider 6 H's: hypovolemia, hypoxia, H+-acidosis, hyper/ hypokalemia, hypoglycemia, hypothermia

Consider 5 T's: Toxins, tamponade-cardiac, tension pneumothorax, thrombosis (coronary or pulmonary), trauma

- Irregular and A-fib: Control rate with diltiazem or beta blocker (caution in CHF/ severe obstructive pulmonary disease).
- Irregular and A-fib with pre-excitation (WPW): Avoid AV nodal blocking agents; consider amiodarone 150 mg IV over 10 min,
- Irregular and torsades de pointes: magnesium 1–2 g IV load over 5–60 min, then infusion.

bpm=beats per minute; CPR=cardiopulmonary resuscitation; ET=endotracheal; IO=intraosseous; J=Joules; ms=milliseconds; WPW=Wolff-Parkinson-White. Sources: *Circulation* 2005; 112, suppl IV; *NEJM* 2008;359:21–30 (demonstrated no benefit over epinephrine and worse long-term neurological outcomes).

NOTES

Stay Connected with Tarascon Publishing!

Monthly Dose eNewsletter
—Tarascon's Monthly eNewsletter

Stay up-to-date and subscribe today at: www.tarascon.com

Written specifically with Tarascon customers in mind, the Tarascon Monthly Dose will provide you with new drug information, tips and tricks, updates on our print, mobile and online products as well as some extra topics that are interesting and entertaining.

Sign up to receive the Tarascon Monthly Dose Today! Simply register at www.tarascon.com.

You can also stay up-to-date with Tarascon news, new product releases, and relevant medical news and information on Facebook, Twitter page, and our Blog.

STAY CONNECTED

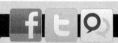

Facebook: www.facebook.com/tarascon
Twitter: @JBL_Medicine
Blog: blogs.jblearning.com/medicine